MORTAL MUSINGS: WAITING FOR DAWN

MORTAL MUSINGS: WAITING FOR DAWN

MEMOIRS OF A CANCER VICTIM

JOHN SELBY WAIT

Copyright © 2019 John Selby.

This edition published in 2019 by BLKDOG Publishing.

No part of this publication may be reproduced, stored in a retrieval system, or transmitted in any form or by any means, electronic, mechanical, photocopying, recording, or otherwise, without written permission of the publisher.

All rights reserved including the right of reproduction in whole or in part in any form. The moral right of the author has been asserted.

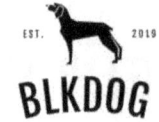

www.blkddogpublishing.com

Dedication

There are so many people to thank for their love and support throughout my battle. My wife, Holly, is forefront in my mind, my heart and my thoughts. Her love, care and undying support gave me strength and reason to continue my fight. This was also true of my two wonderful children, Matt and Elizabeth (Lizzie). Time and again they came through when I needed it most. Each making personal sacrifices to give me comfort and support.

My two sisters, Juliette and Cheryl, along with their husbands, Michael and Richard, were very supportive, not only for me but for Holly as well. It is a true blessing to have such a fantastic, loving family. I also am grateful to all my friends and extended family who reached out and provided their love and support.

It is wonderful to have doctors in the family. That was never clearer than with this fight. Juliette was always there with advice and help to both me and Holly. I must especially thank Michael, who was instrumental in getting me into Emory and in seeing Dr. Bilen. Without his efforts, these words would never have been written as I would not have been here to write them.

There are no words of gratitude strong enough to voice my thanks to Dr. Mehmet Bilen, as well as the rest of the Winship Staff at Emory University. All they did was save my life. Dr. Bilen was unfazed by the extremely long odds I faced and never let pessimism enter our conversations or outlook. There was always a Plan B, and a Plan C, and a Plan D... The staff at the Winship centers are truly amazing people, who give love, care and comfort to those of us fighting this horrible disease, as well as our families. I join President Carter, Erik Berry and thousands of others who owe so much to them.

While I am forever grateful to all those above and those who I forgot to mention, I must dedicate this book to all those still fighting the fight. To them I quote Jim Valvano – "Don't Give Up, Don't Ever Give Up."

Dedication ... 5
Foreword ... 1
Prologue ... 7
What Now? ... 8
What's Next? ... 9
Depress Here ... 10
Coping ... 10
Family Ties ... 12
Funny as Pharma ... 13
Never Give Up, Don't Ever Give Up ... 15
This Book ... 17
Background ... 21
Pre Georgia ... 21
My First Brush with Death ... 21
Early Issues ... 23
Columbus, Here We Come ... 27
The Move ... 31
Allergic to Georgia ... 35
The Spine ... 35
Testee Situation ... 40
Kneeding Help ... 41
Back to Back ... 42
Shouldering the Load ... 43
First Signs ... 44

- Meanwhile 51
  - Biblical Event 51
  - Jesus Saves 52
  - The Week That Was 54
  - More Medical Mess 56
- Southern Hills 57
  - The Study 57
  - The Meeting 60
- S.H. Management 63
  - A Sad Start 63
  - Roger and Out 65
  - Renovations 68

Cancer! 69

- Indigestion 69
- Diagnosis 73
- Emory Winship Center 78
- First Treatment 87
- A Critical Time 97
  - Fateful Day 100
- The Call 101
- Immunotherapy 113

Impact on My Life 119

- Overall Impact 119
- Stress 123
- Exercising the Demon 127
- Becoming Conway 130
- Golf 133
- Work 138
- Social 143

Emotional Impact 148

- Love, Fear and Depression 148
    - Love 148
    - Fear 150
    - Depression 154
- Other Emotions 156
    - Anger 156
    - Guilt 157
    - Patience 158

Death's Door 160

- Time to Go? 160
    - Dad 160
    - Short Cuts 165
- Bucket List 166

Coping 172

- External Strategies 173
    - Support Groups 174
    - Professional Help 176
- Internal Strategies 178
    - Denial 178
    - Distraction 179
    - Venting 181
    - ADHD 182
- Perspective 185

Self-Reflection 191

- Accomplishments 193
- Wisdom vs. Intelligence 197
- Self-Image 202
- Temper and Patience 206

Ethics and Idealism 213
    Bachelor Parties 215
    Charity 225
    Ethics 226
Other 227
    Master Persuader 227
    Taking Criticism 230
    Self-Centered 231
    More Faults 234

Trust and Relationships 235

Business Partnerships 235
Misplaced Trust 240
First Marriage 241
    The Wedding 242
    Kids Cometh 243
Pat 245
Holly 256
Pets 260
    Waxahachie 260
    Pumpkin 261
    Lucky 261
    Peanut 261
    Ferris 263
    Beau 263
    Charlie 265
    The Three Sisters 267

God and Me 269

Feeling Philosophy 269
    Western Civ 269
    Why are We Here? 276
    Is There a God? 276
My Relationship with God 278
My Heritage 284
Kansas City 291
    Of Pride and Prejudice 292
    Early Driving Lesson 294
Ad Astra Per Aspera 300
    Jan 302
Encore 305
    First Date 309
    Timing 311
Greg 314
    God's Sense of Humor 318
The Miracle 322
It Adds Up 328
Career Track 333
    Into Insurance 339
    Getting into Golf 341
    Really? Real Estate 347
    Becoming a Broker 347
Life Cycles 349

The Nature of God 355

What does he look like? 355
    Expanding our Perspective 356
    A Dark God 362
    Beyond Comprehension 363

Good vs. Evil: The Devil Made Me Do It 364
    Yin and Yang..365
    A POLITICAL PERSPECTIVE.........................368
    Pure Evil 372
    Angels and Demons..372
Inner Voice 374
    Temptation..382

The Afterlife..384

Nature of the Afterlife...384
    Eternal Life 385
    Emotional Survival 387
    Morality 388
    Moment of Death..390
The Afterlife Being..391
Evidence..394
    Religions...394
    Spirits..396
    Nature of Ghosts...399
    Near Death Experiences 401
    Faith and Logic...402

Why? 404

Why are We Here? 404
Why Me?..409
    Why? What Purpose? 410
    What are the Lessons? 414
    Repeating Class 414
    Purpose of Life 416

    Consequences.. 419
            Immortality..421
           Universal Truth...421

Epilogue 424

    June 2017 424
    July – August 2017 430
    September – November 10, 2017... 436
    November 10 – December 2017 444
    January - February 2018.. 451
    March 2018.. 458
    New Year's Eve, 2018.. 465
    Social Security 478
    2019... 480

FOREWORD

December 2018
Virtually everyone has been touched by cancer. You either have cancer, had cancer, or will have cancer, or had a close friend or relative who has or had cancer. Cancer is the second leading cause of death in the US, accounting for just under one in four deaths (22.5%). It's a terrible disease made worse somehow because it's our own body rebelling against us.

My first intimate brush with cancer came when it claimed the life of my grandmother on my mother's side, who died of bladder cancer. But I was very young. And because she lived in England, I had only met her once. So, while it saddened me, it did not have an enormous impact.

The first time it really hit me hard was when I lost someone close to me. Nancy was a long-time employee of mine. She was one of two employees that worked at the mailing service when I purchased it in 1986, converting it into IBS Mail Marketing. She remained with me as the company grew to over twenty-five employees. She got sick about the same time I had put the business back on the market. The breast cancer claimed her quickly. I was shocked both with losing someone who was much more than an employee, but a friend; and with the speed at which the cancer worked.

Yet, I never thought I would get cancer. For one thing, I had none of the risk factors. Other than my grandmother, whose cancer was blamed on the fact she was a heavy smoker, there is no history of cancer on either side of my family. And I don't smoke . . . never have. Nor am I aware of my being exposed or consuming any known carcinogens.

Nonetheless, here I am with cancer. And not just a run-of-the-mill cancer. Nope, I have to have a particularly nasty one called Renal Transitional Cell Carcinoma (TCC, also called urothelial carcinoma). It is not renal or kidney cancer. Rather it is a type of bladder cancer that forms on the kidney instead of the bladder. Medscape defines it as "a malignant tumor arising from the transitional (urothelial) epithelial cells lining the urinary tract from the renal calyces to the ureteral orifice." About 5-7% of the urothelial cancers (bladder type cancers) are TCC. Lucky me.

Further, when I read about the risk factors for TCC, which include such things as smoking, working with chemicals, extensive use of analgesics, etc., I have exactly none of them. So, neither my doctor (who specializes in TCC) nor I have any clue as to why I would develop TCC. It was just meant to be.

The cancer is always fatal unless treated. The primary treatment is to remove the tumor, which usually means losing the kidney as well. In this case, the five-year survival rate (if caught at Stage I) is about 73%. But that was not an option in my case, as I was stage IV when it was discovered – with tumors in my chest, including areas that were not operable. The five-year survival rate with people in my situation? **0%**. And that's assuming the kidney and main tumor had been removed, which is not the case for me.

But that does not mean it won't happen. New treatments are coming on-line at a rapid clip. Indeed, the immunotherapy treatment I am currently on, which has had tremendous success (so far) was not even approved for TCC when I was first diagnosed with the disease some four months prior. (One of the advantages of being treated at one of the top cancer facilities in the country, Emory University, is access to the latest and greatest treatments).

As I am writing this, it has been twenty-seven months since I learned I had cancer. And it has been about eighteen months since I heard the miraculous news that the tumors in my chest had disappeared and the main tumor had shrunk greatly. But it has not disappeared. I am still undergoing immunotherapy treatment every three weeks, requiring me to make the two-hour drive to Emory University. But I don't mind. They saved my life.

Everything changes when you have cancer. It affects almost everything you do, and certainly affects how others (especially your loved ones) interact with you.

Like most people, I never thought I would die. Ok, I knew intellectually I was not immortal and knew that I would *eventually* die, but that construct was simply too foreign for me. I honestly don't remember ever really thinking about my own demise. I planned on seeing the new century come in − not this one, the next. Now suddenly, the prospect of my doom was right there in front of me and coming fast! Needless to say, it caused a significant shaking up of my priorities and was a serious challenge to my faith.

In this book, I will talk about my fight with cancer, from its beginning right up to where I am today. I will describe the events, as well as my own thoughts and feelings as I went through them. I will also discuss the impact on my family and friends. I will talk about various coping strategies I have employed, and some I haven't. I will try to use humor throughout, because, for me, humor is a significant coping mechanism.

But I will also talk about my "deeper" thoughts. Because being suddenly confronted with the prospect of eminent death certainly causes you to think about what comes after. As they say, there are no atheists in the foxhole. But I am not here to preach, but rather to inspire people to think about their own faith, and their relationship with God. My approach is more philosophical than religious.

I am writing this book for several reasons. First, I am hoping that by sharing my experiences, I can help those who are going through a similar process – either themselves, or a loved one. I am also hoping to stir the imaginations of all readers, and stimulate the "deep thoughts" about faith, God, philosophy and religion. (Don't worry, I'm not going to get "preachy," but rather guide you through my own questions and possible answers). But I am also writing this book because it helps me cope with what I am going through.

I call myself a cancer fighter. As I am writing this, I am also cancer *survivor*. But that status may have changed by the time this book is published and certainly by the time you are reading it – such is the nature of this terrible disease. (Of course, my death may be great for book sales . . . but I think I would prefer slower sales!).

But I do think it may be interesting for the reader to see how my thoughts and emotions have changed throughout this process. When I started writing this book, my prospects for survival – even making it another few months – was poor, at best. Thus, some of the chapters are a bit "darker" than others as I faced near certain death, although I would never admit it.

I thought about putting it all in chronological order but realized that that would make a lot of the themes chaotic.

Instead, I have settled on putting dates on the chapters and subchapters to reflect when they were written (at least initially, as I have gone back and done some editing). At the end of the book, I have an epilogue that *is* a chronological log of events and thoughts I've experienced after main parts of the book were written.

A quick note about the names used in this book. I have changed many of them to protect the guilty. To make it clearer, I will put an "*" after the first mention of a name that has been changed. The rest will remain as is, at least until they threaten to sue.

I have organized the book into sections. I begin by providing you some background information on myself, my medical history, my family and my work. While some of this may seem self-indulging, there is a point to it as will become clear when I talk about my relationship with God. The next section talks about the cancer and its treatment. It also talks more about what was going on in my life at that time, which only added to my misery.

I next talk about the impact cancer has had on my life, affecting every aspect. I discuss its emotional impact. I follow that with a discussion of what it's like being on death's doorstep and knocking. Next is a section on coping strategies – those I used and some I perhaps should have.

As self-reflection is usually called for when facing the prospect of meeting your maker, I have a section on a rather brutal self-evaluation. I hope St. Peter skips that section.

The following section is about trust and the major relationships I have had. Trust is very important to me, but I have both broken that trust and been victimized by it.

All of the previous sections tie into the next section, which is about my relationship with God. This section will surprise most of the people who know me, because few if any ever suspected the depth of my faith as I never discuss religion, nor attend church. I follow that section with a philosophical discussion on the nature of God.

Perhaps second only to thoughts of those you leave behind, when you are facing eminent death you naturally start thinking about what, if anything, comes after. That is the topic of the next section, the Afterlife.

My final philosophical section tries to answer the question Why?

The last section, the Epilogue, is a chronological diary of major events that happened to me following the writing of the main text of the book. It goes from June 2017 through April 2019.

Before going any further, I have to say I probably would not be here to write these words if not for the love and support of my great children (Matthew and Elizabeth) and especially my wonderful wife, Holly. This cancer has deeply affected her, as it has me. Yet she has risen above the emotional cost to herself and provided me with the love and attention I have needed to fuel my desire to survive. She has always been there for me, even when things seemed darkest. She has been strong when I know it was very hard for her to do so. I need to survive if only to prevent her from suffering more from my loss. I love her deeply and can never thank her enough for all she has done.

Prologue

May 2017
My life changed forever early morning September 17th, 2016. That was when I found out I likely had cancer. Twelve days later, a biopsy confirmed I had renal transitional cell carcinoma -- a particularly nasty, aggressive and currently incurable cancer carrying an extremely poor prognosis. A week later I found out it had metastasized, spreading from my kidney to my chest and lungs. It was inoperable. I was Stage IV, where Stage V is six feet under. In short, my life expectancy was suddenly measured in months, not decades.

To be fair, my wonderful Doctor at Emory, Dr. Bilen, never said I was going to die soon. Instead, he outlined a Plan A, then a Plan B if A didn't work, and Plan C if A&B didn't work, etc. But he also told me realistically I would *never* be rid of this cancer. The best we can hope for is to extend my life, perhaps by a "year or two." Those last words came like a sledgehammer. I was 62. A year or two would not even get me to Medicare. This was not my plan . . . and that was if I was "lucky." (With two doctors in the family, my sister and her husband, who happens to be a noted oncologist, I was already aware I was facing very, very long odds, and that was *before* we knew I was Stage IV).

For a person who never really considered the concept I might cease to exist, this news was rather disturbing (ok, I may be understating this a bit). And that's part of the story I want to tell. How does one cope with unexpected eminent death?

WHAT NOW?

When I first heard I was Stage IV, I was forced to ponder the prospect of not living forever, perhaps not even seeing Christmas. As I never fully embraced the concept of self-mortality, this came as quite a shock. What would happen to my wife? My kids? And what would happen to *me*?

The thought of dying soon naturally changed my priorities. Maximizing my time with my family and close friends became a primary focus. Work slid down the totem pole (although it was still important . . . just not *as* important as previously). Retirement planning (I was 62) was no longer a priority, as it was highly likely permanent retirement would precede work retirement. And perhaps some of those trips I have dreamed about taking should be given a higher priority since there may not be a lot of time left to enjoy them. Admittedly, I was also thinking, why save for the future when there might not be any? Shouldn't I be spending what little time (and money) I had left enjoying all I could out of life?

Yet those hedonistic thoughts conflicted with my family first mentality and upbringing. After all, what would happen if I spent everything, thinking I was going to die in six months then had the audacity to survive and live another ten or twenty years? Especially given I now faced ever mounting medical bills. To be honest, I was not that concerned about my family's financial needs after I was gone as my kids were both adults and doing well and my wife had a good career and I had sufficient life insurance to make sure she was taken care of . . . but not too well, I didn't want to give her any incentive.

WHAT'S NEXT?

In addition to thinking about what to do with the rest of my now-shortened life were thoughts about what happens afterwards? Does it just end or is there something else? Is there an existence that survives the end of life? Is there an immortal "soul"? And, if so, what exactly is the nature of that soul? Will it carry the memories and emotions from my physical existence? Where will it be? Is there a heaven or hell? And if there is an afterlife, what does that mean about our current life?

I would also ask, "why me?" But that would almost always be answered, "why not me?" Was I really so special that I was going to be immune to death? But it did lead to the next question, "why now?" Is there a reason, beyond simple chance, I would come down with cancer and do so at this time in my life? After all, I do not have a family history of cancer. Nor do I have any of the known precursors or causes of my specific form of cancer. So, it does seem strange I came down with it.

Naturally, this leads to the big question, "What is the purpose of *my* life?" While I have entertained these philosophical and theological thoughts throughout my existence, there was a new-found urgency to them.

As these are all questions we must face at some point in our lives, I am hoping my discussing them openly can perhaps shed light on your own quest for answers.

DEPRESS HERE

December 2016
Since I was a young child, I always believed I was "special" . . . meant for greatness. Whether it was from being responsible for an amazing scientific breakthrough or perhaps becoming President, I believed my life would be recognized by others as historic. Even though I realized later these ego trips were a product of my very unhappy childhood, I never truly gave up on them. So, it was certainly disappointing at age thirty, none of my dreams had materialized, not even close. It was even more disappointing at age forty, then fifty, and eventually sixty. Now here I am at age sixty-two and faced with the realization I had achieved everything I was likely to ever achieve, and these achievements were nowhere close to what I imagined.

Under these conditions it is quite easy to get very depressed. Now add to it the depressing thought of maybe not living to see a New Year. You're already depressed about the sorry state of your physical body and that you can no longer physically do things you used to do. You're depressed with the thoughts of not seeing your grandkids grow up (or even being born!) You're depressed with the thoughts of leaving your wife alone and how hard that would be on her. You're depressed you haven't completed your bucket list. You're depressed because you haven't even started your bucket list. You're even depressed about being depressed.

And you're mad. You're mad at how unfair it all is. Why me? I've tried to be a good person. And things were seemingly finally coming together for me. Why did you (God) have to take it all away so suddenly?

COPING

Like I said, it would be easy to get depressed and angry. And I will admit there have been a few times where I have allowed myself to do so . . . But I refuse to give into it. I refuse to allow myself to remain depressed or angry. I realize neither getting depressed nor angry is going to change reality. It is only going to make it worse – for both myself and those around me. Besides, I still do not accept I am really dying, despite the evidence to the contrary. Denial is a powerful tool!

For another, I try to maintain perspective. Everywhere I look, there are people in a lot worse shape than me. I become acutely aware of this every time I go to the Winship Cancer Center in Atlanta for treatment. I see the brave faces of people who are facing the same fate as myself . . . many in worse physical shape. I can't let them down. I can't let them see I have given up, because it makes it easier for them to do the same. In the words of the late Jimmy Valvano, "don't give up, don't ever give up."

I also have my faith. I am not conventionally "religious" as I do not regularly go to church. Nor do my beliefs conform to the constraints set by traditional religions. Nor do I profess my faith to others. But nonetheless, I have a profound belief in God. Further, I believe he has been proactive in my life. Because of this, I know there is a reason for my illness. I even know there would be reason for my death, should it come to that. I may not be able to fathom what that reason is, but that does not mean it doesn't exist.

There have been many, many times in my life where I have been angry at God . . . only to discover something even better emerged. In short, I could see (after the fact) the reasons behind the bad stuff that kept happening to me. At least I could see some of the reasons. I still have no clue as to what the master plan is. I just know there is one.

FAMILY TIES

One thing the cancer has done is it brought my extended family much closer together. My family had both physically and emotionally been separated over the past two years. My daughter lives in Richmond, Virginia and my son in Los Angeles. Two years ago, my wife and I lived in the Dallas area where my two sisters, Cheryl and Juliette, and my father lived. My mother had also lived in Dallas before passing in 2001. Then Holly, my wife (#2 – she doesn't like to be referred to as my "current" wife), got a wonderful career opportunity resulting in us moving to Columbus Georgia. Shortly thereafter, my sister Juliette and her husband moved to Portland, Oregon to be closer to their kids, especially their daughter who was going through a tough time (she would later get a divorce). Then last summer (before I discovered I had cancer) my father died. So now my family is scattered across the United States, with at least 500 miles separating the closest ones. But after we discovered I had stage IV cancer, suddenly everyone made it a priority to come and visit me. The family was united in their concern for me.

I must say I greatly appreciate the attention I have received. I love having my family come and visit. But at the same time, it also comes with a bit of guilt. After all, I don't think I'm dying, so why are they all making this fuss? You almost hate to disappoint them by getting better because they spent all this time and money fretting over me. Oh well, I can get over it.

FUNNY AS PHARMA

May 2017

While the topics covered here, death and cancer, are very serious, I do try to see the lighter side. Humor has always been an important part of my life. It has often served as a coping and defensive mechanism. It has helped me through some bad times and tough situations. It also made it easier to deal with other people as I am otherwise socially awkward and always have been.

They say laughter is the best medicine. Boy I sure hope so. If it's true, then I think I will be cured as I do find humor almost everywhere.

I get most of my sense of humor from my mother, who was English. She had a wonderful sense of humor, including the typical "English sense of humor". Mom was always the life of any party with ever-present jokes (usually dirty) and funny stories to share.

This may sound bad, but it wasn't until my mother died, we (my sisters and I) discovered dad had a great sense of humor as well. Not right then, mind you, but soon afterwards. While my mother was alive, my father was happy to be in the background, rarely saying anything. He was content to let her shine on the center stage, as he loved to watch her perform. But when she was no longer here, his personality emerged – and it turns out, he had a pretty darn good sense of humor as well. We should have known this, though, because it was dad's sense of humor that appealed to my mother in the first place.

Let me relay a quick story about my dad's sense of humor. It will tell you a lot about both my parents. This event occurred when I was very young.

My mother loved Christmas, but not the religious aspect of it (she was Jewish after all). No, what she really loved was the presents – specifically *her* presents. It was my mother who insisted we open at least one present on Christmas Eve. (She wanted to open them all, but we resisted.) Yet, she could not even wait until Christmas eve. Nope. She had a nasty habit of finding dad's presents to her and opening them early, without dad's knowledge.

One year, she opened her present early to discover dad had given her a lovely pair of shoes. She loved the shoes, but when she tried them on, she discovered they were the wrong size. So naturally, she took them back to the store to exchange them for her size. But there was a problem, they did not have the same color in her size. So she took a different color, but it was the same style and at least the shoes fit. When she returned home, she meticulously rewrapped the gift so dad would not know about her prying.

On Christmas morning, when she opened her present, she naturally feigned great delight and surprise about her wonderful gift. But the most surprised look was on my dad's face.

The next year, mom once again went hunting for my father's present. She found it well hidden, but not well enough. She was pleased to find it was both large and heavy. Naturally she set about opening it, even though it was meticulously wrapped.

After carefully unwrapping the present, she found a box, which she naturally opened. But inside this box was another box, also meticulously wrapped. Not one to give up that easily, mom unwrapped that one as well, only to reveal yet another beautifully wrapped present. This went on for five or so layers, until she discovered a wonderfully wrapped item that could only be a jewelry box. Quivering with excitement, she proceeded to open this box as well. Inside was just a note. It read: "This is what you get for peeking! Love John."

Now mom had a real dilemma. Does she admit she peeked? Or does she spend hours meticulously rewrapping each present and putting it back together. She chose the latter. But dad knew.

It seems I inherited my humor from both my parents, which means I appreciate most forms of humor (except *2 Broke Girls* – bad acting just obscures any humor otherwise present).

NEVER GIVE UP, DON'T EVER GIVE UP

Back to cancer. I was a great fan of Jimmy Valvano's – at least after he retired from coaching. When he coached, we lived in the Triangle (Raleigh, Durham and Chapel Hill NC) and I was a huge fan of UNC (University of North Carolina). This does not diminish my loyalty to my alma matter, University of Kansas, one bit as KU is and always will number one in my heart (as far as colleges go). In fact, it was my love of KU that made it easy for me to fall in love with Carolina. For one thing, UNC was where my wife (#1) did her residency (which is why we moved there in the first place), and she later worked there. But there were so many similarities between the schools, starting with the college towns/bedroom communities where they can be found – Chapel Hill and Lawrence – both liberal oasis in very conservative states. Both with big hills and wonderful universities. Both located near major cities and their respective state capitals. KU and UNC are of comparable size. Both have long histories, with UNC being the first public university in the US and KU being the first west of the Mississippi.

But what really attracted me was the fact both schools have a very rich (and successful - #2 and #3 in all-time wins) tradition in my favorite sport- college basketball. Plus, there was a lot of cross-pollination between the two schools (e.g.

Dean Smith, Dick Harp, Roy Williams - twice, Larry Brown, Jerod Haase, etc.). Later, my son, Matthew, would be born at UNC's hospital, then twenty-two years later, graduate from UNC with a degree in Physics.

While rooting mostly for UNC, I followed all the Triangle teams (UNC, Duke and NC State). When my wife became a faculty member I started rooting more for Duke. I would cheer for Duke against everyone – except Carolina and KU. That meant I would be rooting *against* NC State when they played UNC and Duke. This would also later change when my daughter, Elizabeth, wound up attending NC State – and graduating valedictorian (proud papa). However, that was much later. When Jimmy Valvano coached State, he was coaching the enemy. (At least among the Triangle schools). As a Carolina fan, I drew some pleasure in the shoe scandal that would signal the beginning of the end of his coaching career.

But when he came down with cancer, everything changed.

I remember watching his famous ESPY speech live. It moved me to tears as I watched, even though at that time, I not only did not have cancer, I didn't even know anyone with cancer. But now, his speech has taken on so much more meaning. (If you have not seen it, please google it.) I especially remember two main quotes: "If you laugh, you think, and you cry, that's a full day." Boy, have I had a lot of full days lately! And his most famous -- "Don't give up, don't ever give up." And I won't.

I also live by another expression of English extraction and made popular in the US by the music group, *Fun*. I am referring, of course, to "Carry on." It doesn't matter what life throws at you, our job is to "carry on" . . . to continue our work, our loves, our life . . . no matter the circumstances. (I don't abide by another British expression . . . "keep a stiff upper lip." While I realize it means to not show your emotions and go forward, keeping a stiff upper lip would also mean not smiling. And the world needs more smiles. I know I do.)

THIS BOOK

I am not famous. I have not accomplished great things, at least not yet (there is always hope). I do not have a gazillion followers on social media. I am certainly not an active social media person, with about sixty-eight Facebook friends. I'm not on Twitter or any other network. So why would you be interested in my musings? Perhaps because I am a rather ordinary person (hate saying that), who is facing an extraordinary circumstance – a pending (though currently suspended) death sentence. How does one face one's own demise – especially at a relatively youthful age? (Ok, I'm taking some literary license here). Perhaps some of the thoughts arising during this reflection can be of assistance and/or comfort to those facing similar situations, and even those who are not, as the questions are bigger than one's own existence.

There really are three themes to this book. This first is coping with terminal cancer. I go into great detail about my treatments, experiences, consequences and thoughts.

The second is philosophical/theological – what happens after we die? This broadens into a more general discussion about why we are here in the first place.

The third, though, is faith. Which has been a huge part of my life and a focus of my ability to cope. However, those people who know me will be surprised at this as I am not a church goer. Because of this, I do spend a lot of the book on what may seem self-indulgent as I reflect back on my life. Please forgive me, but I believe it is important to understand what I have been through in order to better understand why I have such a profound faith.

You may notice changes of tone and mood as you go through this book. This is because my cancer is a very active disease, especially when I was writing this book. At times, my situation looked very promising, but then as pain got worse, it appeared my cancer was worsening. As much as possible, I am trying to incorporate this active timeline into the text of the book, so you can learn more about what I experienced. For example, as I am writing this paragraph, my future is very unclear. In September (2016), when I first learned of the cancer, it seemed hopeless. Then when the chemo started being effective in November, I became more optimistic. Then we found out in January the tumors were growing again, back to bleak. We switched to immunotherapy and that seemed to be working. In fact, the tumors in my chest had disappeared and the main tumor on my kidney had shrunk considerably.

But then the pain started back. When I started writing this, the pain was modest and could be easily explained by reasons other than the tumor growing again. But the pain has steadily gotten worse. So here I am on May 25th, 2017, writing these paragraphs being very much afraid the tumors are once again growing. I will know soon enough – next week, on June 1st, I will be undergoing new scans. They will reveal the truth. And I will incorporate those results into this writing. (The epilogue contains a sequential log of events after today, and my thoughts, emotions and reactions to these events. I am hoping it will be a long section.)

Writing this book has been therapeutic. Not only because of the cancer, where it helps me cope, but also because I find at the ripe old age of sixty-two, my memories are starting to fade. I am having more and more difficulty remembering the past and this is very troubling. So, I am hoping the process of writing this book will help refresh those memories.

It is funny how the mind and memory work (or don't, as the case might be). I will want to write about a subject, be it a person or event in my past, and for the life of me, only to find I can't recall it. (Faulty disk drive). The details are gone. But then, a few days later I will be lying in bed and **POP** there it is. I will also have different random memories come flooding in when I'm trying to go to sleep – in no particular order. I have learned if I don't get up and write these down, I will never get to sleep. Nor am I likely to remember them in the morning. But because they are random, I must create spots for them in the book. At least that will be my excuse if you find some of this writing choppy. It's because there may have been several days, weeks or months separating when I wrote one paragraph to the next.

Enough of the excuses. I hope you get something out of reading this, beside perhaps it being good sleep aide (even then, I suppose, I can say it was helpful.)

Mortal Musings

BACKGROUND

PRE GEORGIA

May 2017

Throughout my life I have been a very, very lucky man. Notice I said "lucky" and not "fortunate". This is deliberate because luck runs both ways . . . good and bad. And I certainly have had my share of both. I will talk about both kinds in this book. As cancer is the prominent theme, I will begin with some relevant background.

MY FIRST BRUSH WITH DEATH

Getting a death sentence forced me to come face to face with my mortality. Previously, I rarely, if ever, thought about it. Well, there was one time when I thought briefly (like seconds) I might die. That was when I fell down a mountain.

We (my wife at the time, Ann*, and our two kids, Matt

and Lizzy) were driving around in the mountains of North Carolina near Asheville when I saw a view I really wanted to capture on my camcorder. But not from the street. That would be too easy. (We didn't have cell phones back then. If you wanted a video, you used a camcorder that recorded on VCR tape.)

I pulled over and grabbed my huge camcorder (this was in the 1990s when the camcorders weighed about twenty pounds and used full-sized VCR tapes). I wanted to use the camcorder as it had an awesome zoom lens. I hiked into the woods a few hundred yards to the edge of this cliff. Getting as close as my acrophobia would let me, which was still a couple of feet from the very edge, I hung onto a limb while raising the camcorder to record. Suddenly, the ground beneath my feet gave away. At the same time, I discovered the branch I had chosen to grab was not up to the task. It promptly snapped, sending me on my way. I'm sure it looked very comical should anyone had seen it (God must have laughed out loud), but it wasn't funny for me . . . then.

I wasn't given the chance to reflect on whether the cliff was terminal, as I only fell a couple of feet, landing on my butt. But my adventure was not over. I had fallen onto a steep, and very slippery slope. I immediately started sliding, gathering speed. With my arms and legs flailing in the air, I rapidly approached nothingness. I traveled several yards before suddenly being launched into the air while still lying on my back. When I went airborne, I had no idea how far I would fall as my eyes were skyward. But I knew there were cliffs there several hundred feet high. I did not know if I was on top of one or not, but I did know I was close. So, for a brief time, I realized I might just have come to the end of the line.

I hung in the air for what seemed like an eternity – but

was probably only a second or two – as I pondered my mortality. Yet my life did not flash in front of my eyes. I was somewhat disappointed by this. I guess by the time I called up the tape, I hit the ground. I fell about fifteen feet, landing in a soft bed of vegetation. This turned out to be the classic good news/bad news scenario. The good news was I was not dead. And while I was badly bruised and shaken, I did not appear to have broken anything major, other than my pride. The bad news was I had fallen onto a bed of poison ivy! And I was very allergic to poison ivy. I was on a small shelf, probably about fifteen feet wide. However, I did not venture to its edge to see how deep the cliff was. Once was enough.

Amazingly, I found the camcorder lying a short distance away. Miraculously, the camcorder, though banged up and dented, still worked!

Using vines and small footholds, I climbed out. I then slowly limped back to the car, where my family was still waiting – totally unaware I had nearly met my maker. I had survived relatively unscathed, although my clothing was not as lucky.

When we got back to the hotel, which fortunately was close, I immediately took a shower to wash away the itch juice. No doubt, this saved me from a severe outbreak of poison ivy. More importantly, my immortality was once again, reassured.

EARLY ISSUES

Over my life I have had very few physical problems – or so I thought until writing this chapter. I have never broken a bone. The most serious illness I had (other than the various childhood diseases, measles, mumps, chicken pox, etc.) was mono in college (and that was bad).

The biggest issues I had prior to my sixtieth birthday

were being effectively blind in one eye and deaf in one ear. (My wife claims I am half blind, half deaf but totally dumb.) My vision problem is bad keratoconus – or bulging of the cornea. I can't even read the big E with my right eye. It could be surgically corrected (replacing the cornea), but since my vision in the left eye is good, I have never done it. I tried contacts but hated them. Nor did they really help because the brain still effectively blocked the vision from that eye, so I really did not notice any improvement unless I closed the left eye. And I hated putting them on! Effectively, I have lived with one eye since I was thirteen. (The keratoconus though is responsible for my one superpower. Because the focal length for my right eye is about 2", my right eye acts like a microscope as I can bring tiny things right up to 2" away from the right eye and see it well and, because it's so close, in greater detail than possible with the unaided left eye. Although it does freak people out a bit when they see me do it.)

I am very fortunate the keratoconus stayed mostly in my right eye. (Notice the good luck, bad luck theme – bad luck I have it, good luck it stayed in one eye.) It is almost always bilateral – affecting both eyes equally. And while I have a very mild case of it in my left eye, it has not significantly affected its ability to see . . . thank goodness (still 20/20).

Having only one good eye has its consequences. Ever since I was old enough to look up into the sky, I've wanted to fly. I wanted to be a pilot, like my father (even though he gave up being a pilot long before I ever came into this world.) When I was fifteen, I even took ground school for being a pilot.

But because my brain is blocking most of the vision from my right eye, I don't have great depth perception. (I also can't make out hidden pictures because they depend on bilateral vision, which I don't have). And, apparently you want to have excellent depth perception if you're going to be a pilot – certainly your passengers want you to have it. Fortunately, binocular vision is only one of the many clues our brains use to figure out depth, so I really have not had any other issues – like with driving. (I will use the fact I have only one good eye to explain whenever I miss a basket while playing basketball, but I know it has far more to do with a lack of talent.)

And since I'm righthanded, it is especially awkward to not have the use of my right eye or right ear. If I wanted to shoot with a rifle, for example, I must shoot lefthanded as I need to use my left eye. Good thing I'm neither a hunter nor soldier!

The deafness is also on the right side. It started about when I turned forty. It is not complete, but my hearing is certainly much, much worse in my right ear. (It may help explain why I always want to drive, as it puts my wife on my deaf side . . . just kidding, Holly. I do want to live, after all). As with my eyesight, it is very unusual to go nearly deaf in one ear, without an apparent physical cause (like an injury or tumor). Lucky me.

My lack of good hearing affects me more in my daily life than my impaired vision. When people are sitting to my right, I have a tough time hearing them. If I'm lying on my right side (such as in bed), I can't hear much of anything. This can be useful, if I'm in a noisy environment, but can be upsetting if my wife happens to be talking to me and expecting me to reply. In fact, my hearing probably bothers her as much as it does me. There are many times I'm sure she has told me things, thinking I've heard her, when in fact I haven't. That can be problematic, needless to say! (She often complains I don't listen. But that is not *always* the case, sometimes I simply don't hear).

Another major medical issue I had prior to sixty was gall stones. Oh boy. This happened in my mid-forties. It was the most painful thing I had ever experienced. During one attack, which happened over the Christmas holiday when we were visiting with my in-laws (first wife). My mother-in-law, who was a nurse, was initially afraid I was having a heart attack. When I didn't die, I think she realized it was probably gall stones.

Fortunately, it eased off quickly or I would have wound up in the hospital. But it was enough to scare me. I ended up having my gall bladder removed. This is the only organ I have had removed (that I know about) as I still have my tonsils and appendix.

However, I did use the surgery to address another issue. At the time, my wife and I had discussed my having a vasectomy. But, admittedly, I was more than a little scared about the snip, snip. When the gall stone surgery came up, I asked if it was possible to do the other procedure at the same time. They could and did. Problem solved.

The main lifetime ailment I have is ADD (attention deficit disorder) or ADHD (attention deficit hyperactive disorder). I really had it bad when I was a kid. I still have it, but now it's controlled. But back when I was young, they had a different diagnosis for it. They called it "bad kid syndrome" without the "syndrome". The treatment was typically a spanking (if home) or seeing the principal (if at school). I will talk about this a lot more later . . . along with all my dental issues. But that's another story.

Getting older, especially as I neared (and passed sixty), really changed my physical profile (I'm not just talking about my protruding belly here, but my medical concerns). It's funny thinking back. There was a commercial on several years ago featuring two old men at a pool comparing scars. I laughed, not realizing a few years later, I would feel like one of those men – with the scars to prove it.

It started with my knees, with bad arthritis. I had arthroscopic surgery on my right knee four years ago, with the expectation my left knee would be next. (It hasn't happened yet. My current orthopedic surgeon, though, feels I will eventually need both knees replaced. For now, cortisone shots give me several months of relief). Then my vision went to crap. It got so bad I could not make out any highway signs. Turns out I had cataracts. So, I had cataract surgery right after turning fifty-nine, but only on my left eye as I did not see the point in fixing the cataracts on my right eye. But what an amazing experience that was. Not only did it clear up my vision, but it surprisingly also corrected it. I no longer needed glasses.

But things really accelerated downhill when we moved to Georgia.

COLUMBUS, HERE WE COME

Holly left first. She moved to Columbus in April of 2015 to become Executive Director of the National Civil War Naval Museum there. This was as close to a dream job for her as we could find. Holly loves Civil War history, even using it as a topic for her master's thesis at Florida State University. Before taking the job in Columbus, she had been the Executive Director of the Pearce Museum in Corsicana, Texas.

The Pearce Museum had two main galleries – a Civil War gallery featuring a collection of over 15,000 original documents from the Civil War – mostly letters; and a Western Art Gallery. Holly took this job so we could move to Texas back in 2008 because I wanted to be closer to my family – mainly my Dad who was 88 at the time. Unfortunately, Holly hated this job and Corsicana, mostly due to the University politics of Navarro College, which owned the museum.

So, when the job in Columbus became available, she jumped at it as it not only was a wonderful opportunity at a fabulous museum, but it also represented a return home for her. Holly was born and raised in southeast Georgia and almost all her family and friends were still either in Georgia or Florida. Now we would be five hours from her childhood home of Waycross and three hours from Tallahassee, where she spent most of her adulthood and where many of her best friends remain. Since she moved to Texas for me, it was my turn to return the favor and move with her to Georgia. Fortunately, I can do my work as a golf course consultant from anywhere if there is internet and a major airport nearby. Holly moved in April 2015, when she started the job. She was hired in early March, which did not give us a lot of time. We immediately drove to Columbus from Corsicana the second week in March to find a place to live. We were initially thinking of renting an apartment for her until we could sell our albatross of a house in Corsicana (more on this later). However, apartments were relatively expensive and would limit the number of pets we could have. This was a big deal because at the time we had two dogs and eight cats (all rescue). While most would stay with me until the house sold, it still brought up the problem of needing to find a house quickly once we sold ours. Fortunately, we got lucky on that trip and found a house we liked for sale but vacant. The owner agreed to rent it to us for a year with a second agreement to sell the house to us once we sold ours.

I was going to remain in Texas to 1) maintain the property and 2) try to sell the house. I was the listing agent for the home (I did residential real estate part time). The house we had in Corsicana was large, over 4,500 sf in size, with an additional 400 sf outbuilding I used as my office. It sat on three acres of land. We knew it would cost us a lot of money to maintain if I was not there. (Besides, I loved driving the garden tractor around.) We also believed I was the best person to sell it – certainly the most motivated. Because it is easier to sell furnished homes than vacant ones, and they tend to get higher prices, it was decided to keep most of the furniture in Texas. We mistakenly thought it would only be for just a brief time, as the Dallas real estate market was red hot then.

Sadly, that heat extended only to the Navarro County line as we soon discovered. The result was Holly moved into a 3,000 sf house with virtually NO furniture, other than a TV and a couple of chairs. We bought a mattress, a table and a few other necessities, but mostly it was a barren home. After all, we fully expected I would join her in a few weeks. She took the two dogs, both to keep her company (and safe) but also because I travel a lot and we did not want to have to continually board the dogs when I traveled. Cats didn't care if I was there or not, as long as someone came and made sure they were fed and kept the litterbox clean. Luckily the sister of one of Holly's former employees was up for that task.

While we had what we thought was a wonderful house in Corsicana, it was still in Corsicana. And apparently, most people outside of Corsicana felt about Corsicana the way my wife did. (Corsicana did have its nice features, but it always seemed a bit odd to us. It was like the 1950's never left. And if you weren't born there, you never were fully accepted.) So, while houses thirty miles north of us were getting multiple offers when listed and selling for over list price, we were averaging less than a showing a week. And we were priced under market value, although considerably higher than what we had purchased it for just a couple of years earlier. (When we moved to Texas in 2008, we initially moved to Ennis, about twenty miles north of Corsicana and closer to Dallas. We rented a house we planned on buying. But the owner sold it before we could. We then bought a house in Waxahachie six months later. While we loved Waxahachie, the forty-five-minute commute to Corsicana was terribly hard on Holly, so we decided to relocate in 2013.)

Unfortunately, Corsicana agents apparently did not appreciate a non-Corsicana agent (I was based out of Waxahachie) listing a house in their turf. And the Corsicana agents knew how much we paid for the house and just could not get their heads around the fact we made a lot of improvements to the property and the market had gone up significantly. So, the only offers we were getting were ridiculously low.

In the meantime, I made trips to Georgia about every three to four weeks. Each time, I drove the 12-hour trip. And each time I would take a cat. In fact, I would take two. It still took a lot of trips. The last trip I had three cats, which I put in a dog pen I set up in the back of my Ford C-Max (no, I hadn't heard of a C-Max either until I bought one. I love it though. It's a hybrid hatchback). The previous three trips with cats had been relatively uneventful. After about an hour of meowing, they would eventually settle down and remain quiet for the rest of the trip. But not this final trip. Nope.

It was my fault for leaving Cleo and Pumpkin till last, our two "noisiest" cats. Those two never shut up for the entire twelve-hour trip! It was the most miserable car ride I had ever had in my life, up to that point. Two would later surpass it, although technically one was in a truck. But I'm getting ahead of myself.

Finally, in early August, after several price reductions, we got an acceptable offer that was still nearly $70k (or 25%) over what we paid for the house three years previous. Naturally, the selling agent and buyer were not from Corsicana, but from North Dallas. Our house would easily sell for twice as much there, so they certainly appreciated the value. However, the buyer, who was self-employed in the oil business, had a credit issue. As a result, they wanted to do what we were doing in Georgia – rent the house for up to nine months while he got his credit straightened out. Because he owned a company in the oil industry and made a lot of money, I was not worried. The other issue was that they wanted to move in by September 1st, giving us less than three weeks to move.

While a career in museums is gratifying in many ways, financial is not one of them. And while the National Civil War Naval Museum was a terrific opportunity, it paid a lot less than what Holly was making in Corsicana – which was not much. Further, they only offered $1,500 to help us with moving expenses. And because money was always an issue for us, especially since we had not really *sold* the house but were renting it, we had to move ourselves. Hello U-Haul.

THE MOVE

We had so much stuff we decided to move in two stages. My poor daughter, Elizabeth, just happened to be visiting with me in early August. As a result, she got roped into helping us with the first move. We hired movers at both ends to do the heavy lifting -- loading and unloading. Holly drove back from Columbus to help pack the truck, which was the largest U-Haul had to offer. We made the twelve-hour trip in one day, with me driving the truck and Holly driving her car. Lizzy alternated riding with each of us. It was late when we arrived, so we just went to bed. Poor Lizzy had to sleep on an inflatable bed, which quickly deflated. Alas, it was not the most comfortable night for any of us (especially Lizzy). Fortunately, the movers came to help us unpack and move in the next morning.

I did not get to stay long in Columbus as I had to return to pack and take care of the house. Then it really got crazy. Shortly after returning to Corsicana, I took off for a business trip to Omaha. I left on the 23rd of August and returned on the 26th. On the 27th, I rented another truck from U-Haul. While I had hired a moving crew to come and help, they arrived nearly two hours late. In the meantime, I was hauling stuff around and doing last-minute packing – mostly of my office.

Unfortunately, I have a bad back . . . mostly thanks to my mother's side of the family. Almost all her siblings had bad backs, and I was lucky enough (along with my sister Cheryl) to inherit this condition.

The first time I had a problem with my back was in 1983 when I was working as a district manager for Scriptomatic, a manufacturer of addressing machines. This job had me traveling North and South Dakota, Nebraska, Kansas, Missouri and parts of Iowa, Illinois and Kentucky . . . all by car. I kept the machines in my trunk, meaning I was constantly lifting these relatively heavy pieces of equipment in and out of the trunk. One day, my back exploded with pain. It was so bad that I could barely walk. Standing was very painful. So was lying down. The only comfortable position for me was a reclining chair – where I would sleep.

My sister Juliette, who is a doctor, got me into see one of her friends from med school, Dr. Captain Grey, who was also in Lawrence. He was terrific. He first put me through a battery of mostly very painful tests (like a spinal tap). Then after my agony was nearly complete, he gave me an epidural. Like a minor miracle, the pain immediately ceased.

My back did not bother me again until about eight years later when I was living in Durham, NC. My wife, Ann, was a

Child Psychologist at Duke. At the time, Duke had a wonderful benefit for staff – all medical treatment at Duke hospital was free! (This benefit did not survive the turn of the century, but it was wonderful while it lasted). This time, the back did not hurt me as badly as it did in '83, but it was bad enough.

This became my first experience with the electronic coffin tube known as an MRI. (Over the next few years, I had six MRI's – including my back, neck, shoulder and head.) They prescribed physical therapy, as an alternative to surgery. The pain abated, but it took about six months before it disappeared.

I had one other bad bought of back issues in the early 90s, with the same PT and six months before it went away.

It did not go away completely, though. I always had to be careful when lifting things. And the back would bother me if I stood still for more than a few minutes (long lines are a killer!). But I did not have another acute episode – until that fateful date in August 2015.

By the time the movers finally arrived, I was literally withering on the floor in agony. I could not help them even if I wanted to. I'm sure they appreciated that. Sadly, these movers were not the fastest in the world. They also had given me poor advice on the size of the truck I needed. (I even went up one size from what they recommended, but I should have gotten the biggest one again.) The result was they did not finish until about 10 pm. Worse, they were not able to get everything loaded, so I had to leave stuff behind for our new renter/buyers to deal with.

Meanwhile, I had to get to Columbus! I had a flight out of Atlanta for another business trip on Sunday morning (it was now Friday night). The movers were coming Saturday afternoon. Moreover, I had a hotel reservation in Vicksburg

– about halfway to Columbus - that night. It was too late to cancel, so I was paying for it whether I used it or not. So even though I was in great pain and extremely tired, I had to climb into the cab and drive the six hours to Vicksburg, arriving in the wee hours of the morning. After a few hours of sleep, I was back up and driving the rest of the way to Columbus. (It is the first time I ever stayed in Vicksburg without visiting a casino.)

Fortunately, the back pain subsided after some rest. But it did not abate for long, which brings me back to being allergic to Georgia.

Allergic to Georgia

May 2017
THE SPINE

I am allergic to Georgia. At least that's what I told my wife as all sorts of medical problems occurred after moving to Georgia in August 2015. However, the truth is more likely I was allergic to turning sixty. Yet there was a lot that happened once I crossed that border . . .

In addition to the above mentioned back issue, which technically began before entering Georgia (although Georgia was the reason) my neck started hurting more shortly after I moved.

My neck has bothered me since the mid-1990s. When it first happened, I was advised by the Doctors at Duke I needed to have a couple of vertebrates in my neck fused. But they also recommended trying physical therapy first as surgery was a drastic option. I did, and again after about six months, the pain abated, although it never completely went away. I compensated by simply not turning my neck as much. This has resulted in me having very limited rotation of my neck, which is not good for driving! Now in Columbus, the neck pain had intensified significantly, with tingling and some numbness down my right arm and into my hands.

When I was referred to a neurosurgeon for my back in Columbus, I also had them check on my neck. I had MRIs taken of both. What fun!

In case you are not familiar with an MRI, which stands for Magnetic Resonance Imaging, let me try to describe it. The MRI machine is a big box with a hollow tube running through it. This tube is not very big, but supposedly big enough for most humans. It is about eight feet long and seems only a foot in diameter. (It's wider than that, but not much. When I am inside, my shoulders are squeezed.) You lie down on a flat board, with a too small pillow for your head. For chest area MRI's, a small cage is strapped over your midsection with your arms inside, further restricting your movement. I am told the camera is actually a part of the contraption being strapped on top of you. The board then slides into the tube. How far depends on what part of your body is being examined. But unless they are looking at your feet, chances are very good that your head will be inside, and you will feel like you're in an open-ended coffin. Only you can't see the open end. You are staring up at the tube wall, which is about six inches above your face. This is bad, even if you don't have claustrophobia. Unfortunately, I do. You are in a tube so tight that your shoulders are squeezed, and you are staring up at the top of the tube, six inches above your eyes, and you can't move. But, wait, there's more. Then the scan starts.

You don't normally feel the scan (although sometimes they generate heat). But you certainly hear it! The MRI makes a very loud clanging sound when operating. It is so loud; they must give you headphones or earplugs to protect your hearing. When I first had MRIs done, you just had ear plugs. Now the MRIs have headphones and they will let you listen to the music of your choice (classic rock). But good luck hearing it when the scan starts. Fortunately, each scan does not last more than a minute or two. But there are multiple scans. And it takes several minutes to set up each scan. So, you are in the tube a long time.

I have learned to self-hypnotize myself to get through these MRIs. I can convince myself I am relaxing in a snug bed. However, I later discovered the joys of an open MRI, which were not available when I first experienced MRIs. Unfortunately, not only are they limited in availability, they also provide much worse resolution.

When I arrived in Georgia, Juliette fortunately told me to ask for a "large bore" MRI, which is still a tube but much wider. It's still a coffin – but at least I now have 8" above my face instead of 6". This really helps as I hated having my shoulders squeezed together in the narrow tubes, which really exacerbates the claustrophobia. Between my back, neck and cancer, I have probably had a dozen MRIs over the past year and half – with one scheduled now every three months. Each one is forty-five minutes long because they are doing two different areas – the abdomen and chest. I also need contrast, which is where they inject a dye to better see the good stuff. In addition, I have a CT Scan done of my chest. But those are a piece of cake as they take only five minutes. But I'm getting way ahead of myself. Back to the back . . . and neck.

The neurosurgeon we were referred to, Dr. Bronzeman*, was supposedly the best or at least one of the very best in Columbus. This is when we realized the quality of medicine in Columbus was just not up to the standards we had been used to! (I was spoiled in Texas where my sister hooked me up with great doctors). Indeed, Holly was also having a lot of back pain, so she also saw Dr. Bronzeman at the same time.

After the obligatory hour wait in the waiting room and preliminaries by the RN, Dr. Bronzeman finally made his appearance. The MRI's (which we brought in with us on discs), was loaded into the PC in the exam room, and as far as I could tell, only that. That fact, plus Dr. Bronzeman's reaction, gave us the strong impression this was the first time he had seen the scans.

Dr. Bronzeman studied my MRIs for at least thirty seconds, maybe forty-five, before announcing that I had bad "arthritis" in my back. Ok, I will readily admit I am not a Doctor. But I have been to a lot of back specialists in my life and NONE of them called what I have "arthritis." They used the terms "degenerative disc disease," "bulging discs" and "spinal stenosis." Hearing the more general diagnosis of arthritis certainly caused me to wonder just how thoroughly he was really examining these scans in his thirty seconds. (I guess he is technically right, but still it's not very descriptive.) His recommendation was physical therapy, plus having an EMG done for my neck.

He repeated the process and diagnosis for Holly, whom he told he really didn't see anything wrong. Even though Holly has a spinal deformity from birth and has had constant back and hip problems. So much for the best neurosurgeon in the area. Our impression was he looked to see if he could operate and if that was not an option, he was no longer interested.

Unfortunately, the physical therapy did not help. So, I sought a second opinion from the doctor I was told was the best spinal orthopedic surgeon in the area, Dr. Norchalk*. (That's the thing about the spine. It's the domain of both neurosurgeons and orthopedic surgeons; making it hard to know which one to turn to). We were in for another great experience.

Dr. Norchalk has an almost comical appearance. He looks and talks like Thor. He's about 6'1" and well-built. He's Swedish with his accent intact and long flowing shoulder-plus length blonde hair in which he obviously takes immense pride.

At least he did not say I had arthritis. Instead, he noted I had spinal stenosis of the entire spine. My lower back was so bad, it had almost self-fused as there was so little space left between the discs. Thus, there was no surgical option. My neck, though, he felt he could fix – by fusing four vertebrae. He did say I could try another epidural in my back to see if it would bring me relief. I agreed.

So, in December 2015, I had an epidural performed by Dr. Thor. It was not a pleasant experience. In fact, it was one of the most painful events I have had in my life. Although they gave me a pain killer shot first (which, in itself, hurt like heck), but it either was totally ineffective or he gave it no time to work as I felt every inch of that seemingly foot-long needle going in and staying in. I swear he missed the spot, because I felt nothing but pain in my spine. Then he repeated the process on the other side of my back.

The epidural had absolutely no effect on my back pain . . . other than adding to it for a time. And to my surprise, Dr. Thor never followed up with me to see if it worked or how I was doing. Nothing. Not even a call from his nurse.

Meanwhile, my neck was getting worse, so I relented and went back to Dr. Bronzeman to see what his response was going to be. This time he decided I did have a surgical problem and he would happily fuse three of my vertebrae.

Before making a final decision, we decided to try Dr.

Thor one last time, with the idea of seriously exploring the surgery. We even got so far as scheduling it for three weeks away. But I backed away after talking with my physical therapist, my sister and others. For not only would the surgery put me out of work for at least three months (I could not travel), which would be financially untenable at the time, but it is a very risky surgery. Plus, by fusing three or four vertebrae, I would be putting added pressure on the remaining ones, causing them to deteriorate even faster. In short, it was a no-win scenario. On the other hand, I risked permanent paralysis should I not have the surgery and get into a bad car wreck.

I decided to wait. I wanted to see if the six-month rule was in effect for either my back or neck. Throughout my life, I have had several significant pain events, mostly with my back and neck but also once with my right shoulder. This happened in my forties when we still had free care at Duke. It was also my first experience with the wonderful thing call an EMG. This is a medical test where they essentially make you into an electrified pin cushion – think acupuncture with electric needles. They stick needles in you in various places and then send electrical shocks through them. (I think the machine was developed by the CIA). If the pain from the needle wasn't enough, the shock would do the trick. Yet, despite all these tests (including more MRIs), the doctors could not figure out what was wrong. Instead they just declared it had to be a virus infection and said it would eventually go away. I had never heard of a virus infection that only affected one area before, but they were right. After six months, the pain disappeared. Just like it had with my back and neck pain episodes -- whether or not I did the physical therapy.

TESTEE SITUATION

Unfortunately, the neck and back pains were not the only

things that went wrong with me in Georgia! Indeed, the first problem occurred before I moved there, but after Holly had. In the four months between her move and mine, I drove back and forth every two to three weeks, with cats in tow. It was a twelve-hour drive.

In mid-summer 2015, I developed a very sharp pain in my, uh, testicular area (trying to be polite). I thought it might have had something to do with all the driving back and forth. But it got bad, so I went to see a doctor back in Corsicana. An ultrasound failed to show any problems. (This was a mildly embarrassing situation as the technician doing the ultrasound was a very pretty girl. Naturally I had to pull down my shorts. She then handed me a small towel and told me to cover up "the shaft". As soon as I left, I realized I blew the chance to deliver the best line . . . "I'm going to need a bigger towel." Alas, my brain just wasn't functioning right that day). I was given some antibiotics and sent on my way.

When the pain failed to diminish, I went to see Holly's Doctor in Columbus after I moved. She referred me to a urologist. This became my first experience with Dr. Freud*, who would figure so prominently in my medical future.

We were initially impressed with Dr. Freud, who was very nice and sympathetic. After telling me all the horrible things that could be causing my pain, he declared it was most likely an infection and gave me a much stronger antibiotic. This did significantly reduce the pain. However, it *still* has never gone away completely, acting up from time to time.

KNEEDING HELP

The other problem materializing right after the move was my left knee started hurting again badly. This forced me to again see an orthopedic surgeon – but not Dr. Thor-- this time it was Dr. Tucker. He was excellent. He told me I would probably need both knees replaced, eventually. But in the meantime, we could treat the knee with a cortisone shot. It did the trick! (Both Dr. Norchalk and Dr. Tucker are part of the apparently famous Hughston Clinic in Columbus, which has its own hospital and does only orthopedic work.)

BACK TO BACK

In February 2016, I decided to take a different tack with my back pain as physical therapy wasn't cutting it. I went to see a pain doctor, Dr. Dawson. Holly went with me . . . and immediately fell in lust. Have you seen the TV show, "Rosewood?" Well Dr. Dawson was a real-life version, only he works with live patients. He not only has movie star good looks, but he has a wonderful personality with an excellent sense of humor. And he appreciated the dog and pony show my wife and I typically put on.

To give me immediate relief, he gave me a cortisone shot for my neck. But here is where he was so much different than my other doctors. When I was given cortisone shots before, the doctors would typically give me a shot of a pain killer (which hurt in itself), then wait not long enough and stick the overly large cortisone needle in, to my great discomfort. Not Dr. Goodlooks. He sprayed and sprayed and sprayed this numbing freeze spray on me before hitting me with a needle. I never felt a thing! Why can't other doctors do this?

He also wanted to try a relatively new technology on my back, which essentially involves implanting a device that sends shocks to the spine. But before I could have one implanted, I had to have a psychological exam done and then do a trial with an external device. I guess they wanted to make sure you weren't going to turn the juice way up and try to electrocute yourself. (You may be surprised to know I passed the psych eval).

But by the time it came to try the device, the six months were up. And much to my surprise and extreme delight, the back pain started to ease up. A month later, right on schedule, the neck pain did the same. (Neither has completely disappeared, mind you, but both are tolerable. I just must be careful – not lift heavy things, avoid standing for extended periods and doing extra chores . . . at least that's what I tell Holly).

SHOULDERING THE LOAD

But Georgia wasn't through with me. As the back and neck pain started dissipating, my right shoulder started throbbing, including numbness and pain down my arm. I was referred to a shoulder specialist, Dr. McClusky, but his first available appointment was four months into the future! So more physical therapy and suffering were ahead. (FYI, the shoulder pain did disappear again after six months, but will still occasionally flare up from time to time. I have a torn rotator cuff).

All of this happened within the first year of moving to Georgia.

First Signs

May 2017

This brings us to the fateful night of June 10th, 2016, a day forever altering the course of my life. (And still within my first year in Georgia). And it started totally innocently. I did something I have done several times a day my entire life – I peed. However, what emerged was something completely unexpected – grape juice. I was peeing grape juice – at least that's what it looked like. My urine was a dark, dark purple. There was no burning or pain . . . just purple pee. Let me tell you, it was completely shocking to see grape juice coming out from there! At first, I thought maybe I had eaten something that turned my pee that color, even though I could not imagine what it might have been.

The weird thing was the next time I peed -- it was normal. Same with the time after that. But then, grape juice. So now I was really concerned. I realized it probably wasn't grape juice, nor was it from anything I ate, but rather I had a *lot* of blood in my urine. And that was scary – especially given the amount needed to turn it not reddish, but deep purple.

The next morning, I called my doctor who got me in

later that day to see her physician's assistant, Alicia. I didn't mind as I liked her better as I thought she was more thorough.

The lab in her office confirmed the presence of urine in my blood. (The sample I gave wasn't the grape juice, but there was still enough blood in the regular sample). She palpated my abdomen. I yelped as I felt a very sharp pain when she got to the kidney area, which was totally unexpected as I had not felt any pain up to that time.

She scheduled me for a CT scan and a whole mess of blood work. (Over the course of the next several months, my arms became pin cushions having so many blood tests. I really don't know how addicts or diabetics do it. I certainly would not want to have to stick a needle in myself all the time. By the end of the summer, my veins started hiding from the phlebotomist, making it very difficult to get the samples. One notable time left me with a purple arm for several weeks as she apparently missed the mark).

I certainly did not realize it at the time, but the fatal mistake she made was to order a regular CT scan, rather than one with contrast. If she had done that, things might have been a lot different – as the regular CT scan showed nothing amiss.

The grape-juice urine was not a regular occurrence, but sporadic. It would happen once then I would go several days before another occurrence. The frequency increased throughout June but started slowing in July and eventually stopped by late July. I did not know it at the time, but it likely stopped because my left kidney ceased functioning.

Later that same week, two other symptoms appeared. I believe they were related to the grape juice, but could not convince any doctor:

Insomnia: I have had insomnia at various times throughout my life. However, it has mostly been where my mind was simply overactive. And it always responded very well to a *low* dose (5 mg) of Ambien. It may last a few days, but then disappear. One 30-day supply of Ambien would last me at least a year. However, this time it was *very different*. My mind was not the issue at all. My body was. It felt like I had "restless *body* syndrome." I simply could not get my body to relax or stay still, even though I became *extremely fatigued*. I tried everything, upping the Ambien all the way to 30 mg, using over the counter meds, even Bellsomril. But *nothing worked*. For about six weeks, until the end of July, I averaged less than two hours of sleep. Many nights I got no sleep at all. I became a walking zombie. I began to understand how Michael Jackson might have felt he needed Propofol. Believe me, if I had access to it, I probably would have tried it as well. I was that desperate, even knowing the risk. When you're that sleep deprived, you would do almost anything just to be able to get a restful sleep. I can see why it is often used as a form of torture.

The sleeplessness led me to make some *really* bad decisions – especially in the middle of the night. I could not sleep, but I was so fatigued I could not think or do anything constructive (with normal insomnia, I often get up and work). But this time, that was impossible. I was simply too fatigued to do anything, even read . . . or sit still. I was miserable. I tried mixing sleeping pills – over the counter medicine *plus* the Ambien. This was *not* a good idea. I will give you two examples. I had to go to Tallahassee (about three hours away by car) for a consulting project during this period. The night before I was to leave, as had been the case most every night, I could not sleep. So, at about 3:30 am, since I was still awake and knew that was not likely to change, I decided it was a clever idea if I just went ahead and left for Florida. This was most definitely *not* smart. Indeed, it was a very, very *bad* idea. I was so fatigued I could hardly see to drive. I was extremely lucky I did not kill myself or someone else, although I did hit a curve and did minor damage to the car. I was fortunate that was all that happened.

I pulled over about halfway and was able to get in a fifteen-minute cat nap, which really helped. (I had another fifteen-minute cat nap on my way back home later that same day. Luckily, there were no other incidents.) Adrenaline kicked in and the consulting part went fine – at least I *think* it did.

The second incident followed a similar pattern. It was about 3 am and I had not slept. So, I thought it was a great idea to drive over to Walmart (which was open twenty-four hours) and get another type of sleep medicine. The next day, I had no recollection of driving to Walmart, or driving home, for that matter. I vaguely remembered picking the medicine off the shelf. And I don't remember paying for it, although I'm sure I did. At least, I hope I did. I may have gotten two hours sleep that night.

Left Shoulder/arm pain: At the same time, I started feeling muscle pain and weakness in my *left* arm. I initially attributed it to overusing the left arm due to the right shoulder pain. But it never let up; instead it kept getting worse over the next six weeks. I then developed numbness in my left hand. I eventually had another EMG done, but it did not show any nerve damage, so it wasn't being caused by my neck issues. (Fortunately, the needles they use today are a lot thinner, so the EMG was not nearly as bad as first one.) To this day, I still do not know what caused this pain.

As an aside, none of my doctors have ever been able to explain these symptoms, or why they all occurred simultaneous with the grape juice. There does not seem to be a medical explanation. Notably, they went away over time – although it took several months. However, they did not disappear for good, as they both have made guest appearances from time to time. But the severity has not risen to the level it did that summer.

My personal belief is my body was trying to get through to me something was terribly wrong even though I was not showing any other symptoms related to what was wrong, other than grape juice pee. (The more logical explanation is it was caused by stress. Yet I have been under tremendous stress many times in my life – like every day since Jeff moved away in 7th grade, and never experienced anything like this).

After getting the CT scan results, I was referred to my urologist, Dr. Freud, who I saw on the fifteenth of June. He was very casual about my situation, noting this "was not unusual" and it was "likely nothing to worry about." He suspected it was due to infection and prescribed an antibiotic. At the same time, he scheduled two procedures -- a Contrast CT in his office for 6/28 and a cystoscope in his office on 7/11. (Obviously, he was not that concerned as he scheduled these important diagnostic tests for over nearly a month period.) A follow-up visit was not scheduled until 8/18.

Juliette had warned me about having a CT scan at a doctor's office, noting they were often inferior equipment picked up used. When I went in for the scan, I made it a point to ask the technician about the equipment and she assured me that it had just recently been updated.

I was told the CT scan showed "signs of an infection." He changed the antibiotic to a stronger medicine. Although I did not know it at the time, this turned out to be a very fateful, and very wrong diagnosis.

I thought the EMG was bad, and I certainly knew the epidural done by Dr. Thor was horrible, and definitely the gall stone attack was extremely painful. But these were a walk in the park compared to the cystoscope, which must be Greek for 'torture device.' Why they insist on doing this procedure with no pain killers is a complete mystery to me. Certainly, I would have paid almost anything for some had I known the pain I was to experience! I know I would have told them where the gold was buried. Heck, I would have gotten it for them.

Basically, the cystoscope consists of sticking this much too large tube up your much smaller pee hole. The tube has a camera on the end, which I swear must have been the size of my Nikon. He then continued to ram this tube up as I withered in agony. I know the guy must be a sadist. Holly got to watch the entire procedure.

I would like to say the pain was worth it, but given he found nothing wrong, I am not so sure. Anyway, he was more convinced it was just an infection. And given the incidence of the grape juice occurring was becoming rarer, I could not argue. Except I still was experiencing the insomnia and shoulder numbness. So, I knew something was amiss, just not sure what.

I went back to my regular doctor, who referred me to Dr. Patel, a nephrologist (kidney specialist). I really liked him as he was very understanding and sympathetic and had a good sense of humor. Again, he ordered a bunch more blood work and a 24-hour urine test (such fun, peeing into a bottle for an entire day—thank goodness, I work at home. And that I'm a guy). He also had an ultrasound done in his office.

The blood work revealed a *slight* decrease in kidney function and a couple of other quirky things – low vitamin D3 and phosphorous. The latter was new and totally unexpected. I never had that issue before. So, he asked me if I had any recent changes in my diet. I thought about it. No, my diet was as bad as always with one notable exception. I had stopped drinking Diet Coke.

Dr. Patel informed me diet coke was high in phosphorous. Now I had been addicted to Diet Coke. I drank *at least* six cans a day. It was all I drank, except an occasional beer. But when the blood thing occurred, I decided to give it up cold turkey. When he told me I was low in phosphorous, I assumed it may have been a reaction to having a major phosphorous source removed from my diet. So, I decided to start drinking them again – but only one or two a day this time around. (Footnote: My phosphorous level is now normal).

The bottom line, though, is Dr. Patel could not explain the blood and certainly not the insomnia or shoulder issue. But by this time (early August), the grape juice had stopped, and the insomnia was better, so I just figured whatever had been the matter had run its course. Boy was I ever wrong!

MEANWHILE

While all this medical stuff was going on, my personal life was in turmoil.

Our financial situation took a major hit the previous fall. As you may remember, we had our house in Corsicana under contract to be sold, with the buyers renting it. But then came October 23rd, 2015. That was the day the sky fell – literally – on Corsicana.

BIBLICAL EVENT

Prior to that day, the record rainfall for Corsicana was 9.5 inches, which occurred in 1899. But on October 23rd we had **22 inches** of rain at my house (as measured by my neighbor) in a 24-hour period and 28 inches over 48 hours! (It made national news -- you may remember seeing a picture of a train that had been derailed by flood waters. That was a half mile from my house.)

The rain did not come down straight, either. It blew at all angles – sometimes coming in sideways. We had a metal roof, which I loved. The previous fall, we had a storm with golf ball sized hail. *Every* house in our area needed a new roof as a result – except us. But even a metal roof is not built for having over two feet of rain blowing in sideways over forty-eight hours.

Because of the sideways rain, the roof leaked in about a half-dozen places. But that was not the worse problem. Our house sat at the top of a hill. But the area around the house itself was flattened down. Again, it was not designed for twenty-eight inches of rain. The massive amount of water accumulated in the flat areas around the house and water then poured in from both the back porch and front garden areas, which simply could not drain fast enough. Earlier that summer when I was living there, we had an 8" rain, which was near record level then. Yet we had no leaks or flooding.

Our renter/buyers freaked. Or rather the New York wife (who was about twenty years younger than her husband) did. She accused us of lying about the house, that it leaked in the past and all this crap (none of which was true). She apparently thought the house should have been built to withstand damage from a storm more than twice as bad as any in recorded history. (To give you an idea, the average annual rainfall for Corsican is forty inches. We had 70% of the annual total in two days.)

Bottom line, even though we were going to fix the house, add more drainage, and paid for them to stay at a hotel, the buyer/renters cancelled both contracts and left, threatening to sue. (They didn't, but we also did not get any other compensation from them for breaking the contracts as I could not afford to hire an attorney).

JESUS SAVES

Not only did we lose our renters and, more importantly, buyers, we had to fix our house. That is when Jesus saved us . . .

a lot of money. Did I mention that Jesus was my former neighbor in Waxahachie who was also a contractor? He also was likely an illegal alien, but he was a great contractor who had done several jobs for us and for my real estate clients. Not only did he do great work, but he was also inexpensive. This was critical because my insurance (Allstate) was not going to cover many of the repairs because they considered it "flood damage," which was not covered. (It is considered "flood" because the water came in from the yard. So even though we were on top of a hill, we still had "flood" damage because the patio and the garden area could not handle draining over two feet of rain.) But our adjuster was wonderful to work with. And between what they did pay for and Jesus, we were able to get most of it repaired for the amount of the insurance check.

Still, it took several weeks to repair. We also decided to make additional improvements, including all new kitchen appliances, to make the house more attractive for potential buyers. All total, we came out of pocket about $5,000, which was not bad given the circumstances. But as we did not have $5,000 in the bank, it was not good, either. As my wife says, that is why God invented credit cards.

Worse, we were now paying two mortgages, one in Columbus and a much higher one in Corsicana – plus the maintenance and upkeep costs, including utilities, for two homes, without the rental income to offset it. This included hiring someone to mow the three acres. And now we had no furniture there, so we had to show it vacant making it harder to sell. And we did not have the service of the best listing agent (myself). As you guessed, it proved very difficult to sell.

Coupled with my business having slowed down to almost nothing, it created a significant financial hardship. I am self-employed. In addition to the golf business, when I was in

Texas, I used my real estate license to sell residential homes to help supplement my income and smooth out the inevitable slow periods. I did the same when I lived in Jacksonville. But when we moved to Georgia, I did not get my Georgia license as I had my fill of residential sales.

Unfortunately, the consulting business is highly variable. Sometimes it gets very busy, but other times, its dead. As a one-man show, I typically work only one or two projects at a time. But now I had none. Bad time for the business to go into a slump – when our expenses doubled, and our income sharply dropping (loss of rental income). It did not take us long to go through our savings.

The government initially saved our asses (a few months later). Because Corsicana was declared a federal disaster area, we qualified for assistance from FEMA. However, since we did not *live* there at the time, our house was technically considered a rental property and not a personal residence. As a result, we could not get direct assistance (free money) but were able to get an SBA loan at an extremely attractive rate. Making it more attractive, it was not tied to the house. When we eventually sold the house, we would not have to pay off the loan. We will, however, be paying for it over the next fifteen years.

But with the mounting medical costs adding to all our other expenses and the lack of a steady income on my part meant by June 2016, we were in deep financial doo doo. By the end of June I'm not sure which is a worse mess – my body, or my bank account.

THE WEEK THAT WAS

Then, as it has so many times in my life, everything unexpectedly changed suddenly and dramatically – in this case, in the course of a week. The first bit of good news was my company was awarded its first management contract with

John S. Wait

Southern Hills Golf Course.

Then we got the news we waited so long to hear – our house was under contract! We finally had a buyer. (While the sales amount was substantially less than we had the year previous, we still made a nice profit on the home.) This triggered my wife and I to rethink buying the house we were in, which needed a lot of updating, and see what else was on the market. Good thing, because we found the house of our dreams – in the same neighborhood as the house we were renting. And, with the equity from our old house, we could put 20% down, meaning no PMI on the mortgage. We would pay $400/month less than on the house in Corsicana, even though the purchase price was about the same.

Lastly, I received good news on the medical front. The CT scan Dr. Freud ordered revealed no major issues and seemed to confirm his diagnosis of an infection. This was a tremendous relief! I later discovered just how wrong he was, but at the time, it was good news and I had one heck of a week.

With the management contract, I once again found myself driving back and forth to Texas. I drove for two main reasons. First, it was cheaper which was important since I was not getting reimbursed for expenses (I included it in the monthly fee), and money was still tight. But second, it gave me more flexibility as I could stay longer if needed. During these trips, I would also go to Dallas, about 90 minutes away from Gladewater (between Longview and Tyler). I would stay with my sister, Cheryl, and would also visit my father, who was in an Alzheimer unit at a nice assisted living facility a couple of miles from her. The trips would last anywhere from several days to over a week.

MORE MEDICAL MESS

Meanwhile, over the next two months (July and August), I would continue to see a variety of doctors, including changing my primary care physician. Over these months, I saw two different primary care physicians, a urologist (Dr. Freud), a nephrologist (Dr. Patel – three times), an orthopedic surgeon for my knee (another injection) plus a different orthopedic surgeon. The latter I saw for my *right* shoulder, which was not really bothering me anymore (six months), but he would not look at my *left* shoulder which *was* bothering me as my original appointment was for the right and he refused to change arms. (Grrrr) I had to make a second appointment for the left shoulder. (My right shoulder pain is due to a partial rotator cuff tear, which I knew about as I've had it for nearly ten years. But he never could figure out what was wrong with the left. Instead, I waited for the six-month rule.) In addition to all the doctor visits, I also had physical therapy for my back and neck twice a week.

With each doctor visit came more tests, usually blood (pin cushion arms), but also a couple of MRIs (shoulder and neck), another EMG and a CAT scan.

I went back to Dr. Patel in late-August. By this time, I was doing much better. No more blood in the urine, no insomnia, even the pain in my left arm/shoulder had been reduced significantly. My blood tests did not reveal anything alarming (other than the phosphorous and Vitamin D3 and *slightly* reduced kidney functions). The ultrasound of my kidney revealed nothing alarming. So, he scheduled a follow-up for six weeks later. I never made that appointment.

SOUTHERN HILLS

THE STUDY

March 2017

I was initially hired to try and sell Southern Hills in the spring of 2016. But when I inspected it, I realized 1) the owner would not get anywhere near what he wanted; 2) the golf course was horrible, but it had a nice clubhouse and the land was spectacular; 3) the owner had a significant real estate development around the golf course which was to be the major source of income, but the current course was a detriment not an asset to sales and the development too was failing; 4) a great golf course could be built on the site which would make the real estate much more valuable and easier to sell, and 5) the real estate development was targeted to upper middle-income, with several million-dollar homes, yet the golf course was priced at the bottom of the market. As a result, both suffered. So instead of listing the course, I was able to convince them to hire me to do a feasibility study for improving the course. For this project, I brought in the other two amigos – Jeff Brauer and Paul*.

Jeff is a noted golf course architect. His designs have twice won "Best New Public Golf Course" by *Golf Digest*, putting him in rarified air among golf course architects. He is also a past president of the American Golf Course Architects Association. Jeff and I have worked together on numerous projects, starting in 2001 when he and I both subcontracted with the National Golf Foundation (NGF) for a project in Dallas (Indian Creek in Carrollton). Over the years, Jeff and I have become very close friends.

I have known Paul for over twenty years. He was the superintendent of a golf course in Pinehurst that became the inspiration for me getting into the golf business and later became my first golf course consulting client (it previously was my first golf course client when I was with John Hancock, selling financial services.) Paul is an excellent agronomist. In fact, Paul's first job in agronomy was interning at Augusta National after graduating top of his class at Penn State.

Paul and his partner, Barney*, left soon after I started doing business with the golf course to set up their own company, Signal Golf*. Signal is a golf course management company also doing golf course construction. Initially, they also offered golf course consulting services, for which they usually brought me in as a subcontractor. Barney eventually left Signal, but Paul has done well since then – managing a few courses while concentrating on construction projects. I have used Paul several times as my agronomist on consulting projects. (Agronomy is the one area of golf operations I know little about – and I know it. So, I bring in the best when a project includes a golf course maintenance review).

As an aside, I came up with the name "Sirius Golf Advisors" back in 1995, when I first started doing golf course consulting. To my knowledge, Sirius radio did not even exist back then. If it did, I certainly had not heard of it. I named the company "Sirius" because I was an astronomy buff (in my childhood, I had wanted to be an astronomer – a dream I carried with me until college calculus – but that's another story) and Sirius is the brightest star in the sky. Plus, it can be pronounced "serious", and thus became a double entendre. I even got a toll-free number that was 888-Sirius6. This was great until Sirius radio came along. Suddenly, I start getting a lot of calls for Sirius radio! (Their number is 888-Sirius1, but if you spell "one" out, it is the "6" on the phone). For a while, this was extremely problematic as not only was I getting a lot of their calls, I was *paying* for them because with "toll free" numbers the receiver pays for the calls. Fortunately, the volume of their calls has dropped dramatically. Where I was getting several a day, I now only get them occasionally. (Note: I have since dropped the 888-number given so few people now pay for long distance calls and I was getting very little use out of the line.)

I have sold golf courses since getting my real estate broker's license in 2004. However, this has never been a point of emphasis for me as I much prefer the consulting projects. As both professions are time consuming, I have to make tough decisions as to how best to allocate my time. My priority has been to do the consulting projects first, then when they slow down, I start paying more attention to the brokerage side.

For this project, Jeff looked at the design and layout issues while Paul tackled the maintenance problems. I did everything else.

During the evaluation, I spent a lot of time with Roger*, the General Manager at the course. I was impressed by him -- despite him leading a very unprofitable operation. I felt he was trying hard to reverse the tide. He and the Superintendent had only been there a year. The superintendent, another Barney*, had an impressive resume including being the head superintendent at a very high-end course in the mideast. Both were likeable and cooperated fully with our study.

The more I learned, the sorrier I felt for Howard. He had been screwed every which way possible by the people he hired – not just the previous managers who were horrible, (not only were they incompetent, one got Howard to significantly alter the course much to its detriment), but his contractors (the guy who did the residential lot layout did a horrendous job. It appeared he never visited the site.). And even the state as they widened the highway running alongside the course from two to four lanes, without adequately accounting for drainage. As a result, the course had significant flooding issues. I really wanted to make this work for him. He deserved a break.

After a careful and detailed analysis, we determined the market would support a higher-end facility and an investment in improving the course would be well-spent. However, we recommended the middle (in terms of cost) of three possible scenarios.

THE MEETING

At the end of June 2016 during the previously described miracle week, I drove to Dallas to meet with Howard and his family. Jeff, who lives in the Dallas area, met me at the hotel where they were staying, and we joined them for breakfast. Howard and his wife were visiting their daughter, Melanie who had a precious baby boy. Her husband, Adam, had been my contact for the study. After breakfast at the hotel, we drove to Southern Hills to review our ideas for the course.

Howard loved our study and agreed with our conclusions. Except for one thing. He wanted to know if we could route the golf course through the undeveloped part of the property, so it would create more golf course lots – meaning building new holes in the large undeveloped areas of the development. This would mean much higher costs than we had proposed even with the "high" end as we had been very cost conscious in our analysis. Yet Howard does not like doing things half-way.

We loved the idea of going into this undeveloped land which was on the opposite side of the existing development from the golf course. There was, however, two points of access allowing us to connect the holes on either side, so that was good.

Jeff and I were both impressed by Howard, as well as his family. Melanie (Adam's wife and Howard's daughter), was both beautiful and had a wonderful personality. She was a residential real estate agent in North Dallas and was helping her father sell the lots in the development after they got rid of the do-nothing agent they had previously.

It was also during this meeting I pitched Howard on the idea of letting us manage the course for him. I did not think we had a chance, but I also knew how badly he needed us. I just wasn't sure *he* knew that.

When we looked at this virgin land, we discovered it was, if anything, more striking than the original layout. We knew we now had the chance to do something special – create a course that could easily become the best in East Texas and potentially earn national recognition. Now we would have a course able to attract golfers from not only all over the region but pull them in from I-20 and even generate some play from the two larger metro areas – Shreveport and Dallas. It was that good a property and Jeff is that good an architect.

Howard believed in us. He hired Jeff to do the design work, Paul to do the construction (on my strong recommendation) and I was hired to manage the facility. Paul was also going to be my junior "partner" on the management contract as he had the management company infrastructure that could be helpful, plus I needed him to oversee the course maintenance.

Technically, the real estate development was not part of the management contract. But that didn't stop Howard from involving me in a major way. It would occupy most of my time as we sought to get sewer to the development.

S.H. Management

A SAD START

My first trip as head of the management team was the third week of July. It was to be a week bookended by tragedy. On Saturday the 16th, two days before I was to leave, I got a call from Cheryl. My father died.

Dad had been living in the Alzheimer's ward of an assisted living facility for the past few years. It was located just a couple of miles from Cheryl. For the past nine months, he had been on hospice care. He simply wasn't eating. He was also 96. So, his death wasn't unexpected. Indeed, in many ways it was a relief because none of us liked seeing him suffer or be a fraction of the wonderful man we knew him to be. But no matter how old you are or what the circumstances, it is a sad event when your parent dies.

It would have been nice to have seen dad one last time, but I had a feeling the last time I saw him just a couple of weeks previous, at the end of June, it would be my last. And since I was heading that way anyway, the timing at least was convenient.

I left the next day, a day earlier than planned. I went

straight to Dallas without stopping so I could assist my sister with some of the final arrangements on Monday. (Cheryl had to do the bulk of the planning as she was the only one of us left in Dallas. She did a great job.) Tuesday through Friday I spent at the course. Friday afternoon I drove back to Dallas and picked up Holly at the airport. We stayed at a hotel near Cheryl, along with Juliette and Michael who also flew in Friday. On Saturday morning, Matthew, flew in. (Lizzie was not able to come). Later that afternoon, we had a "remembrance" for dad at Cheryl's, in lieu of a formal funeral. The event itself went wonderfully. It was a relatively small group as Dad outlived most of his golf partners and siblings. But his brother, Merle and his son Merle Jr. made it down (Merle still lived in Protection, Kansas where they all grew up. Merle Jr., though, lived in the Ft. Worth area.). Cheryl also invited several of her friends, many of whom knew dad from the club where they all belonged (Brookhaven).

But the days leading up to the event held some drama. Cheryl and I had a big to-do. She did not want me to speak at the event. I wanted to talk about Dad's history, especially his early life and his service in WWII – after all, I had helped dad write a book about it (*"From Dusty Plains to Wartime Planes"*). She was worried I would "bore" the crowd, especially her friends, who she thought would be more interested in hearing golf stories. Tempers reached a crescendo at the family dinner the night before the remembrance when I broke down and even Cheryl's daughter got furious at her mother. The entire family was on my side. Cheryl finally relented, and I spoke and everyone – including Cheryl – appreciated it.

Holly rode with me on the way home. We stopped on the way at Southern Hills, so Holly could see the course (she agreed about how beautiful the property was). We stayed the night in Vicksburg, as was my custom.

When we arrived home the next day, we discovered one of our cats, Clifford, had died. He was one of, if not *the* favorite. We loved that cat. He was a huge (big, not fat) cat with fluffy mid-length golden fur that was the softest I ever felt on a cat. He was the friendliest cat and had a habit of doing cute things. He was also our disabled dog's, Beaudegarde Dog's (a pit-bull mix -- more on him later), best friend. He would always lay down with him and keep him company. He had done this ever since Beau came into our lives two years previous.

I found Clifford in the guest bathroom. It was our belief Clifford had eaten something poisonous outside just before Holly left. Ironically, he was one of only two of our cats allowed outside (we had eight at the time, plus two dogs, all rescue). When I saw his stiff body, I broke down completely. All the sadness from the week just overwhelmed my stoic façade.

ROGER AND OUT

As I mentioned, I really liked Roger. He was sharp, helpful and seemed eager to learn. And he obviously loved the place and was very loyal to Howard. In fact, my first act as manager was to give him a modest 5% raise in recognition of his effort. The underlying message I wanted to give him was I believed in him and did not want to replace him.

But I also recognized a lot of the harmful policies in place were either put there by Roger or endorsed by him. Further, all Roger's previous golf experience was at low-end courses. He had no experience running or even working at a facility of the quality we were going to become. He had a lot to learn.

There were other issues as well, which I will not get into

here. (I could literally write another book on the entire experience – get it, *literally* write . . .)

But perhaps the biggest issue I had was Roger simply would not communicate with me even though I was his boss. Instead of him regularly checking in as one would expect, I always had to initiate the contact – despite my many requests.

On my second trip, I also grew a bit suspicious of how Roger was handling the money. I discovered they had a weekly game there, when non-members were playing *without paying any green or cart fees*, just money that went into the prize pool. This meant the golf course received *no* revenue from these golfers. And Roger, personally, was handling all the cash. Further, staff were routinely ringing in players at a much lower rate at other times than what they should have been. This raised a lot of red flags.

Howard loved Roger. And I could understand that. He was the first semi-competent manager he had. Plus, Roger did everything Howard asked and did it immediately. I was not given that same courtesy. I realized quickly Roger needed to really change if he was to be our manager after the renovation. I also let Howard know my concerns and he said he supported whatever decision we needed to make.

Unfortunately, Howard was part of the problem. He too seemed to ignore the fact he hired me to manage the facility. Instead, he continued to go directly to Roger with any request or questions, cutting me out of the loop. As a result, Roger was doing jobs for Howard that I had no knowledge of and that would interfere with my own requests. Obviously, this could put Roger in a difficult position. His response was to ignore my requests.

Finally, I got tired of it and told him he needed to check in with me daily. At first, I only asked he submit a daily report on business activity – a simple request any manager should expect. Initially he was good at it, but after a couple of weeks he would skip a day, then two then three. By early October, he was weeks behind. I had a long talk with him during my second October visit, but it did not stick.

On my November trip I made it crystal clear he was not performing to expectation and needed to improve if he wanted to remain manager going forward. I also changed the request from emailing a report (which he was no longer doing anyway) to calling me daily when he was at the course. I asked him to do this every *morning*. And for while it seemed to work, except he would call in the middle or late in the afternoon.

Another problem with Roger was he had significant health issues, mostly stemming from birth defects. Further, he had no health insurance. While we could not afford to offer a group health policy to the employees, I did get Howard to agree to give Roger a raise to cover the cost of an individual health insurance policy (Obamacare). I then persuaded Roger to enroll in the program in December during open enrollment.

In the meantime, we lost the one staff member who impressed me. I felt she could be developed into our marketing manager. Unfortunately, we were not able to offer her full-time work until we were close to reopening. She could not afford to wait and was offered a full-time job in her hometown with good benefits we simply could not match.

Roger recommended we hire as a replacement Natasha*, who worked as their marketing person at his previous course. In addition, her husband was in the restaurant business, so she was already plugged in to the banquet and wedding business, an emphasis of our new club post renovations.

Roger brought her in for me to meet during my October

visit. I was very impressed and endorsed hiring her. We could only bring her in part-time, but that's all she wanted. We both understood her position would become full-time in summer, prior to our grand opening.

I apologize for this digression, but the reason for it will become clear.

RENOVATIONS

Back to the renovations. In our feasibility study we recommended a plan calling for $2.5m in renovations. Our high-end proposal was for about $5m in renovations, including around $250k in upgrades to the clubhouse.

Howard had other ideas. He likes to go first-class. On virtually every recommendation, he would want to do more, and spend more. This included doing a major clubhouse renovation that would cost nearly as much as the course. He more than doubled the cost of our high-end scenario.

We planned to start the project in September but permitting and engineering issues delayed the start until mid-October. We began construction by clearing the undeveloped area that would become six new holes. As we did, it became clear the new course was going to be very special.

My November visit was timed to coincide with what was to be the final golf tournament as "Southern Hills Golf Course." After the event, we would close nine holes for construction. The remaining nine holes would remain open until the first of the year, at which time the entire golf course would be closed. But I'm getting ahead of myself. A lot would happen first.

CANCER!

INDIGESTION

March 2017
On September 6th I took what became my most fateful trip to Texas (Southern Hills). I would not return home until the 13th.

Whenever I returned to Texas, I had to have Mexican food. While there are many Mexican restaurants in Columbus, they just do not measure up to what I left back in Texas. And I love Mexican food. So naturally the first night back in Texas I went to On the Border in Longview for dinner. It was wonderful. But upon returning to my hotel in Kilgore, I had wicked (an expression I picked up from my first wife's Boston family) indigestion. This is highly unusual as I rarely get indigestion. (And it's even more rare for me to get nauseous -- I can count the number of times I have thrown up in my life on one hand . . . plus a finger or two.)

The indigestion got so severe, I went to the store and bought a big bottle of Tums. I had probably taken Tums once, maybe twice before in my *life* – and that was about the only thing I had ever taken for indigestion, besides drinking 7-Up. After taking several Tums, drinking a 7-up and swallowing a sleeping pill, things settled down enough I was able to sleep.

I had a minor stomachache the next day, but not bad. I took another Tums and headed to work. I forsook my Diet Coke and lemonades (the drink I started subbing for Diet Cokes), in favor of Sprite (they did not have 7up at the course). I was fine.

That night, I decided it would be great to have Pizza for dinner . . . another indication of my lack of intelligence. Perhaps not surprisingly, the indigestion returned, with a vengeance. More Tums and another sleeping pill and I was good.

Over the next few days, though, the pain kept intensifying and the Tums, which I was now taking wholesale, just weren't doing the trick. Nor was it going away, but instead lasting all day long. Unfortunately, this was a big week for us as the owner, who lived in New Orleans, was coming up and we were having a member meeting to go over renovation plans. We were also meeting with the clubhouse architect to discuss the clubhouse. So, leaving was not an option.

By the third day, I realized this was not indigestion. I figured I had some kind of stomach bug. Fortunately, it wasn't affecting me anywhere else. But it wasn't going away, or even moderating. Remember, all the other symptoms I had in June had virtually disappeared, so I never considered there could be a connection.

By Saturday (the 10th), the day of the meetings, I was really hurting. I muscled through, but the pain kept getting worse. One of the biggest problems with the pain was anything jostling my stomach, even a tiny bit, caused a sharp intense pain in my abdomen. And, unfortunately, one of the things that really jostles my stomach was riding in a golf cart. I had never appreciated this until that Saturday when I had to ride around in a golf cart. I felt every single bump.

After putting in a couple hours at the course Sunday morning, I started the trip home. I would typically do the trips back and forth over a two-day period, staying overnight in Vicksburg, MS, which was about half-way between Dallas and Columbus. I normally stayed free in Vicksburg as I happen to enjoy gambling, so I was able to get a free room at the casino hotel. (I am a penny-ante gambler, playing the penny slots. I have a $100 stop-loss on any given night. But I enjoy it). By now, the pain had grown to a significant level. For only the second time, I never visited the casino. Just went to the hotel room and crashed. Fortunately, with the aid of Ambien, I was able to sleep.

I made it home the next day, but it was a miserable trip. The Tums I was inhaling had no effect. And by now I was also extremely constipated, adding to the misery.

Over the next few days, most of which I spent in bed, my pain continued to intensify. My wife and I were convinced it was because I was so constipated, although she thought it might be my appendix, even though it was on the wrong side. I tried various laxatives to treat the problem to no effect. I was miserable.

By Friday, the pain was reaching intolerable levels. I decided to take drastic action. However, being Friday night and a full moon, I knew it would be a very crowded ER. Thus, I decided to wait until morning, when I thought it would have mostly cleared out.

I could not sleep as the pain was so intense. Finally,

around 5 am I woke my wife and had her take me to the St. Francis Hospital ER. Fortunately, my prediction panned out. We did not have long to wait to get in to see the doctor.

The doctor, who was young and friendly, did a cursory exam before ordering a CT scan. He had me drink some stuff to add contrast. It did not taste good but was better than the chalk I drank for the colonoscopy I had the prior year (as well as when I turned fifty). He also informed me the Tums I had been taking was likely causing my constipation. Grrr. Unfortunately, that was not causing my pain.

After an hour or so, I was taken upstairs for the CT scan. About an hour later, my ER doctor returned with the news no one wants to hear. There was a large tumor on my right kidney. It had also spread to a nearby lymph node. In short, I had cancer.

Diagnosis

Holly was distraught, but I remained calm. As long as I can remember, I always remain calm in the face of disaster. I think it's because I have so much experience in getting bad news. For whatever reason, I tend to get extremely calm and rational – freezing my emotions while letting my brain take over. So, I started asking him questions and even cracked bad jokes (humor has always been my main coping strategy). When he left, I was comforting Holly. Somehow, the tumor made sense to me. It explained a lot. And while it may not directly explain the insomnia and left shoulder problems, I suspected these were simply my body trying to get through to me there was something terribly wrong. Since none of my doctors have come up with another explanation, I still believe this was the case. Especially since both disappeared completely after my diagnosis.

I did not take the cancer as a disaster. I took it as a challenge. I was going to beat this thing, I was confident. Bring it on!

The ER doctor gave me a prescription for Percocet (what a wonder drug!) then sent me on my way. I was really surprised. I fully expected to be admitted to the hospital and immediately get an oncologist or surgeon consulting me. But that was not the case. I was sent home, with no follow up. This just shows how much medicine has changed over the years – mostly, I presume, due to insurance requirements.

Oh, by the way, the constipation problem resolved itself later that day. And how.

The Percocet took care of my pain nicely. For the first time in nearly two weeks, I was not withering in pain.

A quick word about Percocet. I am and was then, aware of the dangers of taking an opioid. I only took the pills when I really, really needed them. And I stopped taking them as soon as the pain became tolerable. But there were times when they were the only thing that worked – and I did try other prescription pain killers.

First thing Monday morning, I called Dr. Freud's office. He immediately ordered another CT scan, this time it was to be done at an ambulatory center instead of his office. (He said his tech was not in that week). The CT scan was set for Tuesday, with a follow-up appointment in Dr. Freud's office on Thursday.

In the meantime, I naturally called Juliette. Remember, her husband, Michael Savin, is also a doctor. In fact, he is a well-known hematologist/oncologist who is currently the medical director of the cancer institute at OHSU in Portland.

After the CT on Tuesday, I got two copies of the scan. One for Dr. Freud and one for my sister, which I fed-exed so she had it Wednesday. As a result, Juliette and Michael diagnosed my condition as renal transitional cell carcinoma, before my appointment on Thursday. So, I knew what I likely had when I saw Dr. Freud.

Dr. Freud, though, was not as willing as my sister and brother-in-law to make a diagnosis. While he thought it was cancer, he was not sure if it was renal, transitional cell, or something else. He also said he went back and reviewed the

CT scan he had done on June 28th and told us the tumor *definitely was not there at that time.* He then ordered a biopsy to be done "as soon as possible."

I was to learn "as soon as possible" does not mean the same as "stat." I was thinking given this huge tumor in my gut had apparently grown so big in such a short time, it would warrant immediate action. But "as soon as possible" in doctor speak, means "as soon as it is convenient for you to do so." Which in this case, meant waiting a week. "Stat," on the other hand, means "drop everything and do immediately."

It was hard for me to believe, however, this tumor developed after the June 28th CT scan done in Freud's office. After all, the blood in the urine occurred on the 11th. So, I requested a copy of the June 28th CT scan from Freud's office, which I overnighted to my sister. She had one of the radiologists at her hospital look at it. He reported not only was the tumor present on the scan, but *it was rather obvious –* and the tumor was also present on the lymph node. Dr. Freud (or is that Dr. Fraud?) blew it. I was soon to discover just how badly.

Ironically, the next day (the 23rd), I was scheduled for a brain MRI from Dr. Miller (my new primary physician). This had been ordered a month earlier, well before we knew of the cancer, and was mostly precautionary as we still did not have an explanation for the arm/shoulder pain on my left side or my insomnia. But now it had taken on more meaning. I was scared it would reveal the cancer had spread to my head.

The MRI was to be done with and without contrast. But a blood test taken prior to the MRI (another pin cushion) revealed my Creatine level (a measure of kidney function) had shot up to over 2.0, indicating significant kidney issues. (Remember, a month earlier, the Creatine level was fine.)

Because the contrast dye is hard on the kidneys the contrast scan was cancelled. Fortunately, the non-contrast scan revealed nothing (insert joke here _____).

The biopsy was done at St. Francis by an anesthesiologist. It was a simple procedure, although I had to go in the day before to get all the pretests done. I can't remember if I was knocked out for the biopsy or if they just gave me the funny juice that makes you completely unaware of what is happening. Either way, the biopsy went off without a hitch and I felt nothing.

My sister was able to get the biopsy results before we heard from Dr. Freud. It confirmed what we feared – I had renal transitional cell carcinoma. Not good. The day after the biopsy a nurse (or receptionist, I'm not sure which) called from Dr. Fraud's office. She *congratulated* me on the fact I did not have renal (kidney) cancer. That's like being congratulated for not having a cold, but instead having pneumonia. Renal cancer is easily treatable, rarely metastasizes and has a relatively good prognosis. Renal transitional cell carcinoma, on the other hand, is the opposite. She then said Dr. Freud would like to schedule me for another procedure – I can't exactly remember what she called it. But it involved sticking another camera inside me, this time going up through the renal canal. He was not, as I would have expected, referring me to a cancer specialist.

By this time, I had already known Dr. Freud blew the original diagnosis, so there was no way in heck I was going back! Fortunately, using his great connections, Michael was able to get me into the Winship Cancer Center at Emory University in Atlanta. He knew the head of the program who recommended I see Dr. Mehmet Bilen. Dr. Bilen specialized in transitional cell carcinoma and other urothelial cancers. I saw him two days after the biopsy with results in my hand.

(Renal transitional cell carcinoma is really a type of bladder cancer, except it forms on the kidney and not the bladder. It is very aggressive and has an extremely high mortality rate.)

Emory Winship Center

May 2017
Holly and I were impressed the first time we entered Winship Center, which is located next to the hospital on Emory's campus in Atlanta (all the medical buildings are connected by tunnels). Finally, I was going to see a non-Columbus doctor.

We were both scared and extremely nervous, for obvious reasons. We had absolutely no idea what to expect. But we never imagined what we found.

Upon arriving, we were greeted by a valet. We declined that first time, as we were unsure of the cost. Holly dropped me off then went to find the parking garage, which apparently was a major hassle. As the valet only cost $8 plus tip, we became regular users thereafter. (This continued until I learned that 1) Holly had parked in the wrong garage and the right garage was actually convenient, and 2) the infusion center would pay for the parking garage, but not for the valet. Unfortunately, I didn't discover these facts until we probably spent $150 in valet parking.)

When we entered the building, we were immediately greeted by a very friendly receptionist, who guided us where we needed to go. Everyone we met that day was extremely nice and welcoming, always asking what they could do to help. Maybe it was the petrified look on our faces making it obvious we were there for the first time, but certainly we could not have been made to feel any more comfortable in a very uncomfortable situation. It was almost like we were checking into a luxury hotel – one filled with men and women walking around with bald heads.

When the nurse ushered us back to Dr. Bilen's examining room, she gave us a bunch of business cards saying, "this is my card, this is Dr. Bilen's, this is . . ." Telling us to call anytime we had a question or concern. What a contrast to how I was treated in Columbus!

Holly and I immediately liked Dr. Bilen (pronounced "Beelin"). He was wonderful – calm and reassuring with a great personality. He spent a lot of time with us that first day. In fact, every time I have seen him, he never seems to be in a rush – willing to stay as long as necessary to answer questions or give needed reassurance. It turned out, Dr. Bilen was new there, having just arrived about six weeks previous from M.D. Anderson in Houston. M.D. Anderson happened to be where my son received his master's degree in Medical Physics.

Dr. Bilen did not believe surgery to remove the kidney and lymph node was the right action at that time. Instead, he felt chemo was the best first strategy. But he would consult with the Tumor board that included a urologist, etc., after receiving more test results.

He scheduled a bunch of procedures for me on the 13th of October – two weeks away – with the first chemo treatment the following day. Given the two-hour drive each way, it was (and still is) highly desirable to get as much done in one trip as possible. It not only helps with the commute, but it means Holly having to take one day off instead of two. I needed Holly to go with me as I was not to drive after chemo treatments. The reason why it took two weeks before I could begin any treatment was insurance. You are dying of cancer and it still takes two weeks to get approval for treatment. Grrrr.

Among the many things scheduled: blood work (pincushion), a hearing test, a PET scan with contrast (another needle), another visit with Dr. Bilen, a minor procedure to install a port for my chemotherapy, which would also involve a needle (for the anesthesia) and my first chemo treatment. The hearing test was because chemotherapy can affect hearing.

The port is a device attached to a major artery allowing the chemotherapy drugs to go directly into the blood system. It is installed under the skin. In my case, it is on the upper right-hand side of my chest about halfway between my neck and arm pit. Before each chemo (and later immunotherapy treatments), I would go to the blood lab where they insert a needle into the port and attach a tube with a bunch of valves used to take blood samples and later for the chemotherapy treatment (called "infusion" for infusing the chemicals into the blood). At last, my arms would no longer be pin cushions! (That's not entirely true as I would later find out). Now it was my chest. But at least the needle does not hurt toooo bad going in. (While the port is under the skin, it sticks out, looking like I have a tiny box under my skin.) The funny thing is, since there are several hours between the lab and the infusion, you are walking around with the apparatus, with various tubes running out of it, strapped to your chest. Fortunately, I could hide it under my shirt.

While all this was going on, I had another issue becoming a concern. My vision was deteriorating rapidly. I was afraid the cataracts had returned.

When we first moved to Columbus, Peanut (our shiatsu)

accidentally clawed me in the eye. This resulted in my first ever trip to an ER for myself, at least since I was six (the second was for the indigestion above). They were very nice and gave me eye drops and referred me to Dr. Cynthia Nix, an eye doctor who happened to be a cornea specialist. She treated me for the scratch (more eyedrops). She not only was very nice and competent, but also happened to be very attractive (as far as my diminished eyesight could see, that is. She was my eye-candy equivalent to Dr. Dawson for Holly). It took several months for the scratch to stop bothering me. So, when my vision started to get bad, I went back to her.

By the way, I absolutely cannot stand having anything put in my eye, including contacts (which I tried as a teen) and eyedrops. The nurses and tech at the ophthalmologist always have a fun time trying to get these drops into my eyes. Anyway, Dr. Nix told me I had a film growing over the lens, which was common with cataract patients. It was easily treatable with laser surgery. The only problem was my blood pressure was too high for them to do the procedure without getting the consent of my primary care physician. I was able to call my doctor's office when I got home. They got me in to see Dr. Miller's PA, who prescribed blood pressure pills. My eye procedure was subsequently scheduled a few weeks later, for the 27th of October.

Now we come to the 13th of October and the return to Winship for all those procedures and pincushion treatment. As it was an all-day venture, it meant driving into Atlanta during the morning rush and then getting to experience the joys of the evening rush going home. I honestly don't know how people do this every day. It's bad enough I must do it two-three times a month. I'm spoiled. Being self-employed, my morning commute is about 50 feet, and I only need to dodge two dogs and seven cats. The worst accidents I see are on the floor – but they do require I stop and clean them up.

First up was the blood work. Here the most interesting thing was the waiting room. For I was now surrounded by people who all had cancer in varying degrees and types, otherwise why would they be at the Winship Cancer center? It was fascinating looking at all the faces. Some were clearly depressed. But most were just like those in any other waiting room, only with more bald heads. I also discovered there is a strange comradery among cancer patients. We all share a common enemy after all. We felt welcome among the group.

After the lab came the PET scan, which stands for Positron Emission Tomography. The PET scan is attached to a CAT scan (computed tomography – and no, I don't know why they do not have a DOG scan, although they do have LABs). The combined device looks like two huge donuts attached to a long tube. However, it is not as long as the MRI coffin (at least it does not appear to be), and the opening is larger. Given I have had over twenty MRIs in my life without a bad reaction, including six in the past year, this shorter, wider device should present no problems, right? *Wrong.*

Prior to the scan, I needed an IV put in (this was the second of three needles going into my pincushion arms that day.) The IV was for inserting the radioactive sugary fluid into my veins. Apparently, tumors are very thirsty for this solution and light up under the PET scan.

Remember when I said I don't panic? That I always remain cool, calm and calculating in the face of a disaster? Well, that all went out the window that morning. For the first time in my life (that I can remember anyway), I felt real panic. I did not want to go in that device.

Yes, I am claustrophobic. But really, an MRI is much more intimidating in that regard. This was something different. I was petrified. And it came from nowhere. Prior to entering that room, I was not the least bit nervous. Yet as soon as I got in, I was hit with this major panic attack. I twice laid down on the platform going into the device, only to get up.

I was finally able to calm myself down with their help. After several minutes I was able to lay down and keep still enough to start the procedure.

There are two scans involved. The first is a regular CAT scan which serves as a reference for the following PET scan. As such, it is very important not to move at all between the scans. The CAT or CT scan is very quick, taking about a minute. This was a full body scan as they were looking for any tumors that might have sprung from the original. Next came the PET scan, which is much slower, taking approximately thirty minutes to complete.

We were about ten minutes in when I had another panic attack. At the time, my head was sticking out the opposite end of the scan. Because my head was out, it was not claustrophobia bothering me.

I was panicking and I did not know why, which only made it worse. I started yelling. One of the techs (and I really wish I could remember her name as she was wonderful), came out and sat next to me. She was able to calm me down, not only with her reassuring words, but by putting her hand on my shoulder. Somehow that human touch made all the difference. She stayed with me for the rest of the exam and as much as possible retained a physical contact with my head. With her help, I was able to finish the exam. Fortunately, throughout all this I had not moved enough to ruin the scan.

So why did I panic? I am convinced the panic attack was caused by my subconscious because deep down, it knew what the scan would find.

My wife and I ate lunch in the deli on the first floor, before going upstairs to meet with Dr. Bilen to hear the results. The news was not good. In fact, it was about as bad as you could get. The cancer had spread throughout my chest. There were at least four other tumors, including two by my lungs in places surrounded by nerves and thus inoperable. Now surgery was completely off the table.

I was my calm self throughout the news. I already had my panic attack. I think Holly was in shock.

In all honesty, as he was telling me the horrible news, all I could think of was the bad joke about the guy who goes to see his doctor after contracting a terrible disease. He asks the doctor how long he has to live. The doctor replies, "10." The patient instantly asks, "10 what? 10 years, 10 months?" The Dr. replied, "9 . . ."

I kept waiting for Dr. Bilen to do the countdown. But he refused to bite. In fact, he would not tell me what my realistic lifespan had become. He obviously did not want me to have a defeatist attitude. (I would discover later doing my own research and talking to other doctors my prognosis was probably that, with treatment, I *might* make it to Christmas, given the spread of the disease and how rapidly the tumors were growing. Holly later confirmed Juliette and Michael told her it was a real possibility and to prepare for the worst. If not for that 'indigestion' that would most likely have been the case.)

One of the best things about Dr. Bilen is he always has a Plan B and C and D. He told us we would first try chemotherapy. If that didn't work, we would do immunotherapy. And if that didn't work, there were clinical trials. And they were constantly coming up with new treatments, so even though historically this was a bad cancer, there was always hope. But he also told us, there was _no_ cure. I would *never* be rid of the cancer. The best we can hope for is to stabilize the cancer and gain extra time – perhaps a *few* years.

This really brought into focus just how costly the misread of the June CT scan done in Dr. Fraud's office had been. If he had caught it as he should have, it would have meant surgery could have been practical. They would have removed my kidney and lymph node, along with the tumor. While I still would likely needed chemo, they would have had a great chance to stop the cancer before it spread.

Not only would this have prevented me from going to stage IV, and thus greatly imperiling my life, it certainly would have saved me from a lot of agony – as well as a lot of extraneous testing! (Yes, I believe I was the victim of malpractice. And I wanted to sue, but that is another story, which I will share later.)

After our cheerful visit with Dr. Bilen, it was time to head back to radiology for my port installation. Once again, I had to get an IV and another needle stick. By this time, I was really glad to be getting the port to avoid all this needle work. Ironically, the nurse had a heck of a time getting the IV started. My luck I had a new nurse (or intern), who was having difficulty finding a good vein (I wonder why! All the good ones had been taken). Finally, her supervisor came to the rescue. I wound up getting stuck three times for the one IV – making it a total of five for the day. (The port did not completely save my pincushion arms, though. Unfortunately, you need to go to a cancer lab for them to access it. Blood work for my regular doctor still requires the ol' needle in the arm routine. And if my scans were done before my labs at Emory, they would use a needle in the arm for the contrast. I now make sure to get the labs done first!).

I received a 'power port,' which meant it in addition to the infusion, it could be used by techs for future contrast work when they needed to put dye in my system. (Apparently, this requires a larger needle). I called it a super port and told them it should give me superpowers. It didn't. But the procedure went fine. The worst part was having the nurse shave my chest hairs around where they were to put the device. Well, it could have been worse . . .

While the port is under the skin, it protrudes a bit. So, I now have an area in my upper right chest that is about $\frac{1}{2}$" square sticking out like a sore thumb. And it is sore (or at least very sensitive), even today, eight months after it was put in.

First Treatment

The next day was my first actual chemotherapy treatment. To be honest, I really had no preconception about the chemotherapy procedure. I knew it involved taking a bunch of chemicals, but I never thought about how they are delivered into your system, or the entire process. Well it turns out they are delivered intravenously (at least in my case) – either through an IV, or through a port. There are many, many, different types of chemotherapy with a variety of drug combinations. Every cancer has a different cocktail of drugs used to attack it. Each treatment is highly individualized based on the cancer sex, weight, etc. of the subject.

In my case, the treatment would last six hours the first time and four hours thereafter. My schedule was going to be one treatment per week for two weeks, then a week off, then repeat. Each three-week period was considered a cycle. I would be reevaluated after four cycles or approximately three months.

This first treatment was at the downtown Emory hospital (about fifteen minutes in good traffic from campus), which has a Winship infusion center on the sixteenth floor. The reason I was going there for this treatment was because I had to undergo a hearing test first (the chemo treatment could affect hearing), and the clinic was located at the downtown facility.

The hearing test confirmed the partial deafness in my right ear, nothing surprising there. The hearing in my left ear, though, was still good although slightly diminished. Now onto the fusion!

It was very cold that October morning. As a result, I wore my heavy Chiefs coat I received one year from Sports Illustrated. It is nice and warm with a great hoody. It is, naturally, red with the yellow Chiefs logo.

I grew up in Kansas City. Truthfully, I lived in the suburbs (Mission in Johnson County) on the Kansas side (most of Kansas City, for those of you not familiar, is really in Missouri). And while I moved away from the area in 1984, I remain a diehard fan of the Royals, Chiefs and Jayhawks. I continue to read the KC Star and Lawrence Journal World every day – well at least the sports sections. Thankfully I can now do this online. I used to have the papers mailed to me. The reason I bring this up is what happened to me at the fusion center astonished me.

When I was first called in, I was escorted back into a large room filled with open bays. Each bay had a curtain that could be drawn to close it off and consisted of a lounge-like chair with brown fabric, a regular chair and a TV mounted to a mechanical arm attached to the wall. The arm could be moved in, out, up, down, or side to side allowing the TV to be positioned anywhere in the bay. The lounge chair had trays attached to both arms. There was also an IV pole. At the front of the main room, though, were two chairs for the lab techs to suck out some of our blood. This was the first time my port was used.

To draw the blood, they insert a needle attached to this clear tube device through the skin and into my port. Since it is only going through skin, it does not normally hurt much (much less than an IV). But this first time was an exception given how sensitive the area was, being freshly installed. Once the needle was in, the phlebotomist or tech attaches a hypodermic to one of the valves and "flushes" the system by injecting a saline (sodium chloride . . . or salt) solution. This is followed by another clear fluid (Heparin, an anti-coagulant.) Next, they put in another one with a test tube attached and draw out the blood. Several tubes were filled in this manner.

In this particular case, the tech, who was a young, pretty and very nice nurse, happened to notice the Chief's coat. She asked me if I was a Chief's fan, which I thought was kind of obvious. She then asked if I knew of Eric Berry.

Every Chief's fan knows about Eric Berry. In fact, most NFL fans know about Eric Berry. Not only is he an all-pro safety, but he recently gained a lot of fame with his own cancer fight. In December 2014, *during the season,* he was diagnosed with Hodgkin's Lymphoma.

In short, he started feeling a pain during a game against the hated Oakland Raiders. He was able to finish the game but knew something was wrong as he was having trouble lifting his arm and having chest pains. Four days later, he was telling his team the totally unexpected news. He had cancer.

The amazing thing about Eric was while he obviously missed the rest of the 2014; *he returned in time for the 2015 season!* Not only did he return, but he had another all pro year. Quite an amazing story. And now that I have experienced some of what he had to go through; I am even more impressed!

Well it turns out my technician happened to be a close

friend of Eric's. She grew up with him. (He was from an Atlanta suburb, Fairburn.) I then learned Eric was treated at the Winship center. (I had no idea previously). She told me a story about how, after he returned to football, he flew her and his entire treatment team to Kansas City for a weekend, including a Chiefs game.

Over the next few months, I talked to several people at Winship who either treated Eric or knew his story well. Everyone I talked to could only rave about him. Not only about his terrific attitude and work ethic, but how genuinely nice he was to everyone. One nurse told me a story of how a nurse was struggling to put the IV in and Eric asked: "should I take off my shirt?" to which every nurse within earshot immediately and enthusiastically replied "Yes!". (FYI, President Jimmy Carter was also treated at Winship. I'm in good company.)

After the blood work was completed, I returned to the waiting room. I had about 30-40 minutes to wait until they called me back for the actual infusion. (They had to process the blood work. Fortunately, the lab is right there. It's amazing how fast they get it turned around).

We were led back to one of the bays where I was told to sit in the lounge-like chair. The chair, which fortunately was comfortable, had electric controls allowing me to recline about 70%. Most importantly, the bay had a window, which, given we were on the 16th floor in downtown Atlanta, offered a nice view.

The first "bottle" (really bag) I was given was the pre-treatment. It contained a lot of anti-nausea medication, and apparently, some relaxers as I would end up sleeping through most of the next four hours of treatment.

The bag of clear fluid was attached to the top of the pole. A clear tube, with several valves, connected the bag to an electric pump. Another tube, with additional valves, connected the pump to the tube already connected to my port. (The various valves would allow the flow to be stopped, or allow another syringe to be attached, etc.) It made for an impressive contraption.

Dr. Bilen gave me prescriptions for two different antinausea medicines to take the day of chemotherapy and as needed afterwards. I guess chemo can be very tough on stomachs! Fortunately, as I mentioned before, I have a cast-iron stomach. I rarely needed the extra pills (although this would change the longer I had chemo).

With chemotherapy you are injecting powerful and toxic chemicals, basically poison, into your body in the hopes these chemicals will kill more bad cells than good. While each concoction is tailored to a specific cancer and adjusted to the individual, it is still like using a scatter gun. You just hope some of the bullets find the right target. In the meantime, you accept there is going to be a lot of collateral damage, read "side effects."

As the mix of chemicals and the amounts will vary with the cancer and individual, each "bag" must be mixed by the pharmacists on staff after you have checked into the lab. I assume the main reason they can't be premixed is these chemicals are so expensive, they can't take the chance you will not show up for your appointment. Further, they must wait for the doctor's orders as the dose may have been adjusted, or additional chemicals added. And the doctor must check your blood work prior to putting in the order, to make sure everything is ok (like kidney function). They also must adjust the dosage based on your weight, which they take again right before you go into the lab. What this means is you will often wait forty-five minutes to an hour or more after you have been checked into the fusion lab before you start your treatment.

We got an idea of just how powerful these chemicals were when we were advised about the use of the toilet. Holly was told it was best to "hover" to avoid any possible splashing, in case some chemicals still remained. We also had to wipe down surfaces, etc.

But I was surprised after that first treatment, I did not feel any aftereffects at all. I never did feel any nausea and felt fine. No side effects! I was thrilled . . . I did not realize at the time the side effects were *cumulative* in nature. Be patient, they will come!

No doubt the most noticeable side effect associated with chemotherapy is losing your hair. While the degree and speed of hair loss may vary with the chemical cocktail, this does seem to be common with most of them. I am blessed with very thick hair. This fact is probably what saved me from going bald. But I did end up losing most of it. I wound up looking like my mother, whose hair was so thin she wore a wig most of her adult life.

While I expected to lose hair from my scalp, which I did, I was surprised to find the hair loss was not confined to the scalp. I lost hair everywhere! In fact, my legs began to resemble a swimmer's legs. They were absolutely smooth at the top. (Yes, I lost hair *there* too).

But this, along with other side effects, were to come much later. There were none after the first treatment. But the one effect we were hoping for did come. The pain began to decrease. What joy!

For the second treatment a week later, I returned to the main Winship center on campus. Now the center downtown featured windows with great views, and excellent snacks, including a wide variety of beverages to choose from. (While they do not serve meals, the do allow you to bring food in.

Which, given you could be there for six hours or so, is important. When we were downtown, Holly went down to the cafeteria and brought up a lunch for both of us. This was repeated when we were at the campus center.) So, I was surprised and disappointed to learn the main center had none of these. The fusion center, which was much larger than the downtown center, was in the basement, underground. No windows. The snack choices were more limited, and they only offered a couple of juices for drinks. So much for the luxury treatment. But the staff, as always at Emory, was outstanding. Also on the positive side, the chairs for the infusion were wider and made of leather, making them much more comfortable.

After my second treatment, I started experiencing a side effect of the treatment. And it was totally unexpected. I became extremely jittery, as though I was pumped with Adderall (which I wasn't). Not only was I physically jittery, but also emotionally. I became extremely emotional. Everything affected me, good or bad. Unfortunately, this caused me to snap at people as the least little thing would irritate me and I would react . . . with no filter.

It is hard to say whether the mental/emotional affects were due exclusively to the chemotherapy or exacerbated because I was no longer taking Wellbutrin to combat my ADD. I stopped taking it the past summer as I was concerned it might have been a precipitating cause for my troubles. Either way, I was a mess.

This was extremely unfortunate as I was returning to Texas for the first time since my diagnosis. This was an important trip as we were amid heavy renovation plans, of which I was intimately involved. In fact, we were about to begin construction on the golf course and were planning for the clubhouse. I made the trip during my "off week" in treatments. I had checked with Dr. Bilen and he said it was fine for me to travel if I felt up to it. I chose to fly for this trip, given my physical condition and to greatly shorten the trip.

During this trip, I told the owner, Howard*, about my cancer. I also told him about the suspected malpractice I felt I experienced with Dr. Freud. Howard happens to be a prominent malpractice attorney in New Orleans. He volunteered to take the case on my behalf, for which I was extremely grateful.

I was very tired throughout the trip but okay for most of the workday. But because I was so emotionally strained, I found myself losing patience with staff at the course, including getting mad at the General Manager there. This would haunt me later.

After the fateful trip to Texas, I returned for my third treatment on the 21st of October. But it never happened. I had the blood work then went to see Dr. Bilen, who had bad news. Apparently one of the side effects of chemical cocktail I was taking was it was hard on the kidneys. And since I was down to one functioning kidney, I did not have room to spare. When my Creatine level went up even more, Dr. Bilen decided he would change the cocktail. So, I had to skip a week (insurance). Further, the new cocktail had a new schedule. Instead of on on off, I would be having a treatment every other week. This change in schedule resulted in an unintended consequence.

One thing about getting a terminal cancer, you immediately get more popular. At least that's the way it seems. Suddenly everyone wants to come visit! The prime examples of this was my own family – especially my sisters.

Since 1984, when I moved to North Carolina, and excluding the years 2008-2015 when we all lived in the same metro area (Dallas), my two sisters had visited me exactly three times. Once by Juliette, when she left the day *before* my son Matthew was born, and twice by Cheryl – although both times were also business trips for her (commercial real estate). But now both wanted to come and visit – and soon.

Cheryl decided to come the 27th of October and stay through the weekend. She chose this weekend because my wife had her biggest event of the year at the museum and so Cheryl thought she could provide needed relief for her in taking care of me. Juliette was coming the next week because that was when I was scheduled for chemo and she wanted to meet with Dr. Bilen.

The change in schedule now meant my treatment was the day before Holly's big event. The good news was Cheryl was here, so she could take me as it would have been very hard on Holly to take me the day before the big event. But it also meant Juliette was not going to meet Dr. Bilen.

The day Cheryl was to come was also the day I was having the laser surgery for my eye. But since Cheryl was renting a car, I was not having to drive to Atlanta to get her. The surgery was outpatient and I was able to drive myself home afterwards. Holly came with me, but she had to leave before I had the procedure due to event preparation. So, it was a good thing they were right, and I could drive home.

The laser surgery was pretty neat. I put my head in a head rest and was told to look straight ahead. The device was like the ones I was used to in the eye doctor's office that take pictures of my cornea. I could see the red light of the laser appearing at various spots and could hear the clicking noise of the laser. I got the strangest impression I was in a video game, where my eye was the screen. The doctor agreed with me.

Unlike the cataract surgery where it took a day or two for my vision to recover, the results were immediate. I could see clearly again! It was wonderful.

The new chemo cocktail did not affect me like the first. I did not have the physical or emotional jitteries. And I was starting to feel a bit stronger. This gave me confidence for my next trip to Texas.

A Critical Time

My second trip to Southern Hills after learning I had cancer was the week before Thanksgiving. Although I didn't know it at the time, it would also be my last. This was another important trip as we were having our final golf tournament as Southern Hills (the course was being renamed "The Tempest" after renovation). We were closing nine of the holes the following week to start construction. The entire course was to close the first of the year. This was also the first time I had played the course – although I only got to play a few holes (I played a hole with each group during the tournament).

I drove for this trip. But I probably should not have. I was much more fatigued throughout the trip. Hopefully it did not show up in my work, but I sure felt it.

Shortly after returning from Texas, and the day after Thanksgiving (Nov 28th), I had my fourth treatment. I also had the first set of scans to see my progress. I had a chest CT scan and an MRI with and without contrast for my abdomen. These were both done at the campus Winship. The scans revealed the tumors had stopped growing! This was exciting news, given how fast they had been growing prior to treatment.

However, after that fourth treatment, my physical health started to deteriorate – fast. Following each treatment, I felt worse – even having increased nausea (although I never puked). I discovered the side effects of the chemo are cumulative. It wasn't the cancer making me sick – it was the treatment. The worst issue was fatigue. I was basically worthless. I couldn't work at the computer more than an hour. The fatigue came from becoming more and more anemic from the chemotherapy. Unfortunately, also increasing was the pain.

In addition to my sisters coming to visit, my son also came in November. In fact, in the first year since I've been sick, my son (who lives in Los Angeles) visited four different times and my daughter (who lives in Richmond, Virginia) three. Fortunately, my son makes good money and has a generous vacation allotment. Still, it is a trip from one end of the country to the other. I greatly appreciated both of their support. I also put them to work! I was no longer able to do a lot of the chores around the house I used to, so having them come and help was a great assistance to both Holly and me.

With cooler weather and only nine holes open, December was a slow month at the course. As my partner, Paul, was there most of the month for construction, I felt comfortable not visiting the course during the month. Which was good, as I was definitely not up for it. Sadly, that proved to be a bad decision.

Both kids came for the Christmas holiday. My wife bought tickets for all of us to see the play Scrooge (Columbus has a great theater program). Sadly, I was too ill to go, but the three of them went and had a great time.

The kids accompanied us for one of my chemo treatments. They were not able to stay during the actual infusion as there is only one guest chair. So, Holly took them to a nearby museum while I was being treated. But at least they got to see the fusion center and get an idea of what I was experiencing.

After visiting us, both went to Durham to stay with their mother. Matthew was then going to fly to Aspen Colorado to meet his girlfriend. They and several friends rented a cabin for the weekend of New Year's Day. Shockingly, though, Matt decided he would rather spend that weekend with us than having a romantic vacation with his girlfriend. He cancelled his Colorado trip and came back to stay with us for another three days. I was really touched but felt guilty he gave up such a wonderful weekend for me.

Roger's apparent inability to follow my directions could be possibly be attributed to several reasons. 1) he simply was incapable of doing it, meaning he could not do the job when we transitioned to Tempest; 2) he had no respect for me or my authority, or 3) he was actively trying to undermine my authority in order to get rid of me, knowing I probably would not keep him on. I always tried giving him the benefit of the doubt.

This brings us to January 2017. The last week of the month was the big PGA Merchandise show in Orlando. This is an event where most of the major vendors in the industry show off their goods to the PGA pros, retailers and golf course owners. It is a huge event taking up the entire North building of the Orlando Convention Center – a building about one block long. Roger had never gone. But I told him back in July I wanted to take him, especially since we were reinventing ourselves on the merchandise front. I also invited Howard, as not only had he never gone, but I felt it was a great way for him to learn more about the industry. Besides I knew we had some major decisions coming – like a new Point of Sale System, etc. I also invited Jeff to come, but he later backed out.

By the first week of mid-January, I was feeling rotten and especially fatigued. I was afraid I would not make it to Orlando. I asked Paul if he could attend in my place should I not be able to go. He declined.

FATEFUL DAY

January 20th was my eighth chemo treatment. It was a little more than a week ahead of the PGA show. It was also the date for the second set of scans to determine progress. We spent the morning at the downtown hospital getting the scans, then saw Dr. Bilen after lunch prior to the treatment.

However, there was to be no chemo that day. The scans revealed my tumors were growing again. The chemo was not effective.

To say the least, this was not the news we wanted to hear. I think I took the news well as I was not surprised, given how badly I was feeling. But I know it was devastating to Holly.

Dr. Bilen did not give us time to dwell on the negative. He had another plan ready. We would switch to immunotherapy. But again, because of insurance, it would take two weeks to get it approved. Instead, I would receive a blood transfusion that day to treat the anemia as my level had fallen so low insurance would finally cover it. I received three units, which really did help with my fatigue. It did not eliminate it as I was still anemic, but it helped considerably – to the point that when the PGA show came around, I was ready.

The Call

May 2017
It was late afternoon and early rush hour traffic when we left Emory for home. Naturally, as had become the pattern, I had not heard from Roger. So, I decided to initiate the call. We had a lot to discuss – especially planning for the trade show in Orlando the following week, which I was determined to go to if I possibly could.

After catching up on things at the course, I asked him if he was still planning on bringing his wife (at his expense) to the show as we discussed previously (I was bringing Holly, after all). He explained she could not come due to her work (she was a teacher). Instead he was bringing Natasha.

This really upset me. I was his boss and bringing another employee along, presumably at company expense, should have been a decision I was involved in. I did not yell at him, but I told him in no uncertain terms he was not to go behind my back again with these types of decisions or he would not have a job. (Later I discovered Roger had a way of saving money – Natasha and he shared the hotel room. I'm sure neither of their spouses, nor Howard, knew about this thriftiness.)

Holly, who was in the car and could hear the entire conversation (Bluetooth), thought I handled it well. No one else did.

There is no doubt the timing of that call sucked. After all, not only had I just been through a long day getting poked, prodded, pricked and pushed, but I was also essentially told the final clock was once again ticking down quickly. So, I was not in the best of moods when I had the conversation with Roger. Maybe if I had waited to make the call another day, it would have gone differently . . . but I still would have been upset with him. Ultimately, I doubt it mattered much as I think Roger would have found another excuse later . . .

After we hung up, Roger immediately called Paul and, I'm told, was extremely upset, threatening to quit. What happened next is still a puzzle to me. Instead of calling me to discuss the situation, my friend and "partner" called Howard.

Now Paul is one of the most pious and ethical people I know. I've seen him write checks to owners because he was able to do a construction job for less than he anticipated. He called his insurance company to have them give him less money because he found a roofer who would replace his roof for less than what the insurance company allowed.

I brought Paul into this job. I also campaigned strongly for Howard to hire him for the construction. So, the last thing I expected was for Paul to do something that seemed like stabbing me in the back. Later, he added fuel to the fire by telling Howard about an incident in a restaurant in which I got upset at an overzealous waiter who kept interrupting us when we were having a serious conversation (again, I did not raise my voice at the waiter, but told him to please stop interrupting). He also shared with Howard an email I sent Paul in confidence. So, if Paul was acting on my behalf, as he later claimed, he certainly had a funny way of showing it and it definitely had the opposite effect.

His excuse was he called Howard to warn him that Roger would be calling. He felt it was better coming from Paul than from Roger that he was threatening to quit. [In fairness to Paul, I suspect he felt a stronger loyalty to the owner as he was spending millions of dollars on the project and entrusting Paul with it. And I also suspect Paul was concerned about how well I could do the job, given my health, which I think was the real reason behind my ultimate termination.]

What followed was the most bizarre sequence of events I ever experienced. I have always been able to do a good job explaining myself. But Howard never gave me the chance. On the phone, he would simply cut me off . . . often cursing. And he did the same in emails. Mostly he ignored my emails. When he did respond, it was a short, very terse reply. Howard claimed I had a big problem – that in addition to Roger, employees and members were complaining about me. If this was true, it certainly was the first I heard about it! I later learned the "employee" was Natasha – whom I had only met once during the interview, and that had gone well. I had asked her and Roger to do some competitive work on banquets – which they never completed. And I had little interaction with members, but those were mostly very positive. Again, I later discovered the "incident" referred to was when our most prominent member asked me if the lifetime members would now be required to pay dues. The question surprised me, because I had no idea we *had* lifetime members. No one had told me this critical piece of information. So, I was not able to give him a direct answer but told him we would get back to him. Which we did as I quickly got together with Roger and Howard to decide on a strategy.

It was very clear to me Roger was lying his ass off in order to get me fired, and thereby save his own job. And Paul, whether intentionally or not, was only adding fuel to the flames. (Another oddity. Prior to the 20th, Paul would call me nearly every day and give me updates. We would talk both about the construction and the management issues. After the 20th, Paul never called me. He also did not return my calls except on occasion. This would go on until the end of February.)

Roger never called me again. Nor would he return my phone calls or emails. This was upsetting for several reasons, not the least of which was I wanted to coordinate our efforts at the PGA show coming up. There were specific things I wanted him to look at that were important for the club. (I would later learn this was another thing upsetting poor Roger. He did not want to be told what to look at during the show, but wanted free reign – even though the main purpose of him coming to the show was to view specific things we were going to need with the new facility – like a new POS system, etc.)

I also learned later the timing of this event could not have been worse on another front. Howard had finally heard back from the clubhouse architect earlier that day on the cost of his clubhouse. The architect put it at $4 million. Suddenly, Howard did a complete 180. Instead of spending money like it was Monopoly, now he was campaigning to cut costs everywhere. (The clubhouse plans went back to a modification of what I had originally proposed – but I was no longer involved in the planning by that point). He also said the business plan I prepared in December was "crap" and the projections were "full of mistakes" and didn't add up correctly, which was not true.

Here's the thing. Before putting the projections in the proposal, I sent them to Howard's accountant, Paul, Roger and Barney to review and comment. *None* of them responded or provided feedback. Now six weeks later, Howard informs me they were terrible. (He was told they were bad by Roger and Paul as Howard did not have any expertise in this area). When I went back to look at it, I did discover I had made a simple mistake – one. And it did not significantly alter the conclusions.

Several days went by and I was physically, at least, feeling much better. So, I was convinced I was going to the show. I was also finally able to get Howard to agree to meet with me down there to discuss the situation.

For the second year in a row, Holly and I took advantage of one of those condo vacation offers where they will give you three nights at an Orlando resort for $49 plus sitting though one of their timeshare presentations. Being cheap, and knowing we would not make a purchase, we accepted.

We arrived late Wednesday afternoon. We were too tired to do much of anything, other than going to dinner. We made the most of that, however, by treating ourselves to a Brazilian steak house. Yum! It was my wife's first time. As a pure meatatarian (or carnivore if you prefer), I love them, but to my pleasant surprise, so did she.

Thursday, we spent most of the day at the show. I was still in full-on Tempest mode. We needed a new POS among many other things, and the show represented the best opportunity to review them. I also had a long list of other needs I wanted to investigate.

To my pleasant surprise, I was able to put in six hours on the floor. (This is not enough time to see all the exhibits, but long enough to see the ones I cared about). I did have to take frequent breaks. Holly loved the show as well and spent most of her time with soft goods and nick-knack vendors – some of whose non-golf wares she could use in her own museum gift shop. We did not see or hear from Roger.

The meeting with Howard was Friday morning at the show. Prior to sitting down with me to discuss the Roger situation, Howard, who arrived an hour late, wanted to walk the floor with me. I had several things I wanted to show him, like the POS I was recommending, and these "surf-board" golf carts for individuals I thought would be a great addition. We spent about two hours walking the floor before sitting down in the cafeteria to talk.

While our conversation on the floor was friendly and professional, our talk in the café was anything but. Once again, the wall went up and I was not allowed to speak or defend myself. Instead, I was basically told: 1) I did not need to communicate with Roger anymore (despite my management contract clearly stating he reports to me); 2) I did not need to visit the site, at least for several months (how am I to manage a facility without being there?); 3) I was to work February for half my fee; and 4) I was to spend the month writing a new detailed business plan including specifics for staffing, budget, etc.

I also learned Howard had no idea that: 1) Roger had another job. He had a sign making business and it did take time away from his work at the golf course (I had told Roger he would need to give that up when we transitioned to Tempest around April perhaps adding more motivation for him to see me fired.); and 2) Paul was my partner and on my payroll, which is why I felt comfortable not visiting the site in December. (He should have known this as it was in the original management proposal and we had talked about it several times back when we were hired.)

This would not be a good time to lose my only source of income. While I recently received a modest inheritance from my father, most of it went to retiring debt. The rest would not support us very long and Holly's income only covered the mortgage and some of our household bills. Plus, we were facing ever mounting medical expenses (it's surprising what is

NOT covered by insurance – even the excellent plan we had from BCBS through the City.)

So, I did not argue and accepted Howard's terms. I was to spend the entire month of February writing a detailed business plan. To be fair, a detailed plan was needed – more detailed than the one I already provided. However, what Howard was demanding was more than a business plan, but a combination plan and operations/employee manual.

I had been hoping to get some help in writing it from my managers – Paul and Barney on the maintenance side, Roger on the operations side and Natasha on marketing. After all, they were the ones responsible for executing the plan, so I felt strongly they should be involved in its creation. But that was not to happen. Paul did send some operational manuals helpful in creating job descriptions and procedures manuals. (It is always easier to edit an existing manual than to create one from scratch). However, Paul was also in the midst of construction. And now, because of the clubhouse fiasco, Howard was leaning on him to do more and essentially oversee the clubhouse as well.

The day after meeting Howard was the timeshare presentation in the morning. We followed that with the highlight of the trip – a visit to Universal Theme Park. Neither of us had been to Universal before and we both had wanted to for a long time. We had been to Disney several times (we lived in Jacksonville for several years), but never Universal. We would not have gone this time, either, if it weren't for the generosity of Universal.

This was the first time (and so far, only time) I used my condition to gain a favor. I knew we couldn't really justify the $100+ per person ticket price – especially since I likely could not put in anywhere near a full day due to my health. So, I took a chance and wrote the publicity director a letter explaining my situation and asking if she would consider giving us a two for one deal. Instead, they not only comped us a multi-park pass each but gave us special access allowing us to instantly go to the front of the line at the rides. This latter benefit was tremendously appreciated because there was no way I would have been able to stand in those lines, which for some rides (like Harry Potter) were over an hour long. And this wasn't because of my cancer, but because of my back (although the cancer did not help).

Neither of us are big roller-coaster fans, so we skipped those dramatic rides. But we did love the Harry Potter adventure. Holly was also very excited to do the Minion ride. This one certainly looked innocent enough. It was a 3-D "ride" where you sat in a chair that would move with wind gusts blowing in your face with noises and smells simulating a roller coaster ride, but the seat was really mostly stationary. However, it did move some vertically and horizontally. Amazing technology! And the ride was fun. But it was also very shaky, jerking back and forth – something not good for someone with a grapefruit growing out of his kidney. By the end of the ride, I was in major pain. So, our trip to Universal ended abruptly. It was about all I could do to walk the mile (or so it seemed) back through the park and to the car. We never got to see the 2nd park, other than a brief look in. Oh well. Got to save something for later! I am still very appreciative of Universal's kindness.

The completed business plan was over 300 pages long. And this did not include over 20 pages of spreadsheets. In 20+ years of doing this, I felt it was my best work and was an excellent plan . . . and would work.

Howard did not agree. I really doubt he ever read much of it because he called me about *two* hours after I sent it, blasting both me and the business plan (which, given its length, he could not have possibly read). He claimed it was mere rehashing what I had already told him (it contained a lot of the same information as I had not changed how I planned on operating the facility – but merely adding several more layers of detail, as requested. I included *everything* he asked for). He also ripped into me for demeaning and attacking Roger. This was not true at all. I said nothing critical of Roger in the business plan. I did, however, discuss four contingencies with regards to Roger – as in whether he continues as General Manager, accepts another position (two options), or leaves. This was needed as the GM is a critical piece of the puzzle and we would need to staff according to what *Roger* decided. All of this was discussed only in terms of the organizational chart and payroll.

He also blasted my budget, saying the expenses were totally unrealistic and that Paul agreed. Ok, this got to me on a couple of different levels. First, I felt the numbers were very realistic and were based on ample experience with similar operations to what I was expecting Tempest to become. But what really got me was Paul's comments. This is because I emailed Paul the budget three weeks prior to giving it to Howard and asked him for his comments and input. I repeated the request numerous times over the following weeks. I got nothing. Yet he had the time to give Howard his input.

I respect Paul's opinion, but it comes from a fundamentally different approach. His is much more conservative – concentrating on holding expenses in line while hoping revenue will build. Mine is more aggressive, and revenue based. I hold you only get one chance to create a first impression, so I wanted the club to open with full services, and not wait until business volume builds up, which it may otherwise never do. The thing is, Howard endorsed my approach in the summer and fall. But apparently when he suddenly went into the panic mode over money, he became much more cost-conscious.

I would have been happy to adjust the plan accordingly, but Paul never gave me the chance before presenting it to Howard, and Howard, I strongly believe, had already had his mind made up well before I ever presented the plan. He was terminating the contract, effective immediately.

I even struggled to get the termination fee from him, as it took several weeks of reminding him what was in the contract – which, if you assumed he had cause (which according to the contract, he did not, plus he would have had to give me *written* notice of any defaults with 30 days to correct, and he did not) the termination fee was one month's pay. He sent me ½ months.

While I could have raised hell over this, he was still representing me in my malpractice case. And I realize I could have and probably should have fired him for this, I just couldn't bring myself around to do it. I was still being loyal to him, even if his loyalty to me was clearly gone.

I cannot lie to you. This one really stung. It was another bad blow to the gut (the first being the tumor). As I mentioned before, I have had many personal disappointments and bad events happen to me in my life. But this was a bit different. For one thing, in twenty-plus years in the golf business, this was my first known dissatisfied customer. For another, I really loved this project. And I dearly loved managing, which is something I had wanted to do for a long time –being able to implement the recommendations I had made! Plus, this was my "baby." I came up with the idea, sold it to Howard, had a major hand in developing the project in all facets (golf course, clubhouse, real estate) and even named the course. I was (and continue to be) genuinely concerned for Howard as well, as I had serious doubts whether another operator would do what I knew had to be done for the operation to be successful (in terms of marketing, operations, fee structure, etc. – Operators tend to get lazy and price based on what everyone else is charging instead of pricing to value).

The timing on a personal level could not have been worse. My cancer was getting worse (although I had just started immunotherapy treatments, it was much too early to tell whether they were going to be effective). And I had no other work in the pipeline. Given my condition, it was doubtful if there was going to be any. And the medical bills continued to come in. Plus, of all the people you would think would understand my cancer situation, it would be my attorney! And the person you expected to back me up would have been my partner and the person I brought into the project and a six-figure payday for him.

I think both Howard and Paul felt because of my condition, I would be unable to "live" up to the contract and he had his investment to protect. What really hurt, though, was the apparent betrayal by my friend Paul, who did end up succeeding me as the management entity for the course. (By the way Paul promised me compensation for getting him the construction job, etc. But to date, I have not received any). I still have a hard time believing, despite all the evidence to the contrary, Paul was acting out of self-interest and intentionally undermining me. Indeed, when I got a consulting job with the Northbrook IL Park District for an evaluation study a couple months later, I brought in Paul as my agronomist. I guess I am the definition of "loyal to a fault."

I honestly believe my cancer was the main factor in my dismissal, even though I know Roger was actively working to have me terminated. The fact that December/January I was not able to travel to the course and was clearly struggling, coupled with the financial pressure that my $6,500/month bill was adding to, I think Howard (and Paul) felt I would not be able to contribute as expected and do what was needed. In short, it was a "business decision". The events of January 20th just provided a convenient excuse.

[Update October 2017: Paul took over as the management company. He terminated for cause Roger – as Roger was basically doing the same things to him as he did to me, including not doing the work. He also terminated Barney. Due to weather and other issues, the course did not open this fall as planned, but should be open early summer 2018. And I still have not received any compensation from Paul.]

[Update December 2018: the course did not open until September, a full year late, and without the driving range, which was still under construction. Now Howard is suing Paul. Karma is a bitch.]

IMMUNOTHERAPY

March – May 2017
While the blood transfusion I received on January 20th really helped with my fatigue, it did not help the pain in my abdomen from the growing tumor. The pain intensified with each passing day. My first immunotherapy treatment was February 3rd. The drug used, Tecentriq, had only been approved for my type of cancer a few weeks earlier. It was nice to be at Emory!

With cancer, immunotherapy gets your immune system to do the fighting for you. It does this by making the immune system sensitive to a mutation in the cancer cells.

One of the big advantages of immunotherapy over chemo is it comes with significantly fewer side effects. Indeed, other than a cough I have had since August it might have exacerbated, I haven't had any. It is also much quicker to deliver – the actual infusion taking thirty minutes instead of four hours. And since they did not need to add other drugs to combat nausea and other chemo side effects, I no longer require Holly to take me. This is nice because she was having to use all her vacation time taking me to Atlanta for treatments. We have better plans for those days!

Another advantage of immunotherapy is my treatments were now every third week instead of every other week. This had one unintended consequence. Yes, my sister Juliette came back to visit, this time bringing her husband, Michael – the man who had, in my opinion, saved my life by getting me into Emory. Naturally, they timed their visit so it would coincide with my treatment, as they wanted to meet Dr. Bilen. And this was right when the treatment got changed. So, the week they came, there was no treatment. They still have not met Dr. Bilen (although Michael has talked with him on the phone several times.) The visit, though, was wonderful.

The pain in my abdomen continued to increase through February. Then suddenly, about a week after my second treatment on the 21st, the pain disappeared! That's right, about the same time as I was getting fired from my job (very bad), my cancer pain stopped (very good), indicating the immunotherapy was working! (Really, I will take that trade-off any time.)

Physically, things continued to improve through March. But the true test came April 4th, my fourth treatment and first set of scans following the start of immunotherapy.

Holly accompanied me to Atlanta that day, as she always does when scans are involved. Once again, I submitted myself to the electrified coffin (MRI) and giant doughnut (CT) in the morning at the downtown hospital. We then ate lunch at Romeo's on campus at Emory, a place that has become our favorite Georgia pizza place for its authentic NY style pizzas (read: dripping with grease.) After lunch, we made the short trip to the Winship center to meet with Dr. Bilen (and later have the immune therapy infusion).

Shortly after we were seated in Dr. Bilen's exam room, he entered bearing a grin stretching the width of his face.

Then he shared the unbelievable news. The CT scan revealed *no trace of any tumors in my chest.* They were gone. Just like that. Even Dr. Bilen could not believe the extraordinary results. While we did not have the final MRI results, Dr. Bilen had called the radiologist to get a verbal report. The huge tumor on my kidney had shrunk considerably! We were winning the war. Needless to say, Holly and I were ecstatic.

While this technically did not qualify under the "six-month" rule, it was close. After all. It had been six months since the *diagnosis* when the pain started easing in March. Although it was seven months since the pain intensified, and ten months since I started having symptoms.

The following week I flew to Chicago where I met Jeff Brauer. We were being interviewed for a large consulting project for the Northbrook Park District. Five other firms, all major players in the golf course consulting world, were also being interviewed. As a small firm, we were a major underdog. For this project, though, I decided to change my approach. Previously, I always tried to undercut NGF in pricing, figuring I could easily do so because of my much lower overhead. But this time, I decided to price it high, knowing it might, in fact, be my last project. I wanted to get paid what I thought it was worth. So far, the strategy seemed to be working as we made the cut for the interview.

The interview was first thing Thursday morning, so Jeff and I flew in Wednesday morning. Jeff, a Chicago native, was excited to be back home. We began the trip down memory lane with an authentic Chicago deep dish pizza for lunch (Giordano's). [While I prefer the thin-crust NY style pizza over deep dish, I still *like* deep dish, and this was good!]. We then headed to Northbrook to inspect the Park District's two golf facilities. While there, we met with the Golf Director. This serendipitous meeting was very helpful, as he not only gave us great background information, but it turned out he had written the RFP we responded to and was on the committee interviewing us the next morning!

At Jeff's suggestion, we stopped by Dunkin Donuts in the morning and picked up a dozen donuts for our interviewers. When we arrived, we found a table set up for us in the back of the room, next to the podium. The committee was seated in a U-shaped arrangement of tables. We immediately moved our table from the back of the room, to the middle of the "U".

I decided prior to the interview to forsake a PowerPoint presentation. I reasoned everyone else would use PowerPoint. Further, given some of these firms had their own marketing department to put together very elaborate presentations, we simply could not compete. Instead, we wanted the committee to focus their attention on us. After all, we were the ones doing the actual work, not the marketing department.

During the interview, we pointed out some of the issues we spotted in our brief visit. More importantly, we gave them solutions to these issues.

Apparently, our strategy paid off. We got the job! The three amigos ride again. (Yes, despite everything previous, I included Paul in the proposal as my agronomist, but did not ask him to join us for the interview as I did not think it necessary). I was thrilled, not only at beating the other top firms in the industry, but also because it represented badly needed funds for moi!

One of my competitors, JJ Keegan, did not take rejection very well. Instead, he wrote a long article in his email newsletter blasting the Park District and especially its director for its decision-making process; essentially saying that they must be idiots for not picking him. He also claimed they just went with the low bidder. Sorry to disappoint you Jim, but we were actually the high bidder.

The Euphoria lasted until two days before my next infusion, which was the 25th of April. That Sunday, in bed, I started to once again feel pain coming from my tumor. It was not bad, but enough to let me know it was there. Fortunately, it went away once I got up.

The pain returned the next night. When I went in to see Dr. Bilen, I only saw Greta, his resident. She is great, though. I mentioned the pain to her but did not stress it as the pain was minor and went away when I got up.

Over the next couple of weeks, the pain worsened . . . but never got really bad. Initially, it would disappear during the day, starting to hurt again around 5pm. But eventually it started bothering me during the day. I decided it was time to do something. I called Juliette and asked to discuss it with Michael. Could there be any other reason *other* than my tumor starting to grow again? I also emailed Dr. Bilen. He responded he was not too concerned as long as the pain was minor, and it came and went (which it did).

Then I got a call back from Juliette giving us a lot of relief. Michael told her this was common. It was because as we start feeling better, we naturally get more active. The activity would then aggravate the tumor, thus causing pain. It did not necessarily mean I was getting worse. On the contrary, it could simply be a sign of my getting better and being more active. Sadly, though, the pain has continued to increase, making this explanation less likely. I am now scheduled for scans on June 1st, when we will know for sure what is going on.

So, this brings us up to date. We don't start the Northbrook (Chicago) project until June 7th. It is early May now. So, I am taking the time before I start the project to write this book, as I know I won't have much time after June 7th. Notably, the day before I head to Chicago, on D-Day, I am scheduled for my next visit with Dr. Bilen. This will determine whether the tumor is growing again, or hopefully continued to shrink. I will either be in a great or terrible mood when I get to Chicago.

[Please see the epilogue to learn what happened with the scan – and the study. It will also bring you current on my condition. It is a dairy of my cancer fight, starting June 1st.]

IMPACT ON MY LIFE

OVERALL IMPACT

May 2017

In some ways, cancer has not had a huge effect on my life. I still work – I need to, in order to pay the bills. But I also *want* to, because I enjoy what I do. I also think work is therapeutic as it keeps my mind occupied and focused on something other than personal issues. I still do *most* of the things I did before. Indeed, physically, I am probably *at this moment* (May 25, 2017) more limited by my back pain, which has nothing to do with the cancer, than by the cancer. That was not always the case, as I will discuss.

However, in many other ways, *everything* has changed. I

am certainly more aware of my own mortality – even though I'm in denial I am fast approaching its end. I am more eager to fulfill long-term dreams, like traveling. I am much more emotional and fatigued, which limits what I can do. I am more short-term oriented (naturally, as there may not be a long-term). I have become more philosophical and thoughtful about God and the afterlife. I am decidedly more aware about cancer and cancer research. And I am painfully aware of how the disease has affected my wife, family and friends. I have tried to become a better person, more thoughtful and generous. And, I have felt the need and urgency to write this book!

But I don't really think the cancer has fundamentally changed *who* I am. I have not had an epiphany that completely changed the way I think or act. I am not suddenly more religious as I've always had a strong faith. I have not "converted" or otherwise changed my religion or my beliefs. I would like to think I was a pretty "good" person before the cancer, and I am not certain I've improved that much since the diagnosis (although I do try – especially being more thoughtful, especially to my wife; and more generous to others).

In some ways, I think the cancer has affected others, especially Holly, more than myself. She is terrified of the thought of my leaving her, permanently. Not only because she will miss me, but I don't think she wants to be alone again, and she is not the type who will want to remarry. (I wish she would, because I hate the thought of her being alone as well. But I hope she waits until I'm gone before she does. I really don't even want her shopping around yet.)

She also must take of me a lot more than she used to. There have been times during the disease when I was essentially bed-ridden. During these times, Holly has had to not only take care of me but assume my housekeeping duties in addition to her own. Further, she has had to take a lot of time off work. When I was on chemo, she had to take me to Atlanta for the treatments – which takes a full day. Even now, when she does not have to come, she wants to come about every other time, or once every six weeks.

However, it impacts her in another way as well. No one (other than a sadist) wants to see their loved ones suffer. And she has had to witness a lot of suffering, even if I do my best to hide it from her.

It has had a huge financial impact on us. Not only the additional medical bills, and the travel costs back and forth to Atlanta (about 260 miles round-trip), but it has had a negative impact on my career. It led to the termination of a long-term management contract and prevented me for going after a lot of other consulting work. Even now, when I have been awarded a nice consulting job in the Chicago area, I am fearful of taking on other work. Indeed, I recently turned an opportunity over to the NGF (National Golf Foundation) for fear I was taking on too much. Not only do I not want to overload myself, but I am fearful of leaving my customers high and dry should I be unable to complete the work in a timely manner – or at all.

Scaling back work obviously impacts us financially. But I am lucky that I'm self-employed as it does allow me to work part-time without changing careers. On the other hand, I don't have any benefits like medical leave, sick days, or disability.

I am much more acutely aware of the word "cancer." It seems like I hear it all the time now. Whether on TV – commercials, documentaries, news stories, or part of a plot – or a Facebook post about a friend or their family, or in conversation. It seems everywhere I go, "cancer" is rearing its ugly head.

Moreover, it really, really hurts when I hear about someone losing their battle with this dreaded disease. Before, when I heard someone died of cancer, I would feel sad for them and their families. But now I take it personally. It's like a punch to the gut, every time.

I have a great deal more respect for people who are in a similar position to myself, whether it is because of cancer or some other disease. It is a hard thing to deal with – the reality of your own mortality. While I have taken the denial track as my primary defense, I certainly appreciate how others can get depressed. I also have an immense appreciation for what it does to their loved ones.

Cancer has affected me in another, more positive way. I don't let little things bother me anymore. "Don't sweat the little stuff" has become more than a motto for me. Why worry if dent in the car isn't fixed? Or if the house is not perfectly clean? (Not that I was that great about cleaning before . . .) Or if someone cuts me off on the highway? When you're dealing with the real possibility of not seeing another Christmas, etc., the little things that used to bother you simply pale in comparison. I don't need to waste energy worrying about little things, when I've got some much larger ones to direct my energy.

On the other hand, some little things affect me more . . . like those cancer commercials. Or phone calls and visits from my kids, family and friends. Those I appreciate a lot more than I ever did.

I'm also very into gardening this year. I've always liked to tinker in the garden – I think it's my farmer heritage coming out. But I think it means more to me this year. The process of nurturing growth and life is just more rewarding now and is a healthy distraction.

STRESS

March 2017
One of the biggest impacts cancer has had is the increased stress to both Holly's and my life. There is no doubt having a terminal disease adds a lot of stress -- Not only to the person having the disease, but also to those around them. This is especially true for the spouse and immediate family who now must prepare themselves, both emotionally and otherwise, for life without their loved one.

Stress to the patient comes from many sources. First, you know you have precious little time left. This puts a lot of pressure on you to maximize that time. But how? You are more limited both physically and financially due to the illness. If you want to travel and your spouse is working, there is a limit to how much time the spouse can spend away from work. This is especially true if the spouse is having to take a lot of time of work just to care for you.

There is financial stress, naturally, from all the medical bills and the reduced income. And it certainly limits you as to what you *can* do to distract yourself.

But one of the biggest sources of stress is watching the

impact of your situation on others.

Holly and I are both used to dealing with stress. As a manager of museums in days where public funding is scarce (two months after taking her current job as Executive Director of the National Civil War Naval Museum in Columbus, GA, the city dropped all its funding to the museum, which amounted to 1/4th their annual budget), Holly has continually faced the pressures of her job – especially financial pressures. Add to that my irregular income and the lack of large savings and the various money crises we've been through and it adds up. Plus, she has had to deal with various medical issues of her own.

But this is a different kind of stress. The kind that only comes when you are facing the loss of your life or the loss of a loved one.

I have always had a lot of stress in my life, whether it be personal, financial, social, or business. I've been essentially self-employed for the last 37 years. And that means I have always dealt with an uncertain income. Further, I've never achieved sustained financial success. As I will discuss later in greater detail, my life has been made up of continuous cycles. But during the good years, I've never made enough to carry me all the way through the down years. So, there has always been financial stress. Plus, in my current job, I have a lot of people that depend on me. Owners may risk their entire business based on my recommendations, which may mean also risking their own financial future. The customers of the golf courses are impacted by my recommendations. And, when I'm working with municipalities, which is most of the time, my recommendations may impact an entire City. When I'm doing feasibility studies, I'm dealing with projects that are millions of dollars in scope. And the project's future often hinges on what my report says. That's pressure, more so because I care. (One of the reasons why I believe I have been successful as a consultant is because I take these responsibilities very seriously). Plus, I've also had to deal with other medical issues, primarily my back and neck, that have not only impacted my quality of life, but also my work.

Now along comes the cancer. It not only has added more to the financial and other stresses we already were facing, but now Holly and I both must deal with the thought I may not be here long. At any time, with this cancer, I may only have a few months to live. It's like living with a permanent death sentence temporarily suspended, only you don't know for how long. (So far, we've been lucky with getting continuances, but I'm really holding out for a Pardon).

There have been four things that have really helped me deal with this new stress. First, the love and support I've received from Holly, my kids, my family and my friends. Even old classmates and others that have "befriended" me on Facebook have been very supportive, even though I'm not very good with social media. (Before the cancer, I may have checked Facebook once a month or so. I think now I'm up to once a week.)

Secondly, I am used to stress, as I mentioned before. While this may be a bit more than I'm used to, I think I've built up an immunity of sorts. Being self-employed, with an uncertain income, I have dealt with lots of stress! I believe I handle stress well. I guess practice makes perfect.

Third, my faith. I strongly believe there is a reason I'm going through this, even though I don't have a clue as to what that is. I believe I'm going to pull through it, but even if I don't, I believe there is a reason for it. I don't waste a lot of time and emotional energy thinking "why me?" Instead, I think, "why wouldn't it be me?" and "there *is* a reason for this, I just need to figure it out."

And finally, my father's death last summer. While it made my life a lot emptier, the modest inheritance I received has been a lifesaver financially during this difficult time. I can't help but think the timing was not coincidental. For the first time in my life, I have enough money in savings that we could go without any income (Holly or myself) for six months and be ok. While this is a long way from being enough to retire on, it does provide a good safety net for now. It also provides us with a means for doing some traveling that I long have wanted to do, before it's too late.

Adding to the stress is the frustration we both feel from the fact we might not have been in nearly so bad a position if my urologist had been competent. I may repress most of the stress I am feeling. Perhaps that is why I have started experiencing my anxiety attacks again. These usually come at night, when I am lying down to go to sleep. I talk about this elsewhere, so I won't bore you with additional redundancy here. But I do want to emphasize these anxiety attacks pale in comparison to those the summer before the diagnosis. And, for the most part, I have been able to handle them.

Exercising the Demon

One way I wish the cancer had a greater impact on me is in the desire to exercise. Boy do I admire Erik Berry and his work ethic in dealing with cancer, as well as all the others who have used the cancer to motivate themselves to exercising and getting into a lot better shape. I seemingly have taken the opposite approach.

Unfortunately, I have never been one to exercise a lot. The only time I ever took up jogging was when I was madly in love in college with Jan, who mentioned before she left for Hawaii for the summer (that's where she lived), that she liked skinny guys and that I wasn't that skinny. I'm 6'1" and, at the time, I weighed 185, which was 20 pounds more than I weighed as an undergraduate. Wow, I really wish I was that "fat" now! Anyway, over the summer I got motivated, took up running and lost 15 pounds. Didn't do me any good, though. She still left me. (Although it took nearly a year). I've never jogged regularly since.

I used to keep in fairly good shape by playing basketball. I love basketball. Part of it is growing up in Kansas and being a huge KU fan all my life. But I also love playing it. I've never been that good, mind you, but wasn't that bad either. I used to love going to the gym when I was in my 50's and beating these 20 somethings that were taller and much more athletic than me.

But since moving to Georgia, my back and knees have prevented me from playing. Sadly, they also have kept me from doing a lot of walking, or even playing golf. It's hard to exercise when it hurts to do it, and not from the muscles you are trying to work.

We now have a swimming pool, and I know swimming is great exercise. I also think it is something good for both my back and knees. We have just had the pool uncovered and treated. And it's starting to warm up. So, I will shortly be void of excuses. Not to worry, I'm sure I will think of something. Perhaps it will be the fact my clothes are getting too tight again. When the cancer started, I lost nearly twenty pounds, going from 250 to 230 (which is still about 20 pounds more than I would like). But over the last month, I've gained twelve of the pounds back. During this time, I would justify not eating well with "well I'm not going to be around long anyway, so why should I worry?" Even if what I'm eating takes five years off my life expectancy – the cancer will get me long before that becomes a concern. But now I'm seeing studies that show that exercise can help extend life with cancer. There goes my rationale. Maybe I should take up smoking?

That does get me, though. I would not have been considered as a high-risk for cancer. I have never smoked. I don't do drugs. I don't drink much – maybe averaging one to two beers a week, and rarely more than two at one time. Nor do I have a family history of cancer. My grandmother did die of bladder cancer, but she was a heavy smoker. My mother had tumors, but they were not due to cancer, but to neurofibromatosis type 1 (otherwise known as "elephant man disease.") My father's family are all long-lived. All his siblings have lived well into their 90s, with his sister making it to 99 and one sister and brother still alive. I have over twenty cousins, of which I am the third youngest. The oldest are well into their 70s. All are alive and well. Ironically, I may be the first to go – a race I do not care to win.

About the only vice I've had is diet coke. I will readily admit that I have been addicted to diet coke. In fact, up until a year ago, I was drinking over six cans a day and it was not unusual for me to drink ten. I drank it from breakfast till I went to bed – rarely drinking anything else. Ironically, late last May was when I decided to give it up. I went cold turkey. Right after that is when I had the grape juice pee incident and the cancer was in full flight (although I did not know about the cancer for another three months). It is possible the diet coke led to my cancer, but I have found no such links in the research. That's the thing about cancer – it can strike anyone at any time. No one is immune. (I thought I was and now look at me.)

Becoming Conway

Sometimes I will catch myself walking like Tim Conway's old man character on the Carol Burnett Show – hunched over and shuffling my feet, being passed by a fast snail. This is due much more to my back then my tumor, although they both can cause it. Especially if they are working together (not the kind of cooperation I appreciate). But when I find myself doing it, I try as much as I can to straighten myself up and walk as normal as possible. I don't want to end up that way and I fear if I continue to walk hunched and shuffling, then that's what will happen. Only I won't be paid like Tim Conway to do so. (I remember my dad used to walk like that – just before he became unable to walk at all). I will make an exception, though, if I happen to be parking in a handicap space.

Before you get too excited, I do have a handicap permit that attaches to the mirror. Ok, so it is a temporary one that expired a year ago. I know I could get a new one. But doing so would require me to go back to that horrible licensing place. Unlike the DMV, which at least lets you take a number and then sit and wait for the paint to dry, the licensing place (tax office) requires you to stand in a very long and very slow-moving line. This is something I used to loathe, before I had any back problems. But now, it is pure torture. If I stand longer than about thirty seconds (on good days, a minute), my back will start sending out shooting pains that will grow more intense as I remain stationary. They will not go away by walking, but they don't get worse as fast. The only relief is to sit, which I can't do at the licensing place without losing my spot.

I could probably ask Holly to go for me, or at least go with me and stand in line for me. But she has done so much and taken so much time off from work for me, I hesitate to ask another favor. So instead, I use the old permit and just turn it so it's much harder to see the expiration date. To be fair, I rarely use it. Only when I'm really, really hurting . . . or there are no other parking places anywhere close.

Unfortunately, there are a LOT more people with handicap stickers now. It used to be the handicap spaces were always empty, and you cursed the fact so much of the parking lot was dedicated to spots that were never used. Now I am finding it very difficult to find a vacant handicap spot when I really need one. Yes, sometimes it is able-bodied jerks parking there to save them walking an extra fifty feet. I am so tempted to key these cars! But often it is full of cars with legitimate handicap permits. Sadly, I think the people who are driving and using these spots are often not the people for whom the permits are intended – they simply use them to park close even when their spouse (or whomever the permit was for) is not there.

So, when I do park in such a space, I make sure I am limping when I get out! I don't want anyone to think that I am jerk, even if I am.

[August 2018 update: To be honest, my "fear" of the

DMV extended to more than the handicap permit. I never transferred my license plate to Georgia when we moved to Texas. So, for the past three years I have been driving with an expired license place. I would live in fear every time a police car was behind me. This did not keep me from speeding, mind you. It's just that I became a whole lot more careful about doing so. I kept it under ten mph over the limit, unless I had a caravan of cars in front of me. I did get pulled over once, but the cop was very nice and let me go with a warning.

Finally, last week I took care of the problem by buying a new car. This forced me to get a new license plate and face the dreaded DMV line. However, I learned long ago that if you must go someplace that's likely to be crowded (whether its shopping, going to the bank, or facing the DMV), *when* you go is critical. Mondays and Tuesdays tend to be the best days. And the magical times are 10:30 am and 2:30 pm. It worked, although I got there at 2:25 and there was a bit of a line. When it struck 2:30, though, the line was gone.].

GOLF

April 2017

I rarely play golf anymore. I've only played once since the diagnosis, and that was five holes. Golf is important to me and has been most of my life. It started out because it was something I could do with my dad – about the only thing we did together. It still reminds me of him. Later, I simply enjoyed playing it. But then it became my career. No, not as a player, as anyone who has ever played with me will gladly attest. I am a golf course consultant. I travel around the country helping golf course owners (mostly municipalities) make their golf courses more profitable, and developers and owners determine the feasibility of building, renovating or expanding a golf course. It's a great job, but someone has to do it. (Truthfully, I don't think of it as work, because I love doing it. In this way, I am truly blessed – to be able to do something for "work" that I truly enjoy, and to be good at it.)

I got my love of golf from my father. He was an avid golfer. He would play every Saturday and Sunday when I was growing up. We belonged to a country club (Milburn in Overland Park) and he would occasionally take me out and try to teach me to play. But I was stubborn, and my father was not the most patient person in the world (to put it very mildly). So, I never played much as a youth. But I did enjoy the game.

I started getting a lot more serious after I started my first business, Encore Copy Corps in Lawrence. One of my big customers was Alvamar, one of the local golf courses. They were willing to trade green fees for copies. We both won. But when you are working 100 hours per week, as I often was, you do not have a lot of time to play. I was lucky if I got to play once a week.

After Encore, the lack of time and money further limited my play. I probably averaged less than ten rounds a year. About a third of these were with my dad, when I would go to Dallas to see him. I really enjoyed playing with him, even though I could never beat him! When dad retired early from Sears, he became a real addict. He would often play five times a week. When he wasn't playing, he was frequently practicing. There was a high school (Hillcrest) a couple of blocks from dad's house. He would go there and practice chipping in their large field. This continued as long as he lived in that house (nearly 40 years). Sometimes students or faculty would come over and he would give them a lesson. They never chased him away. All that practice would pay off as my dad developed an awesome short game.

Dad got better as he got older, due to all that practice and playing. He went from a fifteen handicap down as low as a six, when he was well into his 60s. He once had a round where he had just eighteen putts – one-putting every hole. That is a pretty remarkable achievement. But dad was most noted for being a "gamer." He had the ability to really turn it on when it counted, e.g. club tournaments. He seemed to always win his age bracket (seniors, then super seniors, etc.) at

Brookhaven, where he played. Brookhaven, the home course of ClubCorp was also the home course for Jordan Spieth when he was growing up. In fact, Cheryl, who is also an avid golfer, remembers playing with him when he was about thirteen. He was playing by himself when Cheryl's group offered to let him play with them. It was like that old Titleist commercial where the kid with the untied shoes joins a group of older golfers and proceeds to take them to school. Cheryl was so impressed after the round, she told him he was going to be famous one day, and she was right. Dad was not a sandbagger, though. (A sand bagger is one who deliberately pays poorly or only turns in his/her bad scores in order to inflate their handicaps.) Rather, he just had the ability to really focus when there was something on the line. And it seemed like that was the case every time we played, because I almost never could beat him – even when he was in his 90s. (Dad shot his age every year from 71 until 92).

I will never have the passion my dad had for playing golf, especially competing. While I am a naturally very competitive person, I have a big handicap . . . I hate to practice. As in, I never do. The only time you will see me on a range is when I am working (not practicing), or I'm teaching my wife. I guess that explains why I never got very good at playing! But that's ok, I just love *playing*. I love being outside, I love competing with myself, I love the strategy and I really love the challenge. (Which is why I always hit into the woods and traps, because I want to make the next shot more challenging . . . yeah, that's it.)

The most golf I ever played in my life was when we lived in Durham and I was selling insurance. Ann's best friend, Mary Beth, loved to play. We would play together almost every week. During this period, I probably played between 30-40 rounds a year. And I got to be decent, regularly shooting in the low 80s and occasionally the 70s. (Mary Beth also took me to several UNC basketball games a year, including the Duke game every year, because she knew I was a boisterous fan. She was an awesome friend.)

There were a few things that prevented me from playing more – and still do. First, I always felt a bit guilty playing. There were two reasons for this – time and money. Money was always tight, so it was hard justifying paying $30 or more just for my own personal entertainment. I also felt guilty taking so much time away from my family, or my work.

We never could afford to join a country club. This made it harder to play. It also meant I never developed a group to play with. With the exception of Mary Beth, or my family, or when I played as part of my work, the vast majority of my rounds have been played on my own.

Unquestionably, there was a subconscious need to gain my father's approval that helped propel me into the golf business. (I will tell that story later.) If my parents were proud of my previous career choices, they sure never expressed it to me. I always thought I was a big disappointment to them. They always wanted me to become a medical doctor, like my sister. Even when I was in my forties, they kept saying it was not too late.

I still remember clearly when I told them I was accepted into KU's psychology graduate school. I was very excited as it was a difficult program to get in as it was nationally prominent. But my parents seemed very nonplussed about it. When I asked, my mother said: "well don't they have to take you, since you went there as an undergraduate?" (Truth is, that probably works against you.)

I probably would have loved being a doctor, but at the time, I did not want anything to do with it, even though my undergraduate studies looked very much like premed (lots of chemistry and biology). The trouble was, I hated the sight of blood and the thought of taking anatomy was terrifying.

So, when I got into the golf business, I felt my father would be proud. I think he was, but I also think he was concerned I would not make any money at it. And I certainly have not gotten rich off it.

When I tell people I am a golf course consultant, they naturally assume I get to play a lot of golf. And I do know a few consultants who do. I am not one of them. While I probably visit several hundred courses a year, I rarely get to play.

It would have been different if Ann or the kids played. But none of them ever showed an interest.

Holly decided she wanted to learn to play when we lived in the Dallas area. But we never played more than a few times a year. Now the limitations are more physical. It just hurts my back, neck and shoulder too much when I play. And that was before I grew a golf ball on my kidney.

Truthfully, since getting into the golf business in the mid-1990s, I have not played that much golf, and my game has steadily gotten worse. Most years, I was lucky to average playing once a month. During the last few years, I've averaged less than that. And now, I can't play. This time it's due mostly to my back, not my cancer. Also, my endurance is so low because I have not been able to exercise enough. But I am vowing to change all that. I am hoping to start playing again this summer, back and all. But if I don't, so be it. I still get to enjoy going to the courses during my work.

WORK

December 2017

The most obvious way cancer can affect your work is *physically*.

I have already described in detail how the cancer affected my work with regards to the golf course management contract I had at the time. In short, when I was suffering badly – both from the effects of the cancer and the chemo, I found it extremely hard to work. I was just so weak, plus the pain was significant. So, I had a choice, hurt more, or take the Percocet, which really helped with the pain, but made it a lot harder to concentrate. There was a period of about six weeks where I was doing good if I could spend two hours doing my work. And that two hours may be spread over the day, fifteen minutes at a time, with some of it being done in bed on my laptop.

As I noted, the result was that I lost the contract. It would take a few months before I was really working again. But by this time, we had switched to immunotherapy and I was doing much better and thus able to physically withstand the work. (I know, it is such *hard* work sitting at a desk most of the day. But if you can't concentrate, you can't work.)

Cancer, or more likely, its treatment can also affect your *mental* ability to do work. In my case most of my work is mental as opposed to physical. But when you are dealing with extreme pain or extreme fatigue, it makes it very difficult to concentrate. That's in addition to any issues related to medication. Generally, I refused to take anything that would affect my ability to concentrate unless it was absolutely necessary. Unfortunately, there were a lot of times it was. When you can't concentrate it not only makes work harder, the quality may be questionable.

There is also an *emotional* impact. After all, if you only have a limited amount of time left, do you really want to spend it working? It can be challenging to stay motivated.

There is no doubt that cancer imperils your ability to physically, emotionally or mentally do your work . . . especially when the symptoms are severe. But it also impacts it in other ways.

For one thing, there is *time* and not just from when you are too sick to work from either the disease or the treatment. Even now, when I am doing much better and able to put in full days of work, cancer still robs me of a lot of time. For instance, I must trek to Atlanta once every three weeks for treatment. And these treatments are always during the work week (either Tuesday or Friday). Do the math. A treatment every three weeks means losing fourteen workdays a year. This is just under three full work weeks! For most people, this would equate to using up all your vacation and sick days . . . just for the treatments. (I realize that if I were having the treatments done locally, many of them would only take half a day. But I believe the quality of care at Emory makes the extra time investment well worth it).

Being self-employed, I don't have to worry about using

up sick days and vacation days. But then again, if I am not working, I'm not earning any money. No one is paying me to stay home or go to Atlanta.

As I mentioned previously, when I started Chemotherapy, I had been warned about the likely side-effects. But for the first three treatments, I really didn't feel any of them. So, I was starting to feel pretty cocky. What I did not realize, however, is the effect is *cumulative*. The side-effects get worse the more treatments you have. Sure enough, not only did I start losing my hair, but I started suffering from severe fatigue.

It turns out the chemo had a bad side effect of making me anemic. And the more anemic I got, the more fatigued I became. But insurance would only pay for treatment of the anemia when it got what they deemed "severe." Their definition is much more rigorous than mine. I would think having to stay in bed all day would make it severe, but they use a blood test instead. By the time I was finally treated for it, I had two full units of blood and it still only raised my red blood cell count halfway to where it should be.

One of the wonderful aspects of the immunotherapy I'm on now (besides, of course, for the fact it has saved my life), is that it doesn't have nearly the side effects chemo does. But apparently one of the side effects it does have is an increase in pain. So be it.

Cancer affects us *socially* as well. In the case of the work environment, it often changes how coworkers and/or customers treat you (those that know).

I often find myself in a very awkward position. Do I tell people about my cancer? In almost all cases, the answer has been "no." But there are exceptions. I knew I had to tell my boss (the owner of the golf course) about it. After all, there were obvious long-term implications, and this was a long-term contract. (I feel this greatly contributed to the termination of said contract). I've also had to tell people when my treatments are interfering with my work schedule. But normally I don't. None of my customers this summer knew about my situation. I don't think they even realized I was sick.

I am very fortunate I am self-employed. Honestly, if I was working a "regular" job, I do not see how I could have continued. At the very least, I would have had to take an extended leave of absence and just hope the job would be there when I recovered. I feel horrible for those in that situation.

I also have no employees. So, I don't have to deal with coworkers daily. But I can imagine how hard it can be for those who have cancer and a regular job. There is no way, really, of keeping the cancer secret. You're pretty much obligated to tell your boss. But coworkers know you're sick and they are going to ask and ask until you relent. Suddenly becoming bald is also a give-away. Might as well get it over with. But then you must deal with being treated differently.

Some people will treat you as though the cancer is contagious. They will avoid you. Maybe they just feel awkward because they don't know how to treat you. Then others may do the opposite and smother you with attention. In both situations, you lose out. I will talk more about social impact in the next chapter.

However, there is another way in which the cancer affects your work, and that is *psychologically*. Having cancer changes your perspective, which alters your whole approach to work.

For one thing, work takes on a different priority. In my case, work has always been a very important part of my life.

Not only do I enjoy what I do, but I find it fulfilling. Thus, it has assumed a bigger role for me than just a means to an end.

When you are faced with a much shorter time span, time itself becomes much more precious. Thus, you want to maximize its use. This usually means reshuffling your priorities. In my case, it meant work suddenly became less important.

Sadly, I'm not able to retire for financial reasons. But I can "scale back" a bit. I no longer worry about trying to reach certain work goals. There is no work endgame. Instead, I can put my full efforts into whatever project I'm doing, without worrying about future consequences.

However, even if I was able to retire, I wouldn't unless my wife was able to do the same, which she's not. Even if we could lose her income, we could not afford to lose the insurance. (My medical bills in the past year alone have been over $600,000. Thank God for BCBS, which has been mostly wonderful through this entire process). The reason I wouldn't retire is that I find working *therapeutic.*

The more I concentrate on my work, the less time I dwell on the consequences of my situation. And as I focus on a project, I can block most of the pain, which may be part of the reason why I feel the pain so much more in the evening, when I am no longer working.

Social

April 2017
Cancer impacts your social life in many ways – both positively and negatively. On the positive side, you get more attention. On the negative side, people become afraid of you. Ok, maybe they are not scared they are going to catch cancer from me like it was a cold. But people, I think, feel awkward because they don't know what to say or how to act around those who might be dying. I also think people get anxious because it reminds them of their own mortality.

On the other hand, since learning of my cancer, I certainly have heard from more of my friends than ever before. I even had one of my closest friends come visit. (Unfortunately, I don't have any friends close by. Since moving here two years ago, I have spent so much time traveling and working that I really have not had an opportunity to develop a social life locally. But that's ok as I've been pretty much a loner all my life, preferring the company of family and a few close friends.)

I have found myself also reaching out to my friends. But this is also awkward. I really, really would like to see and hear from more of my friends. But, given my circumstances, it just seems weird to do so. I don't want to make it seem like I am seeking their pity.

Thank goodness for Facebook! While I have had a Facebook account for at least ten years (I don't remember exactly when I started), but I have never been very active. Although I would go through an occasional burst to see if I can find any more of my long-lost friends. But other than those rare times, I hardly ever went on and even more rarely posted anything. And by rare, I'm talking maybe once a month or so. (Pausing while the Millennials recover).

But the cancer changed that. I decided to let the world know, so I posted about it. I did so, not wanting pity, but knowing how badly others would feel if I should pass and they never even knew I was sick. That has happened to me before and I know it's an awful feeling. So, this way people can have the opportunity to reach out if they want to.

But I wanted to do more than just inform the world. I thought perhaps I could help those going through a similar process or have family or close friends going through one. That's why I started the *Mortal Musings* videos, which I posted on Facebook and You Tube. Surely some hotshot Hollywood Director would see these videos and immediately cast me in their next blockbuster . . . maybe a new superhero flick, "Cancer Man!" Alas, no one has called.

When I do see people, whether they are friends or acquaintances, who know about my condition, I can really sense *their* awkwardness. After all, what do you say to someone who has cancer? What do you say to someone who is likely to die soon? "Been good to know you?" Ignoring the elephant in the room can seem callous or uncaring but bringing it up could cause anguish – especially on the person asking because no one likes to hear someone else complain!

The truth is, I *have* cancer and I still don't know how to treat others with cancer. Although now I have common ground. Yet I realize people handle the situation very differently. Some want to talk about it, and its therapeutic for them to do so. Others don't want to be reminded of their situation and are adamant about not being treated differentially. Still others are dealing with either great anger and/or depression, which affects not only them, but those around them.

For the most part, people ask "how are you doing?" Automatically I will respond, "great" or "doing fine," because I know that's what they want to hear. They don't want to know about your suffering, or your fear of dying, or fear of leaving your wife and family alone. They want to know everything is going to be ok.

For the most part, that's fine with me. I get no pleasure from sharing my misery. (*Misery doesn't really like company. Misery wants hope, compassion and escape*). So, I say, "I'm fine," and hope they can still treat me like they used to . . . ok, maybe a *little* better than they used to.

Occasionally, though, I will make an exception. I will do this in a couple of situations. If I think the person genuinely wants to know the truth and can handle it, I will tell them . . . as far as they want to pursue. Or if it's family or a close friend who I think can handle it and can offer some comfort when I really need it. I may also admit to some pain when it is terribly obvious that I am feeling some, but I will always follow up with "but it is nothing I can't handle." Which is true.

But sometimes you really do need the comfort. You really *want* to be able to tell *somebody* about what you are going through – both the physical and the emotional. If you don't, you find the emotional stress just keeps building up inside you, until it explodes, which is something no one wants. You absolutely need to vent, but you need to make sure you vent to the right people, who can handle it and understand. But, on the other hand, you don't want to be a burden, and sharing your misery *is* going to create a burden on that person, even if that person is your spouse.

I guess the best approach to dealing with people with cancer is to let them know you're there, you care, and you are *willing* to listen if that helps. You will likely know quickly if that person wants to talk about it or not. Although I will admit my first reaction is always to tell people "I'm fine," when I really would *like* to talk about it but am fearful doing so would create a burden on the other person, which I do not want. Or it would make them think I'm plying for their sympathy, which I'm not.

My advice, then, is if you're close to someone, like a loved one or a close friend, you should encourage them to talk about it. It can really help. But don't come across too syrupy. Knowing you care is what we want, not to be babied. (Ok, maybe once in a while . . .)

I can see the fear in Holly's eyes. I know how hard it would be on her if I die . . . and she's not bashful about telling me! (Although she also claims to know the date and time of my demise . . . at her beckoning.) So, talking to her about what I am going though is a two-edged sword. There is no one in the world it hurts more to know what I'm going through than her. But there is no one in the world who can offer as much comfort as she can.

I end up compromising. At times it is quite obvious when I am hurting, even though I do my best to disguise it (unless I'm parking in a handicap space . . .) When it's that obvious, I will be honest with her . . . or with my family. But not *too* honest. I always try to mediate the news, putting it in the best context I can . . . e.g. "it's not nearly as bad as it was" or "it's likely a byproduct of the treatment – which is a good trade-off for my life!" or "it's getting better."

It's weird. Often, I find it is me offering the encouraging word or the comfort. I must be strong, so they can be strong . . . in case I need their strength later. But by doing so, I think I am helping myself as well. *You can talk yourself into feeling better . . . or worse. I choose better.*

And I am always optimistic, which is not a front. As I said before, I don't accept the fact this cancer is going to kill me. I *will* beat it. But then again, I have *always* been an optimist. The glass isn't just half full with me, it's also one-third full, etc. Perhaps that's why I have been a risk taker throughout my life, because I'm always optimistic about the outcome. (You think I would have learned by now . . .)

While I can and do share my physical sufferings (to a degree) to my inner circle (mostly my wife), I am extremely reluctant to share my *emotional* state of mind. Part of this is because I feel the need to maintain the image of being a rock, because I know my loved ones *need* this for *their* emotional well-being. It's a lot harder for them to perseverate on the negative if I am refusing to.

Plus, I'm a guy. Let's face it. There is still considerable cultural pressure on guys to be stoic. We are not *supposed* to get emotional or to share our feelings. We're to tough it out.

I realize this impasse is why the cancer support groups are so important. It's so much easier to share what you are going through with people who are also going through it. It can be such a wonderful relief and needed support.

EMOTIONAL IMPACT

Love, Fear and Depression

LOVE

October 2016 (from Mortal Musings video)
The cancer has made me more emotional. I have always been very sensitive, especially for a guy. But now those emotions are on overdrive. I am especially affected by things where people have experienced great joy or dealt with death. Even commercials can leave me in tears – especially those dealing with cancer and most definitely the ones about immunotherapy.

It seems like every show I see, including the news, is always dealing with death. A lot of this is because my wife loves crime shows, which seem to think only murders are worth investigating, except Law & Order SVU – one of my wife's favorites (Holly seems especially enamored with shows where the husband is murdered by his wife – should I be worried? It is a bit disconcerting that she takes notes). I think our society has become a lot more desensitized to death and to violence thanks to the media and to video games. I'm not sure this is a positive thing. Well now consider me sensitized.

Learning I had cancer naturally had a strong emotional impact on me. I was sad – not as much for myself, but for how it impacted those around me, especially Holly and the kids. There was anger, but really, not that much. Nor was there any hatred involved. The emotion that really overwhelmed me? *Love*. I could not give or receive enough love. While I did not find any joy in my situation, I did embrace how much love meant to me . . . especially the love of my wife and children, and to a lesser extent my extended family and friends.

As I mentioned before, I have always been an emotional person . . . just the opposite of my father, who was very stoic, rarely showing any emotion (except occasionally anger). Instead, I tended to wear my emotions on my sleeve.

But this cancer thing has really put my emotions on overdrive. I feel like *all* my emotions are on overdrive. Movies, TV shows, and yes, commercials, affect me more than ever before . . . which can be very embarrassing!

I am particularly sensitive, though, to both love and death. I try very hard not to take my love for my wife and family for granted. I don't want to be that guy that goes to the grave with regrets about not telling people how he feels (positively, that is). I also believe I feel the love more intensely than before. And I certainly react much more strongly to situations dealing with death. Which is unfortunate, because it seems that's all that's ever on TV, whether on the TV shows, or the news. And those cancer commercials . . .

Perhaps it's because you know the end is near, or maybe because you are feeling all your emotions more intensely, but love becomes ever more important to you. You feel so much closer to the ones you love – your wife, your family, your friends – even your pets.

To me, this intense feeling of love is what helps give me strength. It also gives me something to fight for, a reason to live.

FEAR

February 2017
There is another emotion I feel more strongly now than ever . . . *fear*. I suppose this is to be expected.

I don't claim to be the bravest of humans, but I also do not recall ever experiencing a real bout of fear, where you are frozen and unable to think or move. I admit I have always been afraid of heights (acrophobia) and closed spaces (claustrophobia), so I certainly know what it's like to be afraid. And I've always been scared to go to horror movies. But this was very, very different. But I was never paralyzed with fear, even when I was in that bloody claustrophobic contraption, the MRI.

Now, it happens at night. During the day, I'm okay. I can keep myself busy, and thus I don't dwell on my cancer or my impending termination. But once I lay down at night, it all changes. When I lay down to go to sleep, the distractions are minimized, and the thoughts and fears come flooding in.

For one thing, my pain always increases at night. It's like sundowner's syndrome that often affects seniors (as it did my father). Once the sun sets, my pain level seems to increase significantly. Truthfully, I don't think the sun has anything to do with it, as it seems to be more correlated with the time of day, starting at about five or six. (As I am writing this, that time does correspond to the sun setting, but it was also true when the sun was setting later). And because my pain is much more noticeable, it is very hard to ignore the source of that pain, and thus, the consequences.

It's not a conscious thing. What happens, I think, is this fear is dwelling in my subconscious, where I keep it repressed. But then at night, it seeps out in the form of an anxiety attack.

It started this past summer − before I even knew I had cancer. But it was obvious something was wrong. People don't go around peeing grape juice, after all. It was shortly afterwards when I started having this terrible insomnia punctuated with these "anxiety attacks." No, they weren't panic attacks in the sense that I had any physical pain with them. But suddenly I would come wide awake (I usually had not gone to sleep, but was in that hypnogogic state where I am about to . . .) And I was shaking . . . mentally, if not physically.

Often, these "attacks" would come with these awful visions of dying in the most terrifying of ways − like being buried alive (my biggest fear). Or I suddenly thought about what my orthopedic surgeon said about my neck − that I was one whiplash away from being permanently paralyzed. Now that statement had been made months earlier and I never gave it much thought, until now. And it was virtually impossible to purge these extremely unpleasant thoughts from my head.

These attacks came almost every night (the insomnia was *every* night). And there was nothing I could do to stop or shorten them. None of the pills (sleeping pills) had any effect whatsoever. I tried to distract myself, usually by playing a video game on my phone. But I was so fatigued, I could not concentrate enough to even do that.

It got so bad I would dread going to bed, despite being extremely exhausted. I even panicked about panicking. These attacks were so horrible, the fear of them contributed to my overall anxiety.

At the time I was convinced the root of the problem was physiological, not psychological. After all, I had never experienced anything like it before. And though it was a very stressful time in my life, the stress was less than I had been through before, with no such symptoms. Plus, the attacks persisted long after the stress was reduced significantly with the award of a new contract and the selling of our albatross house in Corsicana. (I suppose one could argue the stress caused by everything, including the physical issues I was going through, initially caused the attacks – but then the attacks themselves added to that stress, which is why they persisted after some of the outside conditions eased off. And the attacks did eventually go away – about two to three weeks after the "windfall week" happened.)

As I mentioned, this bout of insomnia, with the occasional "anxiety attacks" stopped after about six weeks or so. But then they started up again soon after I got my diagnosis. This time, they were qualitatively different.

For one thing, it was not every night affair like it was then. And instead of thinking of horrifying ways to die, I started thinking about dying much sooner than anticipated, and what that meant . . . not just to myself, but to my family, friends and especially my wife. Although I occasionally thought about suffocating for some reason . . . perhaps because I was aware of the tumors in my chest. Or maybe it was the cat sleeping on my face.

On the other hand, these attacks have not been limited to the nighttime.

The first daytime attack happened when I went in for the Pet Scan, as I described previously. Again, the *machine* was not that scary. It was not nearly as claustrophobic as an MRI. And I really was not *consciously* thinking about the test. After all, I already knew I had cancer. This was just to determine how bad. And it honestly never occurred to me the cancer had spread. After all, it had just been discovered.

But I could not get in the machine. As soon as I sat down on the table, the panic started. It was as though the machine was the edge of a deep ravine and I was being asked to go and stand on that edge and look down. And it came from nowhere. Going in, I wasn't nervous at all about the scan. And now I was embarrassing myself, which seemed to only add to my anxiety.

What happened? I was not *consciously* thinking about the scan itself or what it could mean . . . but apparently my subconscious was! It wasn't the physical scan setting me off, it was what it meant. It was as though my subconscious knew what the scan would reveal . . . that my cancer was, in fact, Stage IV, with tumors throughout my chest, including one key spot that was inoperable. In other words, I was screwed.

Fortunately, the incidence of daylight attacks has been very rare. And as my physical condition improves, I have had fewer at night as well. But boy are they scary when they happen. I can sometimes feel one coming on and try to distract myself by taking a sleeping pill then playing a game or reading a newspaper (KC Star, Washington Post, NY Times) on my phone until it starts to work.

I do believe it's more than just the thought of a life cut short bothering my subconscious. It's the fact it's my own body doing this, and I cannot control it. I also think it's the uncertainty – not knowing what is going to happen. Always before when I get sick, I knew I would get better. And even with the back and neck pain – I know they will get better, even if they will never go away. But again, this is different. The six-month rule was not likely to be in effect.

Another thing I think is happening is the sudden confrontation with the realization I'm not immortal. Since nothing ever serious has happened to me in the past, I guess I assumed it never would.

DEPRESSION

March 2017
Yes, it would be easy to get depressed. Impending death certainly seems like a good reason. And I will admit there are times when I feel depressed.

These bouts tend to occur when I am really hurting badly or when I receive bad news. The worst time came after I was fired from the management contract. That was extremely depressing on so many levels. First, it was a dream job for me. Second, it put us in serious financial jeopardy with little hope (at the time) of it turning around. Third, there was that cancer and dying thing. Fourth, I was physically hurting at the time (although not as bad as I had been). Fifth, it was so incredibly frustrating because I did not think I had been treated fairly at all. Sixth, I truly felt by releasing me, Howard has put this project in serious danger of failing, as I know it will require outside-the-box thinking, especially with regards to marketing, to make it work. Seventh, and most of all, I felt betrayed by my friend, Paul.

I had not gotten really depressed before this. I think it was because I was still in denial. I also felt the need to stay strong for my wife and family.

But when the termination thing happened, it was like all

the bad came flooding in, overwhelming my defenses. I did my best to talk myself out of it, by reminding myself of the cycles and how it was bound to turn around. But given the pending death sentence, it seemed like maybe I really was on the final cycle.

I won't kid you. That really hurt. And the pain still lingers from it. But I was able to control the depression. I think the main reason I was able to do this was because I could see how much it was impacting my wife.

Holly already suffers from chronic depression. It is a hereditary condition for her. And she takes medicine for it, which helps. But when you are already prone to being depressed with no real outside cause, then to be presented with a truly depressing situation, like the prospect of losing your spouse, it can be pretty bad.

So, I have been especially sensitive to how Holly has been handling my situation. And to her credit, she has done amazingly well. I think there are two reasons for this. First, I have tried to be strong and very positive throughout. But she also has been strong and positive. I think she knows she is needed and refuses to let herself get depressed to the point where she can no longer help me.

I think that has been one of the keys to avoiding a lasting depression. You must think beyond yourself and focus on others and how your depression is affecting them. Most importantly, you cannot dwell on the moment or the situation, but focus on fighting. I will talk more about this in my Coping section.

OTHER EMOTIONS

May 2017
ANGER

There is a lot to be angry about. You're mad this is happening to you. Why me? Why now? Most of your anger is directed at God or the Universe, but also at yourself because you failed to accomplish the goals you set for yourself. You're angry at everyone not suffering as much as you, just because.

With all your emotional turmoil, it becomes easier to have that anger erupt and become misdirected at the people you love, or your pets, or your clients . . . That only adds to your problems.

This is an area where I really surprised myself. I never let this anger consume me. In fact, just the opposite. Whenever I felt the anger rise up, I squashed it because I knew it was unfounded. There were a few notable exceptions, such as the time I yelled at Roger about the time I learned of my diagnosis. But fortunately, the incidents were few and far between.

My sudden control was unexpected, given that I have

always felt a deep rage within me. It's like all the times I was teased or tormented as a child lay buried beneath, ready to rise ala The Hulk, should the situation merit. Sadly, there have been times in my life where I lacked the self-control to keep this rage completely restrained, allowing it to emerge and me to lash out – too often at people who did not deserve it.

Maybe it was the prospect I was reaching the end, and thus not needing this rage anymore that has allowed it to dissipate . . . maybe not completely, but at least it's under control. Or perhaps because the cancer has given me a better perspective, causing me to realize those things that would normally trigger an angry outburst just weren't that important in the bigger scheme of things. I will talk more about perspective later.

GUILT

Why would someone who has cancer and is facing eminent death feel guilty? It's because you see how your condition is impacting the lives and emotions of others. They are suffering because of you, and because of your suffering.

This is a real feeling. It is especially strong when I see people making sacrifices on my behalf. Mostly, this involves my family. My wife's suffering is directly tied to my condition. As is her tremendous sacrifice of time. My sisters spent the money and took the time to come visit me. And my kids made several trips to see me at a cost of both time and money.

The best way to cope with this guilt is to make sure they know how grateful I am for their sacrifice. I hope they know.

As my condition changed from eminent death to getting better, my guilt evolved as well. It did not go away but changed from feeling guilty about what I'm putting others through, to *survivor's guilt*. Why am I being chosen to survive when so many others do not?

I feel this guilt every time I hear of someone dying from cancer . . . which is almost daily as I'm ever more sensitive to the subject. It is especially hard when it is someone you know. Facing the survivors is hard because you know they are thinking "why did my loved one have to die while John is still alive?" And I have no answer for that. [*December 2017 update*: This guilt really came into focus this past summer when my ex-father-in-law, who I and anyone who knew him adored, passed after battling prostate cancer.]

I know this guilt will never go away as long as I'm around. But it does help inspire me more. I realize I must make whatever time I have left count. When all things are considered, I can *live* with this guilt.

PATIENCE

I have never been known for my patience (except when I tried teaching Holly golf . . . I was surprisingly very patient then. Perhaps I knew the consequences if I wasn't.) I reserve most of my impatience for myself, when I cannot do something quickly that I feel I should . . . and idiots who drive slow in the left lane.

I am very impatient with traffic. I absolutely hate being held up by something I cannot control. I am not sure which bothers me the most. The fact I'm being held up or that I have no control. But while I may fume in my car and be quick with the horn, I have never threatened another driver or anything like that . . . although my middle finger has occasionally gotten a work-out.

I can also get impatient with people. Especially stupid people. Here I am not talking about people with low IQs. They cannot help themselves and I understand that and am patient with them. (My daughter is *extremely* patient – almost saintly, which is wonderful as she teaches special ed in one of the statistically worst high schools in the Commonwealth of Virginia.) No, I get impatient with people who should know better but for whatever reason act stupidly (like certain politicians).

This is where the cancer has really changed my perspective. I have found myself having incredible (for me) patience. I even have more patience with people driving slow in the left-hand lane! (Although I still consider them morons.)

I am especially more patient with people. I think it's because I have learned not to sweat the small stuff anymore. This is somewhat ironic in that, with precious little time left each moment takes on more meaning, so you might think I would become more impatient rather than less.

I have come to realize I don't want to waste my emotional strength on petty things and things I cannot control. Life is too precious to waste that way.

I also realize there may be reasons why people are acting the way they do besides just to annoy me. They may be suffering from an illness or dealing with an emotional tragedy. It doesn't matter. Because we are all shaped by the events of our lives. And we must do our best to understand that others do not have the same life experiences you do. So, their motivations and reactions are going to be different. And that must be respected.

Death's Door

Time to Go?

October 2016 (from Mortal Musings 1 video)
Understanding we are all going to die at some point, one may want to know, "when is it the right time to go?" Most of us would answer "as late as possible." We naturally want to live as long as we can.

I used to think the same thing. I didn't want to die. I wanted to live a long, long time – even hundreds of years. But that changed this past summer when my dad died (July 2016).

DAD

My father was always a vibrant person. And he was always healthy. Other than the stroke that nearly claimed his life in his 40s, he was the picture of health. It's hard to remember him even having a cold. And I honestly cannot remember ever seeing him sick in bed.

Dad, who was a pilot in WW2, had a phenomenal sense of direction as well. He never got lost.

But that all changed over the past ten years. Gradually he started becoming senile. He would get lost driving his car, even short distances. And then he grew more and more reckless . . . Running red lights and stop signs, etc. It got to the point where he was very dangerous – to himself and others.

My dad had lived alone since Mom died in 2001. He wanted it that way. He refused offers to live with any of his kids. He was very independent and extremely stubborn.

But finally it became painfully obvious to us three kids that he could no longer function independently. He was not only a danger on the road, he was not taking care of himself (or the house) at home. Yet he stubbornly refused any help, or even the mention he needed any. We even hired help for him, but he sent them away.

We made the extremely difficult decision to put dad into a nursing home (senior living center in today's lingo). My sisters found a wonderful facility close to both of them (at the time, they lived in North Dallas as did Dad. Holly and I lived in Waxahachie, about 45 minutes away). But we knew Dad was not going to go willingly, to put it very mildly.

The issue was then how were we going to get him to go? We could not physically force him. And he would not listen to reason. So that left tricking him.

Dad has three children and five grandchildren, but just one great grandchild – the son of Cheryl's daughter Rebecca, who also lived in the Dallas area. Dad absolutely adored Colton, who was about five at the time. Colton was taking karate lessons. So, we arranged for him to give a demonstration at the facility and then invited dad. (The staff was in on the charade.)

But it wasn't that simple. Instead this was a complex operation (think spy novel) requiring intricate timing and coordination. Because we wanted dad to feel as much at home as possible, the idea was to have his bed, his clothes and personal belongings, some chairs and artwork from the house put into his new room *before* he got there. To do this, Cheryl arranged for her to play nine-holes of golf with Dad at Brookhaven prior to taking him to the facility to see the demonstration. (She got the easy part – playing golf, having fun, while the rest of us worked our butts off!) In the meantime, the rest of us got busy taking the bed apart, packing, and taking the bed, a chair, the TV, some pictures, his clothes and personal items, etc. over to the facility and setting up his new living space. We had about two hours.

The plan worked to perfection. Dad and Cheryl arrived in time for the demonstration and Colton put on a "show" for seniors, who all loved it. (Colton was wonderful). After the demonstration, we told dad we had something to show him, and led him to his new quarters, where the facility manager and another counselor were waiting to help us with his transition.

In an understatement akin to saying a category 5 hurricane is a bit windy, Dad did not take it well . . . at all. The staff, though, shooed us away. It was difficult for us to leave and we were all in tears. Dad did not make it easy on the staff, either. He tried to escape several times that night. Sadly, he even got violent.

By the time we had decided dad needed to go into a facility, his memory was already pretty shot. He occasionally digressed into living in the past. Further, his health was deteriorating rapidly, necessitating several trips to the hospital. This from a man who never got sick. I remember during one of these visits, he called Cheryl "Maxine", his oldest sister, and me "Merle," his brother.

Dad likely did not have Alzheimer's. According to Juliette, his symptoms were more similar to Lewy Body Dementia – which is kind of like a merger of Alzheimer's with Parkinson's. Not the best combination.

There was no doubt he needed to be in a facility where he could be cared for. My sisters had discussed him living with either of them – Juliette suggesting he live with Cheryl, and Cheryl wanting him to live with Juliette. (I am kidding, they both volunteered, as did I, although our house was the least suitable and my sisters would not have him living so far away.) However, Juliette and Michael were both doctors who worked long hours, meaning dad would either be home alone or need round-the-clock at-home care. For various reasons, they both decided Dad was best off in a nursing home.

We initially had dad in the minimal care wing where the residents could come and go as they pleased and lived independent lives. But when dad got violent, we realized that was not going to work and accepted the facility's recommendation for him be placed in the Alzheimer's unit, which is locked 24 hours a day. In other words, it's a very nice (and expensive) prison.

Initially, we convinced him he needed to stay there because his house had become infested and was being treated and the facility was simply a nice extended stay type hotel. That worked. And we all came and took him out, whether it was for lunch or dinner, or for a haircut. Dad played a few more rounds of golf, but his health quickly got to the point where that was no longer possible.

Over the next several years, we watched as my father became more and more a shell of the man he once was. Both the body and the mind deteriorated before our eyes. Dad alternated between real time and living in the past. Although he always recognized the three of us kids, he occasionally forgot who our spouses were, etc. Frequently, he imagined he was back at work at Sears, or even back in the military – some seventy years previous.

While it was devastating for us kids to see him like this, dad (after the first couple of months) seemed very happy in his new home. (We later moved him to another facility, and he liked that one as well.) And the staff took great care of him. And while his memory was swiss cheese, dad retained his personality and especially his sense of humor. The staff loved him.

But I could not help but think that if the 85-year old dad (or younger) could see the 95-year old dad, he would say "I don't want to be like that. I would rather die before I lost the memories that defined me and the body that carried me").

In the last year of his life, it had become clear to all of us that Dad had lost the will to live. He wasn't suicidal, but he just did not care about staying around any longer. He simply stopped eating.

Juliette commented that when you hear about all the health foods, etc., adding years onto your life, well these are the years you're getting.

Thus, I found myself asking, "do I really want to live that long, if it means living like that? And putting my family through it?" The answer was "no."

Well, apparently God heard me and took me too literally. He's about to grant me my wish. (Be careful of what you wish for . . .") I should have known to make myself clearer and state I wanted to live as long as possible *until* I became that burden. Not that I wanted to go right away . . .

SHORT CUTS

Ask my family and they will tell you I'm famous for taking short cuts. They are referring to the way I drive, where I will go to great lengths to avoid traffic jams (I hate sitting in traffic). I do love driving, though. Always have. I find it relaxing, mainly because I'm alone with my thoughts. And I like the metaphor of the journey . . . of going from one place to another. And I enjoy the scenery and visiting new places.

But I have always loved taking short-cuts. Long before we even heard of the initials "GPS", I took "alternative routes." Usually this involved pulling over and looking at a map (the printed, fold-out kind) and choosing a logical route. But I also enjoyed occasionally taking a road just because it seemed to be going in the right direction.

It wasn't only driving where I took short-cuts. I have always been all about efficiency. If I think I can do something quicker by doing it a different way than norm, I'm going to try it. When I was in school, this often involved creative ways of doing (or not doing) homework or studying. (While I got good grades, I was not very "studious." I always found a way to do the least amount of work possible.)

But this was one short-cut I did not see coming, nor do I really want to take. I am not ready to die at age 62.

BUCKET LIST

October 2016 (from Mortal Musings 1 video)
Several years ago, there was a movie called "*The Bucket List*" starring Jack Nicholson and Morgan Freeman. It was about two seniors, one of whom had cancer, deciding it was time to complete their "bucket list" before it was too late.

Believe it not, that really was the first time I ever confronted the topic of a "bucket list" – a list of things to do before you "kick the bucket." I had never thought about creating such a list. Nor did I really create one after seeing the movie, either. That's mainly because it was not real to me. Not the bucket list, but "dying." I refused to consider the possibility I was going to meet my maker. (If I was going to "meet my maker," I wanted it to be on *my* terms, not his.) The movie came out in 2007. I was 53.

Now here it is nearly ten years later, and I am suddenly seeing that bucket dead ahead of me. Not only should I be warming up for the kick, but I should be working on filling that bucket. And yet I still find it difficult to come up with a list.

Not that there aren't things I still want to do. It's just

that I have realized most are not ever going to happen, regardless of how long I live. For example, I've always wanted to go into space . . . preferably traveling to a new world (and seeking out new civilizations, boldly going . . .). But that's not going to happen, even though for the first time it may be possible for "regular" civilians (read "not astronauts") to travel commercially into space. One problem, you will basically have to be a billionaire to afford such a flight, even if it were to happen in the timeframe I have left.

Really, there are only two things that I have on my list. Family and travel.

Family has always been extremely important to me . . . both my immediate and extended family. Perhaps some of that comes from having so few friends . . . and none of them within 500 miles of me. All my life, I have always been one who favored being close to a few people rather than trying to have a ton of friends. Growing up, I had one extremely close friend (Jeff) who was more like a brother to me than a friend. I also had several close friends – Greg (who became my best friend when Jeff moved), Andy (who was more like a frenemy – we were close friends, but we also competed against each other for the affections of Jeff and Greg), and my neighbors Bill and Jim, who were brothers but a year behind me in school. (Bill was my age and Jim a year younger).

I developed other friends in school, but they were people who did things with me at school, but rarely beyond. This pattern (and the same friends) carried on through college. Even when I joined a fraternity, I never developed any close friends among the "brothers." Instead, I recruited several of my close friends from high school into the fraternity! And many of those friends have disappeared as we took off to different points on the compass.

Now I find myself with only two really close friends –

both named Jeff. Jeff Gordon, my "brother" from growing up, who I rarely get to see but when I do it's like we were never apart; and Jeff Brauer, who I met through work, but instantly liked. But Jeff G. lives in San Jose, California and Jeff B. in Dallas and I'm in Georgia.

There are several others who I consider dear friends. Most notably Greg, who still lives in Lawrence, Kansas. But he never calls me. I still call him on his birthday. The few times I've made it back to Lawrence we get together, and I still feel the strong affection I've always had. (He called me when he learned I was sick, and we had a wonderful conversation. But he has not returned any of my follow-up calls). I also keep reaching out to Andy, but he has not reached back.

My immediate family – including my two sisters and especially my two kids -- have been terrific. As I mentioned, I am seeing them more than ever before, which is wonderful. But I also miss my extended family, which is concentrated in two places – western Kansas and England.

My dad's family is mostly in Western Kansas. I still have an Aunt and an Uncle left and dozens of cousins. The last time I saw them was about four years ago when I took Dad for his last visit there. This was the summer after we had moved him to the long-term care facility. I knew it would be Dad's last visit, and I am certain he knew it too.

Since Dad moved to Dallas in 1976, I had almost always gone with him when he went to visit Western Kansas, which he did about every other year. He liked having someone to go with him to share the driving as well as keep him company, and I loved doing it. I loved seeing my family and visiting the farms. I also love driving as I find it very relaxing. It usually was just he and I, but twice I included my son Matt, once my daughter, Elizabeth, and once Holly.

Dad had three plots of land. One in Comanche County,

where he grew up, and the other two farms in Logan County. One, I believe, was purchased by his father for Dad from the money dad sent him during the war and the other two he inherited.

Anyway, over the years I have gotten to see my Kansas family a lot. Growing up I saw them more. Not only did we make the trek on an annual basis, but I spent two summers working on my relative's farms. It was a wonderful experience, at least for me and my parents – I'm not so sure about my relatives.

Sadly, though, I have not had the same opportunities with my mother's family, who remain mostly in England (I have two cousins in Australia and one in Israel). Most of them I have not seen since my last trip there in 1976! And I do love them all and miss them terribly. So, a trip to England would certainly be on my bucket list.

My mother was born and raised in London. (She was a war bride). And her family (what's left) all still live there. And I love it there. Except I haven't been back in forty-one years. There have been three main reasons why, and they are related -- Money, time and family.

Prior to getting married in 1984, I simply did not have the money to go to England. From 1976 to 1980, I was in gradual school, in debt up to my ears. After 1980, I owned a small business (Encore Copy Corps in Lawrence, KS), and in debt over my ears.

When Ann and I got married in 1984, we still had no money. Plus, we moved to North Carolina. This presented another issue. My parents lived in Dallas and hers in the Boston area. As a result, whenever we had any time and enough money, it went to visiting them.

Even when I did have more money, time was always an issue. Plus, when the kids came along (starting in 1988), it made it even more difficult. Because this not only created a stronger financial and time crunch as the need to see the now grandparents became even more important, but I could not justify being selfish enough to go by myself. If I went, I wanted to take the family. And that required real bucks – bucks we never seemed to have. It was always just so hard to justify. And it still is. Even now, I am having to put the England trip off to next year because, you guessed it, time and money. I decided the trip to the west coast was a higher priority for me, mostly because I want to visit my son at his home. But I am determined to go next year, with Holly. God willing, I am still here and healthy enough to make the trip!

I know what you're thinking. If I loved my family and friends so much, why don't I contact them more? I never write, and, rarely call my friends (except Jeff B, and that's usually for work) and never my extended family. I don't even post often in Facebook, nor, admittedly, do I read all their Facebook posts.

I wish I could answer that. I just have always been terrible about it. Some of it may stem back to my childhood and my huge self-image problem. I simply could not take the thought of more rejection and was afraid if I reached out and they didn't respond, it would be another rejection and I just did not want to go through it. (The fear of rejection still plagues me today and is one of the main reasons I hate sales, as a career, so much.)

Because I don't want to travel without Holly, both because I love her – and given my condition – I may need her, I am tightly constrained by her availability in planning any trips. As a result, I fear we can only make one long trip (a week or more) a year. And I have decided right now, going to the west coast will be my highest priority (along with a shorter trip up the East Coast to Washington DC, with a long stop in Richmond to see my daughter.) But there is more. Not only has Holly never been to the West Coast, but there are a lot of people to see, along with incredible scenery. Most importantly is my son in Los Angeles. But Holly has close friends who live in Seattle. My sister Juliette lives in Portland as does her daughter, Sarah. My dear friend/brother Jeff lives in San Jose. My dream is to start up in Seattle then drive down the coast to LA – visiting friends and relatives and experiencing the fantastic scenery along the way. (I love taking pictures. And I do that really well – that is, I take a LOT of pictures! Thank goodness for digital photography).

And that's how I plan the two items in my bucket list – traveling and seeing friends/family. I will combine my travels with visits to the friends and family. Should I survive long enough, perhaps there will be the opportunity to see other parts of the world where I don't have friends or family . . . something I've always dreamed about doing. But for now, I am quite content to just seeing my family. I just pray I have the time and capability to do so.

Ok . . . I will admit, playing Pebble Beach and /or Augusta National and/or St. Andrews would also be on my bucket list, if I thought it realistic.

COPING

November 2017

Now that I've talked about various problems suddenly confronting me, it is important to discuss how one *copes* with these issues. Coping strategies, I believe, can be broken down into two categories: internal and external. Internal strategies are things you do alone, while external requires outside participation of one degree or another.

EXTERNAL STRATEGIES

November 2017

I discussed one of the biggest external strategies above, mainly *talking* about the issues – whether to a family member, a friend, a support group or a professional. It is important to have an outlet. Otherwise you are at risk of having these things build up inside you until there is an explosion – which is never good.

The most obvious external strategy involves *being around family and friends*. Knowing there are people who love you and care deeply about you and your situation helps give you the strength and determination to fight. And I am forever grateful for their love and support.

But friends and family can be a two-edged sword. While you soak up their love and support, you also realize how much your situation is affecting them. And that hurts. As a result, you become reluctant to share all you are going through – both the physical pain and mental and emotional anguish – because you know how badly that affects them. By sharing, you realize you are making it harder on them. On the other hand, people like to feel they are helping, which is good. So, you want to let them help. It makes them feel better and is important for *their* coping.

Thus, it becomes a delicate balance of figuring how much you can share without causing them undue misery. You want to share enough to let them know you trust them and to let them know they're helping, without sharing so much it makes them even worse off than they otherwise would be.

It becomes very important to find *other* external support rather than relying on just family and friends. This support can come from several places, such as cancer support groups, church, and professional help.

However, I am not a church goer (as I will discuss in greater detail later). And it would seem hypocritical to me if I suddenly went to church just so I could have someone I can unload my burden on.

SUPPORT GROUPS

There are lots of support groups available for people with cancer. These are wonderful and very helpful. Being with others going through the same thing as you can be immensely therapeutic. It is often very difficult to talk about what you are experiencing unless that person truly understands it – and who else knows better than someone who is also going through it.

These groups also give you a sense of belonging, kinship. This can be extremely helpful, especially since, as discussed previously, your regular social life is in disarray. You begin to wonder to what extent people are treating you differently because of your cancer. You don't have that concern with support groups. You can be honest here.

I have also not used any of them. It's obviously not that I don't believe in them or think they might not be helpful.

So why haven't I gone?

Damn good question. In all honesty, I think it's because to go to one would be an admission that I am, in fact, dying from cancer. People say I'm being brave and handling the news well. Nonsense. I am just in total denial, that's all.

I also think it's because I refuse to admit I need help. To do so would be an acknowledgement of fear, which would then be picked up by my wife and others.

I don't recommend this strategy. As a psychologist by training (I have a master's in psychology and was working on my dissertation for my PhD when I got distracted by opening a business), I fully understand the danger of what I'm doing. Repressing these feelings can lead to a dangerous release . . . as I sadly discovered on January 20th. But I'm stubborn. And I refuse to let the cancer beat me . . . either physically or emotionally.

Not to say that's all bad. I do think having a positive attitude is very important to getting better – which is what doctors also tell me. The fact the positive attitude stems from the refusal to believe I'm dying, to me, does not change the positive impact. I'll take it any way I can. (While I may deny I am dying, I am still doing everything I can to prevent that from happening. That is an important point to remember.)

I also am guilty of poor time management. When I am working, I feel guilty taking time off to do something not work related – such as going to a therapy session. I spend enough time away on things I can't miss such as my treatments. This prioritizing my time for work even applies to playing golf, which is obviously work related. But because playing is fun, I feel guilty about doing it rather than actually working.

When Holly gets home, I want to spend my time with her.

I also had an alternate release . . . I shared my feelings with the world through my videos (*Mortal Musings*). There is no doubt they were cathartic and immensely helpful to my well-being. And since my wife refused to watch them, I did not suffer any adverse consequences from posting. And now I am using this book as my new therapist. I guess that makes you my new shrink . . . so, what do you think, doc?

PROFESSIONAL HELP

Unfortunately, I have never been good at seeking outside help. I'm too stubborn to admit I need it. Emory, though, does provide both a social worker and a psychiatrist at the Winship Center, to support their cancer patients. The social worker not only helps with life adjustments the cancer dictates, but helps you get the support you need, including family and financial assistance, etc.

While I really have not needed the Social Worker (who is extremely nice), I have taken advantage of the Psychiatrist. Admittedly, it took me several months before I did so.

I took Holly in with me to see her. While I certainly had issues I needed to work through, I honestly felt Holly was having a more difficult time. I think this is probably common. After all, the problem is really short-term for me, but Holly will have to deal with the loss for (hopefully) decades. And that can be an extremely depressing thought.

The Psychiatrist was very helpful, even in that first session. Just having someone to discuss the feelings we had was cathartic for both of us. I also think it was good for us to hear each other talk about our emotions. It can be hard to do that when it just the two of you as you are so afraid of hurting the other.

Since that first time, I have probably seen Dr. Baer another four times. When Holly is accompanying me for treatment, she goes in too. And it has been helpful for both of us, which is why we so seldom go. (Right? If it works, stop doing it . . .) Both Dr. Baer and I have tried to encourage Holly to see someone in Columbus. But she is very stubborn (sound familiar?), as well as busy. So, I doubt it will ever happen.

Another excellent external strategy is to *be active*. This can be in the form of going out more, travel, entertainment, exercise, etc. Well, exercise is off the table for me, for several reasons – but mostly because I'm lazy and hate exercising.

The degree that you can get out will depend on your physical situation. But anything you can do that is "normal," even including shopping, can help you cope. It says you are not going to let the cancer "win" and change who you are. And that helps.

For me, it was work . . . when I had it. As long as I had a project to delve into, I felt I was doing something. Cancer wasn't going to defeat me. There has to be a good balance. While work can help keep your mind off the cancer, it can also take you away from what is more important – your family.

INTERNAL STRATEGIES

December 2017
While external strategies are good, I have always been one to rely on myself and my own internal strategies as my primary coping mechanism.

Examples of internal strategies include denial (a big one for me), rationalization, distraction, hope, faith and perspective.

DENIAL

Admittedly, I have used denial as one of my main coping strategies. I don't deny having cancer (I more ignore that little fact), but I do deny I am dying. I absolutely refuse to believe it. And because I use denial so much, I really have not had to rely on *hope* because, after all, if I refuse to believe I am going to deny there is no reason to *hope* that I don't.

I believe my denial ties back to my faith as well. But I will have a lot more to say about faith later in this book. Suffice it to say for now, having a strong faith has been essential in keeping me level-headed.

The trouble is, denial can also be a successful strategy to get you to the coroner. If you take the denial to the extent you deny anything is wrong, then you do not seek treatment or take the treatment seriously enough. That can get you only so far – like six feet straight down.

I practice *practical denial*. While I deny the cancer will kill me, I do not deny I have the cancer or that I need treatment. It's like an atheist who prays. He (or she) may not believe the prayers will do any good, but then again, there is nothing wrong with covering your bases.

DISTRACTION

I use distraction a lot. The main distraction being getting really lost in my work. I think this has helped me in several ways. First, it helps me ignore my physical issues. If I am concentrating on work issues, I can often block the pain – and certainly push away the mental and emotional problems I face. Second, it gives me a goal: "I need to finish this project." This, in turn, can provide motivation, energy and adrenaline needed to push through the obstacles.

Unfortunately, there have been times when work was not an answer. The first occurred starting in late November and stretching through most of January, when I simply was too weak and in so much pain, I was not able to concentrate on work. Sadly, that led to the second issue – the termination of the management contract, which I strongly believe was the result of both the diminished output I had in December, plus the owner's fear I would not be around to see the project to completion.

You might wonder why I did not reduce my fee or take a leave of absence when I got so ill. Good question. But there were several reasons. First, I charged a flat fee that was the same every month. When calculating the fee, I considered December and January being slow, but that would be more than made up by the months leading up to the grand opening, when I would be spending most of my time on site.

But more importantly, I had Paul. As I mentioned before, Paul was my partner in the management contract. And he was on-site on an almost daily basis. Thus, I felt I had it covered pretty well.

So, there were a couple of months where I really did not have a lot of work to distract me. Fortunately, that changed when I won a large consulting contract for the Northbrook Park District in Illinois, and later consulting jobs for the City of Detroit and Forest Reserve Park District in Chicago. These really helped me from June through Mid-November 2017. (Now, I'm taking time off to both recharge my batteries and to hopefully finish this book!)

Another way I distract myself is through activities. Unfortunately, not only the cancer, but issues with my back (which has gotten a lot worse) make it difficult to use physical activities as a distraction. Instead, I rely on television, reading and playing games on my phone. These help the most in dealing with short-term issues like an increase in pain or anxiety.

When I was younger, reading was my favorite escape. I was a vociferous reader from a very early age. Science Fiction was always my preferred genre. I usually went through a couple of books a week – more during the summer. To my wife's great disdain, I still have most of my books (she made me give away a couple of large tubs full when we moved), and they fill many bookshelves. I think I have more science fiction books than most used bookstores.

Sadly, I don't read many books anymore. Part of the blame goes to those damn smart phones with their highly addictive games. Another is there are a lot of good TV programs on and this is an activity that I can do with my wife. We enjoy cuddling together on the couch while watching. But another big part of it is my declining eyesight. It's just hard for me to read small print anymore. I will use reading glasses, but they tire my eyes more quickly. Getting old is hell, but it's a hell of a lot better than the alternative.

VENTING

Another strategy I have employed with great success is finding ways of expressing myself or venting as the case might be. While I have been reluctant to share my intimate feelings with my family or friends *directly*, I have found it much easier to talk into the camera (my *Mortal Musings* videos) or write in this book. I think it has been extremely therapeutic for me to find such an outlet.

Writing as an outlet is not new for me. It started in Junior High (seventh grade), when I was having such a tough time – being teased and bullied on a daily basis. I really stood out in Junior High. I had physical issues – mostly extreme buck teeth earning me the nickname of "beaver" that I hated. But I also dressed and acted differently. I was a geek long, long time before that was a "cool" thing to be. No one had backpacks back then, but I remember occasionally using a briefcase. I even remember having the enigmatic pocket protector (although I used it seldom). And I wore glasses.

It was difficult bringing my SF books to school. For one thing, as backpacks for school were some twenty years in the future, we had to carry all our books. So, there was strong motivation to not bring additional ones. Plus, my teachers strongly frowned on me reading them in class (which I did since I found most of the classes very boring). Moreover, the books only added to my geeky reputation. But that was not what caused me the most grief.

ADHD

The worst thing was I had severe ADHD. Back then, the diagnosis was different. I was a "very active" and distractible child, which usually was shortened to "bad" child. There was no syndrome and certainly no treatment other than an occasional spanking (at home) or trip to the principal's office.

ADHD stands for "Attention Deficit/Hyperactive Disorder." Sadly, I never learned about this disorder until some twenty years later, when I was in my thirties. Until then, I just accepted the idea I had "behavioral issues." For one thing, I could not sit still. My feet wagged like a pendulum and I fidgeted like a drop of water on a greased hot skillet, only it did not disappear in a puff of steam, much to my and my teacher's regret. ADHD also made it hard to filter my output. I often blurted out whatever I was thinking – with frequent unfortunate results. I also had a very bad temper, which may or may not be related.

ADHD also meant I was either highly distractible (if I was not really engaged in what I was doing, like listening to a teacher), or locked into hyper focus where I essentially blocked *everything* out except what I was doing – which was usually reading my SF book. Neither of these were good in a school environment.

Many years later, when I was thirty, I happened to marry a child psychologist. It was after we moved to North Carolina, where Ann was doing an internship at UNC and later worked there (and later still on the faculty at Duke). I can't remember the exact year, but since we moved in 1984, it was either 1984 or '85. Anyway, Ann apparently talked to some people about my situation and one of them turned her on to a book, which she got me. It was called "*Driven to Dis-*

traction." It changed my life.

Reading that book was an amazing revelation. I was in tears most of the time reading it. For that book was describing ME! Until that point, I never realized I had a known disorder. Nor did I realize so many others had the same problem. And more importantly, that it was treatable! Ann got me in to see one of her mentors, a nationally prominent neuropsychiatrist, who put me on Adderall. What a change that made in my life! (I have sense moved on to Wellbutrin). I still have ADHD, but fortunately its impact has diminished with age. But I still need those wonderful pills.

God, with his dark sense of humor, made sure I knew what a real pain I had been to my parents by blessing me with not one, but two kids with severe ADHD. Thankfully God also made meds! If only they had them for the parents.

Ironically with a disorder called "attention deficit," you have "hyper attention." This is when you get in a state where whatever you are doing (like reading, writing or even watching a TV show) will focus all your attention so you literally (yes) will not know what is going on around you. You simply block everything else out. Sadly, this can and often does include whatever my wife is saying to me at the time, which is forever getting me in trouble. (When I was younger, it was my parents and teachers, with equally bad results). I am always accused of not listening. But that is not accurate. It implies I have a choice. I don't. When I am focused on something, I really do not hear anything else. I am completely unaware Holly (or whoever) is talking to me unless they do something drastic to get my attention (Holly has found a punch on my shoulder is effective). Merely saying my name in a normal voice will not do it. I get her frustration, as I experience the same when I am trying to get through to my kids.

While this hyper attention can adversely affect my interactions with anyone, it seems more problematic with women. I think it's because the wiring is so different. I am constantly amazed whenever there is a group of women together, they all seem to talk at once. Moreover, they seem to hear and understand what everyone else is saying! I have enough problems paying attention to one speaker, let alone several. No wonder my wife has such an issue when I can't hear her.

However, hyper attention serves me well when I'm hurting. Because it not only blocks outside distractions, but it also shuts out internal ones – including hunger and pain.

Back to Junior High. As I mentioned, for various reasons, I could not bring SF books into school with me. But no one could object to my writing. For one thing, the teacher assumed I was just taking notes. And it did not require bringing any additional materials. Further, no one knew what I was doing or writing about.

Star Trek had just started on TV that year. Naturally, I was a huge fan right from the get-go. So, it became the inspiration for my own story. I wrote about my own starship and my own adventures.

I only wrote in school. I never took it home, because at home I could read. I just started filling up a big notebook. And I easily got lost in my writing.

I continued to write that book for the two years I was at Milburn. (My parents sent me to a private school for ninth and tenth grades because of how hard a time I was having, even though they really could not afford it). By the end, I had easily filled up over 500 pages of notebook paper. And since I wrote very, very small, this equates to about 1,000 pages for most people. (I still have that notebook somewhere. But I'm not sure even I can read my handwriting).

PERSPECTIVE

October 2016 (Mortal Musings IV)
For me, *perspective* has been one of the most effective coping strategies. Perspective is, in my opinion, one of the strongest tools you can have in dealing with depression or coping when bad things happen. But it is also one of the hardest to develop.

There is no doubt cancer changes your perspective on life. It certainly makes every moment count that much more. Think about the house fly. They have a life span of about twenty-eight days. Do you think for that fly, a single day may take on a lot more importance than it would for us? What about Mayflies? They have a lifespan of just twenty-four hours. For them each *hour* is a huge part of their entire life. Don't you think that changes their perspective? (What a bummer if it was raining that one day . . .)

In the same vein, when you're told you may only have a few months to live instead of the decades you were expecting, it certainly changes your perspective! Now each day, instead of being one of 10,000, it may be one of 100 or less.

This means you pay more attention to each day. It also

means little things are no longer that important. When you may be checking out in a couple of months, are you really going to let a jerk driving slow in the left lane upset you? (well maybe a little). Instead of worrying about the little things, you focus on the most important, because you want to maximize your enjoyment of them. Obviously, loved ones become even more important. But so do things that you really enjoy – like travel. You can no longer put off that big trip until next year, because there may be no "next" year.

I also use perspective as a way of coping. Because the more I appreciate my situation in relation to the universe, the less critical it becomes. Let me explain.

To a child, losing a toy may seem like the end of the world. To a teen, losing a boyfriend or girlfriend is *definitely* the worst thing that could *ever* happen. But as an adult, we realize these things are minor because we have our own life experiences to guide us.

When talking about perspective, I am not referring to just the *perceptual* perspective, but our *life* perspective. All our life experiences go into shaping our own personal perspective, including sensory, emotional, and even imagined. Also shaping it is our personal beliefs. For example, you can take two people, a far left-wing democrat and a far right-wing republican and have them listen to the same speech and they will come away with two very different descriptions of it. That's because each person's perception is influenced (filtered) not only by their own past experiences but also by their own belief systems. In other words, we hear only what we want or expect to hear.

My psychology training way back when showed me just how easily our senses can be fooled, both deliberately and inadvertently. I used to study visual illusions and we all have experienced them. Magicians know they can fool your senses, but so do politicians, advertisers and the media. If they can control the message you receive, they can influence or even control your personal perception of reality.

We also know our perspective is highly influenced by the environment in which we grew up – especially our parents, and to a lesser extent, our peers. The environment not only determines your sensory input, but also likely shapes your internal view of the world.

Sometimes we realize our senses have been tricked, or our perspective manipulated, but often we do not. So how do we know when to trust our perception of reality? My answer is you don't.

When I was in high school, I was on the debate team for a semester. In debate, they teach you to argue both sides of an issue. In competitions you never know which side you are going to have to argue, so you *must* not only know both sides, but be able to persuasively argue each of them.

I have found that strategy to be very helpful in my adult life. I always try to look at any issue from both sides. After all, both sides must have merit if there are people who strongly believe in each. I feel you cannot really learn about an issue, or most importantly, be able to solve one, without learning both sides. And not just learning the facts but understanding how they are interpreted and why.

Sometimes there are a lot more than just two sides. In other words, it is always helpful to be able to see an issue from multiple perspectives. The more perspectives you can incorporate, the closer you are likely to get to "reality."

To do this right requires divesting the natural emotional attachment you have to your own personal perspective. You must realize the validity other realities might have. While this is almost impossible to do, the more you are able to see things from another's perspective the more you appreciate the "breadth" of reality. That is to say, there can be multiple "truths" with equal validity. It just depends on how you look at it. (This is not the same as "alternative facts," however, which are a deliberate distortion of reality.)

Think of it like this. Say you had two people visit California. One went to Palm Springs and the other to San Francisco. For one, California is a hot, dry desert. To the other, it is a cool, hilly place full of vegetation. Who is right? They both are. They are just looking at two different aspects of the same thing.

Imagine you're an alien and knew nothing of humans. You're on the moon and you have a powerful telescopic camera. Don't you think your opinion on humanity may be influenced by where that camera happened to be pointing at the time? Or if they are listening in, what channel they happened to pick up? (What if the only show they had was *The Simpsons* . . .?)

If one person is looking at the back of your head and other at your face, don't you think they will have different perceptions of you? Further, might they use these perceptions to form vastly different opinions of you? Yet both perceptions are valid, they are just *incomplete*. Thus, the more perspectives you can incorporate, the better you are able to perceive the whole. (Yes, this can be applied to politics as well as just about everything in life).

For me, perspective is more than just seeing different sides of an argument or different aspects of an object. It is also important to develop a *temporal* perspective. That is, how a current situation may relate to a past one or impact the future. Indeed, I find developing a temporal perspective is one of the most useful tools in coping with day to day issues. I first learned about using temporal perspective as a coping mechanism when I was in junior high and came home crying nearly every night.

But then I realized others had it worse. And I asked myself, no matter what happened that day, would I even remember it in ten years? a year? a month? If the answer was "no," then it simply wasn't worth the tears that day.

When you combine looking at different sides with a temporal perspective you develop a *holistic* approach, which is what I try to do. It is important to not only understand different sides of an argument, but their place or importance in time – both past and future. In this way, you can make the best decision possible. Using this approach has helped me in my business career.

What is particularly hard to develop is perspective with regards to *ourselves*. We tend to get ego-centric and think whatever we are feeling is the most important thing in the world and others can't possibly understand what we are going through. Yet, what I have learned is that no matter how bad I feel, or how badly things may be going for myself, there are lots of people experiencing much worse. The same is true in the opposite direction. The latter used to be a cause of jealousy for me. I found it very difficult to understand when I saw people who I felt were so much less capable than myself achieving great success – often with the help of extremely good luck. This was especially frustrating as I seemed to get so close myself, only to have something entirely unexpected happen and have it jerked away. However, as I've gotten older, I have realized there is a bigger plan in place, so my jealousy and frustration have been tempered.

While we may intellectually know and understand there are people who are worse off, it's another thing to really *accept* it. We don't like minimalizing what we are feeling, even if that feeling is bad.

An example of using perspective as a coping strategy is the time-honored "count your blessings." Certainly, when I do this, I realize that I am a lot better off than many others going through the same thing. I've got excellent medical care, and good insurance. I'm financially stable. I have a wonderful support structure with my wife, family and friends. I've got a great home and loving pets. And I'm not experiencing the level of pain many do. And because I don't believe I'm dying; I'm not dealing with the emotional impact of an eminent death like others are.

I also have the perspective of having lived through many, many "down" times in my life. And I've survived, coming back stronger. I fully believe this will be the case this time as well.

I am also hopeful that through my videos or this book, I may help others. This, in turn, makes me feel good. In other words, it helps change my perspective, turning a tragedy into a victory.

As I have gotten older, I have also gotten to hear more "life" stories. And this has caused another "epiphany". Namely that *everyone* has led an interesting life. It's just that some are more gifted at telling their story, or have had more grand events, or impacted more people. But no matter what a person's life station may be, when you hear their story you will find if full of interesting events and often unexplainable coincidences or turns of luck that have shaped their life.

These "touches" differ with the individual. While we all have cycles, I have yet to meet anyone whose cycles have been as definitive and repetitious as my own. I conclude from this that we each have our own "life lesson" that we must learn. We all have our own individual purpose.

Self-Reflection

December 2017

I assume it is natural for one who is facing death head-on to do some self-reflecting. Having never been in this position before, I can't say for sure. It's not like I go around asking dying people what they are thinking. But it does seem like a natural thing to do. Regardless, my prognosis certainly has caused me to do a lot of self-reflecting. Perhaps as a preview for St. Peter, so I can rehearse my counter arguments.

No, I have not had my life flash before my eyes – at least not like you hear about when someone is about to die. I am not at that point, yet, either. But since my diagnosis, I certainly have had instances where I remembered vividly various events from my life. Perhaps writing this book has also been a good trigger.

But it is a lot more than simply remembering past events

or feelings. There is a judgmental aspect to these periodic reviews.

While I am not one who believes when we die, we come before St. Peter in front of the pearly gates to hear a judgement on your life that determines whether you enter heaven or take the elevator down. But I do believe there is a purpose to our life, so it is natural to reflect on that life to determine 1) what was that purpose, and 2) did I accomplish the mission given me?

I will be discussing my search for a purpose more in the coming chapters (spoiler alert: I haven't a clue!). But I can talk more about the nature of my self-review.

There appears to be two elements to this review process. The first is reviewing actual accomplishments. The second is to reflect on my individual *development*. That is, have I become a better person?

ACCOMPLISHMENTS

As to accomplishments, well I have had several critical self-reviews of my life achievements – at least once every ten years, when I have a birthday with an "0" in it. These reviews tend to be very depressing, so I try to limit them to once a decade.

When I was young, going back as far as I can remember, I had extremely lofty expectations for myself. Maybe I would become President, or, more likely, make a scientific discovery that would forever change human life for the better. One thing that was never a goal of mine was to become *rich*. I always thought such material goals was beneath me. Good thing, because I've never come close to achieving any. But I also never thought I would become *poor*. And, while I've been bankrupt four times, I have never been in a position where I did not have a roof over my head or a hot meal ready. Close, maybe, but never quite there.

While I think its likely most children have dreams of achieving greatness, to me it was more than a dream. I felt *destined*. I was not sure which direction my life would take me – whether it would be political greatness, or scientific – I was just convinced it would be something big.

Calling these "goals," though, is misleading. They were not goals. Rather, they were simply "givens." I was certain they would happen. This is an important distinction. Had they been goals, I would have been compelled to try to achieve them. That is, I would need to structure my life in such a way it would make achieving these goals easier. For example, if I really *wanted* to become President, I should have become an attorney, like most politicians. I should have run for offices in school, to get experience. I should have been active in political movements, etc. I did none of these things, because it really wasn't a *goal* of mine to achieve.

Becoming a world-class scientist, though, was more of a goal. One that I kept right up until I took a leave of absence right before beginning work on my dissertation. Actually, that's not true. That dream did not die for a few years, when I finally accepted the fact I was not going to return to graduate school.

I never had the goal of being *successful* in business (whatever that means). I always worked hard and did the best I could, but I never set a *goal* of achieving "x," which perhaps is the reason I never achieved it. In looking back, I think it was because I felt I needed to be flexible so when my *destiny* came calling, I would not be so locked up in achieving a specific goal I would not recognize it. It could also be I simply did not want to set specific goals, because I just could not handle failing to achieve them.

Still, I always thought greatness was going to find me, somehow. Yet I felt it was "cheating" if I set out to achieve it. I realize this was really a defense mechanism. If I sought to achieve greatness, then failed, it was because I was not good enough. Thus, by *not* making greatness a goal, I could protect my fragile ego.

Nonetheless, I was always depressed at my ten-year reviews. Because I never believed I had accomplished much. Certainly, I had not achieved "greatness," at least as far as the general public (or my family for that matter) is concerned. The public generally tends to equate success with financial prosperity, which I never had. So, no matter what accomplishments I may have had, I would never be considered "successful." Ironically, I have never set out to be wealthy. That has never been important to me – which is a good thing, considering. Yet, I always thought it was something I would achieve. However, I also realize I am rich compared to most in the world. I do not take that for granted. I do think I am one of the best at what I do– being a golf course consultant – but it's a small industry and few people outside it have any appreciation of what I have accomplished. And while I do feel good about what I do, I also realize I'm not exactly saving the world.

For my "terminal" review, though, I have given myself some slack. Admittedly, I am saddened by the fact I have not achieved anything monumental to mark my period in history. But I also realize material accomplishments are not the measure of man (or woman, I don't mean to be sexist here).

Indeed, when you look at the character of some of the great figures in history, you quickly realize they are usually very flawed people. And it is often these flaws that helped inspire them or enabled them to achieve greatness. Does this mean we need to strive to be flawed, character-wise, so that we can accomplish more? (Maybe that is why I felt destined for greatness, as I already had so many flaws).

If we are to believe our lives have no meaning beyond our lifespan, then I suppose the answer would be "yes." If you want to accomplish the maximum amount of material goals during your lifetime, then you usually need to be willing to hurt others, or at the very least, put your needs above the needs of others, in order to do so. At least that seems to be the message we get when we look at the character of most of our politicians and CEOs. The same is often true of our scientists as well. I don't think there is a more political environment than what you find in academics. (I was extremely disillusioned when I discovered this in graduate school. I always had very high ideals).

I, though, happen to believe there is more to life than our corporal life. I believe there is a purpose for our individual life, and that purpose is likely something we cannot understand, *nor are we meant to*. Think about it. Might knowing our life's purpose cause us to act in ways that may be detrimental to accomplishing that purpose? It's like the Heisenberg's uncertainty principle, which states the nature of an object may change just by the act of observing it.

Because I think there is a purpose to life, I realize this purpose may have nothing to do with material accomplishments. Indeed, I believe it has more to do more with *who we are* than *what we have done*. That is, the development of our character – or soul, if you prefer.

Thus, during my terminal review, I am much less critical of my material accomplishments. Instead, I am much more concerned about the development of my "soul." (Here I use the word "soul" to refer to that aspect of us that perseveres after the death of our material body. I will talk more about the nature of the soul later.)

Rather than waste a lot of mental and emotional energy wallowing over my non-accomplishments, I have reflected heavily on my character. Am I truly a good person? Have I improved over time?

Wisdom vs. Intelligence

December 2017

Most people consider me to be intelligent. But people tend to have different definitions of what makes up "intelligence." Some, I fear, confuse intelligence with learned. Certainly, it does take a degree of intelligence ("smarts") in order to learn more than others. But to me, having a warehouse full of facts and figures does not make one "intelligent." It makes them "smart." To me, I equate "smartness" with the acquisition of knowledge. But to be "intelligent" one must understand how to *apply* that knowledge.

Since studying Plato and Socrates in High School, I have always valued *wisdom* over smarts. Maybe because I realized I was never going to be the smartest man in the world. For one thing, I have a terrible memory. So, storing a bunch of facts and figures is difficult. In nerdese, I have a good processor, but an inadequate hard drive.

Those who know me would certainly agree at least part of my anatomy is very wise as well as smart (the backside).

But I strive to make the thinking part of my body wise as well. That is one of the reasons why I always try to look at an issue from all sides before committing to a given direction.

While I may *try* to do this, I also realize I often fail. In some cases, I may not try hard enough to discover different perspectives. But admittedly, there are some instances where my world view makes it very hard to understand a truly foreign concept (like pedophilia, especially when involving prepubescent children). When I realize I am being prejudicial, though, I try to step back and look for other perspectives, even if it's just to better understand how a person can do such a terrible thing.

I think wisdom comes from two places: what we learn and the ability to view things from different perspectives – especially other peoples. Learning can come from three different sources: education, observation and experience. I guess I could add a fourth, reflection, although one could argue that is just a mix of the other three.

Here I am taking a broader view of education to include not only what we learn in school or work, but what we are taught by our parents, peers and others. These are largely things we have not observed or experienced ourselves but have been relayed to us by others or by various media. Obviously, your native "intelligence" will influence how much you are able to learn and retain. To that degree, intelligence and wisdom are related. However, it is not a one-way street. What we learn can influence our wisdom, but it is our wisdom that helps us separate what is real and what is fake.

When we are young, we tend to accept everything we are told as fact, regardless of source. This is because we simply do not know any better. But as we grow older, we learn not all we are taught is true, and that some sources are much more reliable than others. And some notoriously distort the facts to suit their agenda (cough Fox News cough).

I remember when I learned teachers were not infallible (sorry, Elizabeth). As a young child, I basically worshipped teachers. This was because I was so thirsty for knowledge, and teachers were a seemingly unending source of it. This illusion was shattered for me in the 7th grade.

In 7th grade at Milburn, we had a science teacher named "Mr. Watches." He single-handily knocked teachers off the high pedestal I had placed them. (I continued to respect and admire teachers for the rest of my education – but no longer did I accept what they said as the absolute truth, nor did I ever think of them as infallible again.)

You see, I loved science. I absorbed everything I could science related. When I was in 4th grade (or around there), my grandfather on my mother's side bought me a college textbook on Astronomy (*Flammarion's Astronomy*), because I saw it in a bookstore and really, really wanted it. I absorbed (and understood) that book in a matter of weeks. I subscribed to *Scientific American* from fifth grade on reading each issue from cover to cover. (I continued to subscribe until I was around thirty when I realized I would not be returning to science.)

The science class in 7th grade was my first class dedicated to Science. As such, I was really, really looking forward to it. But I quickly became terribly disappointed as I realized I knew much more about science than our teacher!

I can still remember clearly a question from one of our tests. The question was "true or false, lightning rods prevent lightning." Naturally, I chose "false." When I got the test back, I was shocked he had marked my answer wrong. I grew very angry. I marched up to his desk, pulled out the textbook and showed him where it said specifically, "lightning rods cannot prevent lightning . . .". But it was too late. The bubble had burst forever. Ever since then, I took what a teacher taught with a grain of salt. I put more faith in the textbooks, although I later realized they, too, were not infallible. In this way, though, *experience* acted as a filter for education.

Technically, observation is a subset of experience as you experience the observation. But I make the distinction thusly. By *observation* I refer to those events or action you observe *that are not directly affecting you at the time of observation,* while *experience* refers to those events or actions that impacted you in some way at the time. Both are valuable. However, we can train ourselves to be more observant, paying greater attention to things we are not directly *experiencing.*

I try to apply wisdom in the business world. I will give you two examples. First, I quickly realized how important it is to *know what you don't know*. This can be hard for someone with a fragile ego to acknowledge the fact you don't know everything. (Especially if you're in the White House . . .). But I understood if you wanted to truly be good at something, you not only had to recognize your weaknesses, but to seek people who can fill in those gaps. And you must be willing to really *listen* to those in a position to know more about a particular subject than you. I learned this lesson well during my days with Encore and its why I bring in other experts with me when I consult.

The other thing I learned early on was that in almost all cases, the most valuable asset in a business is its employees. You may have the best idea in the world, but if you do not have a great staff to implement the idea, you are doomed to failure. But it's not just the executive staff that is important. *Every* employee contributes to a company's success – or its failure. This is especially true if that person interacts with the public. Even seemingly menial laborers, like janitors, can influence a business because if the environment is not kept clean, it can create a bad image with the public, which can be difficult to overcome.

Sadly, I have found these pearls of wisdom, which I considered "common sense," are often neglected by the people in charge. And when the business struggles, these same people will always look outward for a reason, instead of looking inward where the true problem often lies.

Whether it is in business, politics or everyday living, I have found "common sense" is really not that common. Too often we try to "cheat" common sense in order to get ahead. It rarely works.

Self-Image

Admittedly, I am not the sharpest observer in the world. I believe part of that is because of the ADHD, which tends to hyper-focus your attention to the exclusion of everything else. Thus, I observe more than most people about what I am focusing on but can be totally oblivious of everything else. (That is, I am the opposite of Sherlock Holmes).

One area where I tend to be an astute observer is in human relationships. I can observe two people interacting and, with great precision, accurately describe what they are feeling about the other. I can usually spot when someone is lying, as well. And this was true well before I took psychology and learned some of the giveaways.

But this observational skill has one extremely important blind spot. While I can accurately describe the feelings of two different people interacting, I am completely lost when one of the people is myself. It's like there is a big blindfold on when someone is interacting with me. It is virtually impossible for me to tell how that person is feeling about me when we are interacting . . . unless they verbally tell me. And then, it is very hard for me to know if they are telling the truth.

Obviously, this has been a big problem for me throughout my life and has impacted almost every aspect of it. I think it is one of the reasons why I have so few friends . . . because I cannot trust my observations of their feelings about me.

Naturally, this made dating an extremely difficult proposition for me when I was young. Further hampering me was my extremely poor self-image. I can thank those two years at Milburn for that. During those two years (7th and 8th grade), it became ingrained in me that I was very ugly (thanks largely to my buck teeth). I felt that was one of the reasons so few people had anything to do with me.

This poor self-image carried through not only the rest of my childhood but continues today. I still find it very hard to accept when people tell me I'm good looking. And I can't stand to look at myself in the mirror . . . doing so only when I must like when I brush my teeth. I comb my hair once a day, which is when I brush my teeth in the morning. I'm probably the least vain person you can imagine.

It was so bad, that when a girl showed interest in high school, I assumed it was a set-up. (Yes, this is true.) Surely if I reacted, I was going to be major league embarrassed in some way. (Thank goodness we didn't have social media back then!) Even when I went on a date, I still wasn't certain of my date's motives . . . which led to a lot of one-time dates.

Also hampering my dating life was the fact I was incredibly naïve . . . about everything. But that's a different story.

Thus, my wisdom still has a blind spot when it comes to relationships that involve me. But I'm trying. I do have considerably more confidence in myself than I ever used to.

Why the blind spot? My guess is there are two reasons. The first traces back to my ADHD. I become hyper focused on what that person is saying (which has been exacerbated by being hard of hearing) that I am unable to note the non-verbal cues of the speaker.

The second reason may be my poor self-image. If you feel yourself unworthy of attention, you may dismiss evidence to the contrary. But whatever the cause, I still have difficulty with it, although I'm better than I was.

I developed a poor self-image honestly. Part of it was having two older sisters constantly reminding me of my failings (though they will counter I was spoiled by my parents . . . just because they always gave in when I pitched a screaming fit.)

My self-image problems, though, really took off in 7th grade. In grade school, I was not the most popular kid by any means, but I wasn't the least liked either. I had several good friends. Plus, I had grown up with most of the kids, so they were used to my "peculiarities."

Two big things happened in 7th grade. The first was going to a new school several times bigger than my grade school. Mohawk was smaller than most area grade schools, with just two classes per grade. But Milburn probably had 1,000 students. As a result, I knew few if any in a given class.

The second big thing was Jeff moving. As I mentioned, he was much more like a brother to me than a friend. His leaving was a big emotional blow.

I stood out for a number of reasons in Junior High. I was a geek, number one. I had severe ADHD (though we did not know it was an actual condition back then), which caused me to behave *differently*, and I had really severe buck teeth. (My orthodontist, Dr. Radke, one of if not the busiest in Kansas City, said mine was the worst malocclusion he had ever seen.) Put these together and I was a target for every bully in the school. As noted,, I came home crying nearly every day.

My parents pulled me out of Milburn for ninth grade

and put in a private school, Pembroke Country Day School or Pem-Day, which at the time was an all-boys school. I did not appreciate the sacrifice they made at the time, because Pem-Day was expensive, and my parents could not really afford it. But it was so much better. Braces helped my appearance (believe it or not – but I had to wear them for five years, plus a retainer for another few), and I was surrounded by other bright people.

But the damage had been done. My self-image was permanently scared.

I have worked hard these past several years to improve my self-image. And I have succeeded to a degree. But I still have trouble taking compliments and I still refuse to look at myself in the mirror. And I do *not* take selfies!

TEMPER AND PATIENCE

I am infamous for my temper. I have a notoriously bad temper . . . and it has cost me dearly throughout my life. It is often associated with my inability to take criticism.

In some ways my temper is a defense mechanism rearing its ugly head when I perceive I am being attacked in some way. I must quickly add, though, that while my temper is bad, and I will yell and even, on occasion, curse, I do not get violent. But apparently, I get scary, nonetheless.

I got my temper honestly, though. My father had a very bad temper. Fortunately, he did not lose it often. But when he did, oh boy. It was a lot worse after his stroke.

If I remember correctly, it was the summer of 1967. My dad would have been forty-seven. Cheryl had graduated high school and was preparing to go to the University of Kansas (all three of us ended up going there.) It's funny. Throughout high school, Cheryl always stated KU was the *last* place she wanted to go. She wanted to get as far away as possible. But then she started dating a senior, when she was a junior. His name was Russ. Guess where Russ went to college? Guess where Cheryl suddenly wanted to go. It worked out though. They eventually got married and had two wonderful and beautiful daughters.

Anyway, we were making the trip a family outing. We were going to start by visiting the Natural History Museum on campus, which is an outstanding museum. One of its claims to fame was its collection of dinosaur bones.

This leads me to another quick side story. Cheryl was notoriously famous for fainting at the side of blood, especially her own. I remember her getting a paper cut on her thumb, then going to the bathroom to wash it off, when we suddenly heard a thump. Yep, she had fainted.

Juliette, though, was not sensitive to blood. Her Achilles heel turned out to be dinosaur bones. Yep, my sister, who went on to become an MD, fainted at the site of dinosaur bones! Well, she did once, anyway.

But back to that fateful afternoon. Dad, who had been a heavy smoker (Lucky Strikes), started complaining of pain on his left side on the drive up. When we got to the museum parking lot, dad, who was driving, could not get out.

Mom had Juliette take me to the museum. Cheryl went with them to the University Hospital, which was just a block away. The problem was that because it was a University Hospital, they could only treat students and staff. The most they could do for dad was give him an aspirin and call an ambulance.

To be honest, I can't remember if mom drove us, or if she rode in the Ambulance and Cheryl drove. All I remember is us following the ambulance to Kansas City and to KU Medical Center, where he was treated.

Dad had a bad stroke. Temporarily, he was paralyzed on his left side. Fortunately, that did not last. But he did almost die. Not directly from the stroke, though. He had an angioplasty, and during the procedure his heart stopped.

Code Blue. But they were able to revive him.

Dad recovered fully physically from the stroke, with no permanent damage. But his personality changed afterwards. He was no longer the patient father we had known, but instead developed a hair-trigger temper.

Dad did not completely give up smoking. But he did reduce his consumption dramatically. He would never smoke indoors again, nor in front of mother, as he wanted her to believe he had given it up. He switched to filter cigarettes, and mostly confined his smoking to the golf course. I think he was in his late 60s before he gave it up for good.

Weirdly, though, I don't remember losing my temper much in junior high, when I was being teased so mercilessly. Then my reaction was essentially to curl up in a ball and bawl. I was too hurt to react otherwise. (I'm sure my crying only added to the incentive of the bullies to tease me.) Besides, I believed them. I was ugly. And I was very hyper. And I did act very differently than they did. The only times I would tend to act angrily were the times I felt I was undeservingly being attacked – like someone calling me "stupid." I knew I was not stupid.

I have had some whopper temper tantrums in my day. As a child, I was famous for them with my family. My sisters accused me of using them as a means to get my way. I really can't argue as it was particularly effective. But I don't remember being smart enough to *deliberately* have a temper tantrum. I just liked getting my way and would get upset when things did not go as planned.

While I would lose my temper with some frequency – and continued to do so up through most of my adulthood – I never get violent. But I do get scary. At least that's what I am told. When I lose my temper, people tend to get very afraid of me. And it has a rather dramatic impact on them.

To be honest, I have never fully understood that. They should know I am not going to be violent, as I never am. (Well, I have on very rare occasions broken something – like smashing my fist into a wall. I think I can count those times on one bruised hand. Although my first wife might disagree.) I also hoped they realized my temper tantrums are of very short duration. And once they are over, they're over. The anger is gone and soon forgotten (by me). I do not hold grudges.

What's more, I see other people losing their temper and they do not get the reactions I get – even though I see them losing control. But for some reason, I just am very scary when I'm angry. And that cost me dearly. I lost a few girl friends over my temper tantrums, including the one that hurt the most – Jan. My first true love and the first girl I wanted to marry. I will have more to tell about this later.

I think one of the reasons I'm so scary when I lose my temper is because there is a lot of rage built up inside me. This rage comes from a lifetime of disappointments and frustrations – dealing with the teasing when I was young, and dealing with all the ups and downs as I got older, etc.

Mostly I get frustrated when I am dealing with things I can't control, like traffic. I know there is this deep fire within me. God help anyone that should cause it to fully explode.

Sadly, there were several things that would cause me to lose my temper. Things like a perceived slight, being treated unfairly, perceived attacks, my impatience, and my kids. It is the latter that I am most ashamed of. I lost my temper too many times at my children, especially Matthew. And I honestly think the reason is because I see them acting in a way that reminds me of myself when I was younger – behaviors that caused me a lot of grief – and I don't want them to go down that same path. I think seeing these behaviors would also call up some deep hurt in myself – touching on that rage. Kids, I am so very, very sorry for all those times I have gotten angry at you. You did not deserve it. (I don't believe my temper outbursts were frequent enough to be considered abusive.)

Fortunately, my kids are a lot better than me. They have grown up to be wonderful, wonderful adults despite my temper outbursts. But then again, they always knew how much I loved them. And they learned quickly my bark was a lot worse than my bite – ride out the outburst and things would be ok. Sadly, though, I managed to pass my temper on to them, well at least to my son. But he seems to handle it much better than I did.

One thing I have noticed with my temper is the little voice inside my head tends to egg me on. When I find myself starting to get mad about something, that voice chirps in and adds all the other aggrievances I have with that person and why they deserve my wrath. Unfortunately, I never had another voice arguing against it.

As I've gotten older, I've become more sensitive to this voice and have realized what it is doing. Sometimes I've been able to short-circuit the fuse. But medicine has also helped.

When I moved to Dallas, my new doctor put me on Wellbutrin, instead of Adderall, for my ADHD. To my great pleasure, it has been a miracle drug as to helping me not only with the ADHD, but also in controlling my temper. I rarely lose it anymore. I would love to say it's because I have gotten older and wiser, but when I went off the Wellbutrin last summer thinking it might be a cause for my problems, the temper returned. Unfortunately, that was also when I was managing Southern Hills and it contributed to my losing my temper at Roger on a couple of occasions.

I am not sure what Wellbutrin does that helps so much. Maybe it slows things down just enough that my "thinking" brain can overrule that voice that's telling me to yell. I don't know. I am just grateful it helps.

I should make a distinction between losing my temper and simply getting angry. To me, losing my temper means losing some control (though not getting violent), but making it difficult to get calmed down or listen to reason. When I just get angry, I can still be reasoned with, not so with a temper outburst. When I lose my temper, I will yell, and I can really yell. When I get mad, I may raise my voice (although I am often accused of "yelling," but those people have no idea what yelling is!). When I lose my temper, I often curse. I rarely curse otherwise, except maybe at a ref on TV or that moron in the left lane.

Related to my temper is my complete lack of patience. I've always lacked patience, most especially with myself. I will get upset at myself if I can't do something right the first time. And even angrier if I fail again. The more I fail, the angrier I get.

I tend to think and move at high-speed. Anything that impedes that speed upsets me. Things like stupid drivers, especially those driving slow in the left lane! Grrrr. I've gotten better, but slow traffic is one of the few things anymore that still sets me off. My time is precious to me (more now) and I hate things that steal it away.

I used to have little patience for people saying or doing things I considered stupid, when they should have known better. That did not serve me well in school. Nor has it served me well in business.

When I was in High School, my biggest fear about being drafted was not going to Vietnam, but that I did not think I could take orders from someone who I did not believe knew what they were doing . . . and that thought scared me. The military "frowns" on people who question authority. Fortunately, I drew a high draft number and then the draft was cancelled, so I never had to face that fear.

I have acquired a lot more patience with people as I've gotten older. Indeed, I am now often praised for my patience and have become a good teacher as a result. I think I have realized I have a lot of faults myself and I cannot look down on others simply because they have them too.

I still get upset at my sports teams (Jayhawks, Chiefs, Royals – yep even though I permanently moved from the KC area in 1984, I still am very loyal to the City and its sports teams. I have continuously subscribed to the KC Star and Lawrence Daily Journal since leaving. It used to be the print editions, but now, thankfully, its digital) – or the refs that are treating them unkindly. I do try to control my outbursts when I'm with others, but a high-volume profanity will still escape from time-to-time. I don't like that, (and my wife especially hates it), but then again, I do think I need some point of release – especially with what I've been through. And if yelling at a flat screen accomplishes that without hurting anyone, then so be it. Besides, those refs deserve it.

I do believe AC (after cancer), I have become much more patient – with people, events, and yes, even traffic. A lot of it has to do with a changed perspective. There is so much to appreciate in life that you can't let little things get in your way of enjoying them. Focus on the bigger picture.

John S. Wait

ETHICS AND IDEALISM

I have always been idealistic, both in terms of human behavior in general and my own, in particular. I have always thought of myself as a "good" person in that I never seek to do another human harm. I have always tried to abide by the Golden Rule – treating others as I want to be treated -- and to be a forgiving soul, never holding a grudge. I may lose my temper at someone, but the next day, the incident is forgotten (at least by me . . .). And I am a loving person.

I have always been a "good" person. I honestly cannot remember ever *deliberately* trying to hurt someone (except for one notable, and very brief, fist fight with my good friend Andy in 7th grade). And, except for the Speed Limit (which I view as merely a strong suggestion), I am perhaps obnoxiously law-abiding ("Mr. goody-two-shoes"). I even abstained from sex until I was a Junior in College because I was told it was wrong (foolishly, I believed it until I realized the hypocrisy of most of those who were saying it.) Of course, I did not have that many opportunities before then . . .

When I was younger, *parents* loved me . . . especially the

parents of the girls I dated. Sadly, though, I began to realize this worked against me and most girls did not *like* "good" boys. Much to my dismay, girls I was interested in always seemed to go for the ones who treated them like dirt. Even realizing that, I could not make myself do it. I would always treat my date with the utmost respect and kindness – which is not necessarily what they were wanting, I would discover. It made things very confusing for me!

I was the guy who was always friends with a lot of girls. And they all treated me as a good friend and confidant. But never as a romantic partner. It was very frustrating.

Perhaps this shines light on another flaw I have. And that is a "hero" complex. No, I don't go looking for an opportunity to through myself in front of a bullet. But I have always been a sucker for a person in need. But not in need of something physical or material, but one who needs "fixing," as in they are going through a traumatic time in their life. Such a situation led to the end of my first marriage, but I'm getting ahead of myself.

I also discovered being "good" did not make one popular. While I was wise enough to know I should not be critical of others, or heaven forbid, be a tattletale, the fact I abstained from most anything considered illegal (like drugs) did not win me any friends. Having strength-of-character was not a trait relished in Junior or High School. I do remember going to one high school party where I had a few drinks – but that was about the extent of my "bad boy" days. (Well, during the summer before I turned 18, my good friend Kim (male) and I would drive to Lawrence to play this baseball game at a local bar. We would usually have a beer to two during the games – they never checked ids back then -- and 18 was the legal age for 3.2 beer. He was 18, but I wasn't yet. And I never drank enough to get drunk).

I never even considered taking drugs. Although that philosophy was shaped strongly by my fear of "losing control." I hated the thought of anything that might imperil my ability to think clearly. This is still true today. While I will have an occasional beer, it is very rare that you will see me having more than two. I can probably count on my fingers the number of times that I was drunk enough to fail a breathalyzer test. And only twice do I remember drinking enough to pass out (both before I was twenty-five). It is also why I will try to avoid prescription drugs that affect my mental acuity, unless the pain is such that it is already impaired. Even then, I do so only as a last result.

BACHELOR PARTIES

One of those few times I got really drunk was a notable bachelor party – but not my own. It was for a high school friend during my Freshman year in college, if I remember correctly. That party was also my first experience with prostitutes. No, I didn't indulge, not then, not ever. Paying for sex is just not my style. But before that party, I had never knowingly *met* a prostitute. And I haven't met that many since, at least, not that I know of. I am still very naïve sometimes.

That was my first bachelor party. I haven't been to many since. And even though I've been married twice, I have never had a bachelor party of my own. At least one I was able to attend. When I was getting married the first time, my soon-to-be brothers-in-law organized a bachelor party for me. Because we were getting married in Massachusetts [I was from Kansas], I did not have any friends at the wedding . . . except one. And he is the reason I missed my party. Jeff was flying in from Los Angeles to be my best man. He happened to be coming in the night of the bachelor party. His flight was due in the early afternoon, giving me plenty of time to pick him up and make it to the dinner and party. My in-laws-to-be lived in Beverly Farms, on the North Shore of the Boston area. With traffic (and there's always traffic), it took about an hour to get to the airport. Keep in mind, this was 1984 – back in the dark days. We did not have the internet, where you can instantly track a flight, or cell phones, whereby someone can call you to tell you they are coming in late. Suffice it to say, I arrived at the airport only to discover Jeff's flight was delayed. At first it was just an hour. But then that hour expired, and it was another hour. This went on for about six hours. His plane finally made it in around midnight. But I'm told the bachelor party went great! I should've been there!

Nor did I get I get to have one for my second marriage. Of course, I was a lot older (54), so a bachelor party did not have the appeal it used to. But that wasn't the reason I didn't get my party (I still wanted one!).

The year was 2008. Holly and I were planning on having a nice wedding, probably around Thanksgiving, where my family and close friends could attend. She even had a nice spot picked and was busy planning the entire event, when fate threw us a wrinkle.

Earlier that Spring, before we were engaged, I had a revelation. I can't remember what event it was that inspired me (perhaps a sappy commercial), but I suddenly realized I really wanted to move to Dallas, to be close to my family. I had not been near them since my parents moved from Kansas City (I was in Lawrence at the time) to Dallas in 1979. My sisters had moved away earlier – Cheryl moving first to Michigan, then Kentucky, then Houston, before making her way back to Dallas after her divorce. Juliette had moved to Connecticut (to do her residency at Yale), then Virginia, before moving to Dallas. So now my father (my mother passed in 2001) and both my sisters were there. My father was 88 and I felt I needed to spend more time with him while I could. I also felt it was important for my kids. Both lived in North Carolina with their mom. So, they rarely got to see their Dallas family, unless I had them fly there for Christmas and I joined them. But this way, they could see their Grandfather and the rest of the crew while also visiting me.

I remember Holly and I were sitting on the beach near Jacksonville (Little Talbot Island), when I brought up my thoughts. I was shocked when she agreed. She had spent a few months in Texas way back when (Laredo) and loved it. And because she had to take care of her mother when she was ill, she really appreciated the need to be close to my father. (Both her parents were deceased. Her father died when Holly was 10. But her mother had died just a few years previous, while living with Holly where Holly could take care of her.)

We decided to take a trip to Dallas later that spring. The idea was to get a notion of housing, as well as to look at potential work opportunities for Holly. Fortunately, I could do what I did (golf course consulting) from anywhere, as long as there was a major airport nearby. Indeed, I thought it would be great for my career because I had done so many projects in the Dallas area. Plus, my good friend, Jeff Brauer, who is a golf course architect, lived there and it would give us a better opportunity to work together.

We drove. I had a golf project north of Houston I wanted to check out. It had accommodations and we got a free night stay from it. By driving, we had more flexibility and it was cheaper. Ironically, by coming in from the south, we drove by Corsicana on the way to my parents. We had no idea it would figure prominently in our future.

It was also during that drive the sheer size of Texas became more meaningful to me. I always knew Texas was big.

But this was the first time it really sunk in. That's because when we got to the Texas border on I-10, there was a sign showing the distances to various cities as you expect to see on the Interstate. Only on this one they included El Paso, which was on the far side of Texas. I can't remember the exact mileage, but I want to say it said 870 miles or so. But I do remember seeing that sign and looking down at the trip meter on my dashboard that I set when we left and saw the odometer read over 20 miles less. We started our trip from Jacksonville, on the Atlantic coast. While we were inland some, it was less than 20 miles. That meant the distance from the Atlantic Ocean to the state border of Texas was roughly equal to the distance from one side of Texas to the other! I would later check a map and realize the same was true going west. It is about as far from the western edge of Texas to the Pacific Ocean as going across the state! That's big.

Holly enjoyed the trip. It was also the first time she had met my family, and they loved her. They were ecstatic with the idea that we might move there. (I deeply regret my mother never got a chance to meet Holly as the two of them would have gotten along famously.)

Encouraged, Holly began applying for positions in the Dallas area. Unfortunately, there are not a lot of opportunities for museum directors, so the choices were few. However, in late June, she got a "hit." It was the Pearce Museum on the campus of Navarro College in Corsicana, about 45 minutes south of downtown Dallas.

Holly was invited to interview in mid-July. We flew there, not knowing what to expect. I had never been to Corsicana (although I had driven past it on I-45). And, because my family all lived in North Dallas, I was not very familiar at all with the areas south of downtown. So, it was a new experience for both of us. Holly was one of four interviewees.

We arrived about an hour before the interview in order to take an unofficial tour of the museum. Boy was that a revelation! I'm not sure what we were expecting, but it sure wasn't what we found.

Corsicana is a town of about 35,000 people. It is in Navarro County, an otherwise very rural area. It is the first county south of the official Dallas-Ft. Worth metropolitan area. Driving through town, we were struck by the fact it appeared to be stuck in the 1950's. This impression would never quite go away, as we later discovered the parochial nature of the people – but I'm getting ahead of myself.

The town hosts Navarro College, which is a two-year school. At the time, though, it was the fastest-growing two-year college in America, with four campuses. It also was the reigning National Juco Football champion. (Ok, another sidebar . . . everything you've heard about high school football in Texas is likely an understatement! Corsicana had one very nice football stadium – it was the high school's. Navarro College also played their games there. Now remember, they were the *National* champions. But when they played, the stadium was sparsely filled – maybe 1/5th of its capacity at best. But when the high school played – and they were middle-of-the-pack in their league – it was filled.

When 'you drive around Texas and see these huge stadiums, you wonder what college plays there. The answer is usually, "none." They're high school stadiums. While we were living there, Allen, a northern suburb of Dallas, spent $60,000,000 on a *high school stadium* with 18,000 seats. Not to be outdone a few years later, Katy, a Houston suburb, built a stadium costing $70,000,000. These are by far the most expensive high-school stadiums in the country. Heck, when I was in high school – Shawnee Mission North, in Johnson County, Kansas – we won the state championship three years in a row. Our stadium was more or less glorified bleachers, and we had a student body of over 2,000.

In addition to Navarro College, Corsicana is famous for the Collin Street Bakery, one of the top fruitcake manufacturers in the country. Unfortunately, I hate fruit cakes, except as building blocks. However, my dad loved them. This made it a lot easier getting him presents as he was otherwise notoriously hard to shop for.

Another thing we discovered that day, it was almost impossible to find a diet coke. I am admittedly addicted to diet coke. Although I've now cut way down to one or two a day, back then that was about *all* I would drink – from first thing in the morning until I went to bed. Naturally, when we got into town, I had to have a diet coke. But everywhere we went, no one sold diet cokes (fountain drinks). They didn't even have Diet Pepsi (a very poor substitute). Instead, they had Diet Rite Cola. Now, I have rarely ever seen Diet Rite as a fountain drink, but here was a town where there was nothing else! (I later discovered the reason -- Corsicana is about an hour from Waco, home to Dr. Pepper. And Corsicana was very loyal to Dr. Pepper. Well the distributor for Dr. Pepper insisted their customers serve Diet Rite, which they carried. If you wanted Dr. Pepper, you had to have Diet Rite.)

The Pearce Museum was named after James Pearce, heir to the Colgate fortune, who donated most of the collection. The museum was housed in the Cook Center, which was also home to the largest planetarium in the state (at that time). (We later discovered the Planetarium was in poor shape – like a lot of things on campus, but that's another story.) Outside the Cook Center were two notable displays. One was a real jet fighter mounted on a pedestal and aimed at the sky. Another was a stature of an Indian Chief. What a marvelous contrast!

But when we got to the museum, everything changed. The Pearce Museum, at the time, had two main galleries – a Western Art gallery and a Civil War gallery. Both were amazing! The Western Art museum has one of the best collections of western art in the country, in a wonderful gallery. The Civil War museum featured the largest collection of Civil war documents west of Mississippi, with over 15,000 documents (mostly letters). The gallery displayed a number of these, including ones from Lincoln and Jefferson, along with some nice artifacts and some really great interactive displays. Both of us were struck with how out-of-place this museum seemed to be. It felt like it should be in Fort Worth, which has a great collection of museums, or Dallas. Certainly not in Corsicana! Now Holly was very excited. She had never worked in an art museum, but history museums were her forte and the Civil War was her passion.

Holly thought the interview went very well. One of the interviewers was Mr. Pearce himself. He was in his 90s, and wheelchair bound. But still sharp as a cookie. Apparently, he went to the museum every day, spending time with the staff. Holly liked him but was leery of having him come to the museum every day! Not only would he take up a lot of valuable staff time, but he would try to impose his will on everything. Nonetheless, it still looked like a great opportunity.

One of the things about the Pearce Museum that really appealed to Holly was they did their best to present an unbiased perspective of the war, despite being in the South. Both the Union and Confederate stories were equally presented. This is also true of her current museum, the National Civil War Naval Museum in Columbus, Georgia. But it was definitely not true of another civil war museum we later visited. That's the Texas Civil War Museum in Fort Worth. When you visit there, you come away not only thinking the South won the war, but that the reason they won it was Texas!

Two weeks later, in early August, we got the news. Holly did *not* get the job! It went to another person who Holly had met at the end of her interview and was unimpressed. (It later become apparent the University and especially the head of the Cook Center, still held some '50s values – including very sexist views.) Disappointed, Holly and I went on with our wedding plans, which were to get married in November, probably over the Thanksgiving weekend so the kids could easily attend. Dallas would have to wait another day.

That day turned out to be two weeks later. The person they hired lasted an entire day before quitting. Holly was next in line. One problem. They wanted her there in *two* and a half weeks.

Back in the spring when Holly agreed to move to Texas with me, she had one condition. We had to be married first. I was a little surprised by that as we were already living together. But I was happy to agree. We were going to be married, anyway. Might as well do it before we move!

But now that promise came with an unanticipated consequence. Suddenly, we only had two weeks to not only plan a major move, pack, put my house on the market (Holly's was already on the market), but, oh yeah, plan a hurried wedding. But that was not all. In order to sell my house, it needed to be fixed up, meaning repainting the entire interior. We could not afford to hire a painter, so the job was left to yours truly.

But wait, there's more. Of the two weeks we had, I spent one of them traveling for a consulting job. This meant that most of the move and the bulk of the packing was left in Holly's hands . . . a fact about which she was not happy, nor has she ceased to remind me about it. It was about as crazy a two-week period as you can imagine.

Nor could Holly take any time off. She felt guilty leaving the museum with such short notice. She did her best to minimize the impact.

Oh yeah, one more thing. We had to find a place to live! That was going to be fun. We flew to Dallas I think two days after Holly learned she got the job. Neither of us were particularly excited about living in Corsicana, though. But there weren't a lot of other choices. The next closest town going towards Dallas was Ennis, twenty minutes north of Corsicana. Naturally, I wanted to be closer to Dallas, both for my family as well as the airport.

During the trip, we went by the Pearce Museum. Holly wanted to meet the staff and get a more thorough look at the museum. Holly also visited Mr. Pearce for what turned out to be the last time. Holly did come away impressed with the staff she was inheriting.

We did not want to live in an apartment. For one thing, finding an apartment that would take five cats was an impossible task. Ideally, we would like to buy a house. But we could not do that until we sold our two houses, which was not going to happen in two weeks' time. So, the next best thing was to find a house we could rent prior to purchasing. That certainly limited the market!

We only had two days to find a house, negotiate and sign. Talk about pressure! But we got lucky. We found a great house in Ennis (30 minutes north of the museum) that was vacant. and the owner was willing to rent it to us for six months, at which time we would purchase the home – assuming our two houses had sold by then. (Turned out to be a bad assumption. Remember what happened in 2008? Remember where it started? Yep, the housing market crashed, and Florida was the epicenter. We eventually were able to sell Holly's house (six months later), but never could sell my house or the house I had purchased as a rental – but that's another story and I have digressed enough, don't you think?)

Ok, back to the side story of the side story of my bachelor party, which was another side story from by self-reflections . . . (I guess I do get a bit distracted from time to time. Ahh the joys of ADHD.)

Holly did not want to get married in a courthouse. She wanted a true service, and she wanted her friends and family to be able to attend. Unfortunately, though, because of the short time constraint, and because school was in session, it meant neither of my kids could attend. Nor could my extended family, or friends. I ended up having my one employee, who had become a friend, Steve, serve as my best man. He was the only one on my side of the aisle. Holly's right-hand person at the museum, Turin, was a minister and administrated the service. We got married at her Lutheran Church in St. Augustine. It was a small, but wonderful wedding. But alas, no bachelor party!

The craziness did not end with the wedding. We left the church and headed down I-95 to Miami. Not because that was where we wanted to spend our honeymoon, but because that was where the Florida State Association of Museums was having their annual convention, and Holly was an officer in the association and had lots to do at the convention. I was at least able to upgrade her room to the honeymoon suite!

We returned from Miami in time to supervise the loading of our furniture onto the moving truck. Then we loaded up our two cars with clothes and cats and took off for Dallas. We had five cats we were taking with us. Holly took the three sisters and I had Cleo and Easter. Cleo, our oldest (five at the time) loved to ride in cars, so she did not have to be in a carrier. But the other four did.

It took us two days to get to Dallas. Notably, this happened at the same time Ike was hitting the Texas coast. Fortunately, I had booked our hotel in Hattiesburg, Mississippi several days prior or we would have had trouble finding a hotel. As it was, the hotel was filled with both people fleeing the hurricane and others (lineman) heading *into* the storm area. After checking in, I told Holly, "grab a cat and let's go" as we headed to our room.

The next night we stayed at my dad's before driving to Ennis the following day to meet the movers. I had to supervise the move-in because Holly had to go straight to work. But she did not have to worry about Mr. Pearce. He died the day after our wedding.

CHARITY

One of my personal paradoxes is that while I try to be a good person, I am not very generous in giving to charity. Nor do I go out of my way to volunteer for anything.

I always rationalize that money is always tight. But that's just an excuse. I know others who have far less who are far more generous.

Rarely do I give to people begging on street corners either. Again, I rationalize that I don't want to support their supposed alcohol problem, even though I have no evidence they have one. There but for the grace of God . . .

The same is true for volunteering. Again, I rationalize I just don't have the time to spare. But I know if it really meant something, I could find the time.

I have been a lot more generous since the cancer. But I still don't volunteer my time, except at the museum. Now if someone directly asks me for something, I will always help. I just do not go out of way to find opportunities.

I offer no excuses. I can and should do better.

ETHICS

Back to ethics. I know there have been times in my life when I have not lived up to my own high standards. But, fortunately, they have been few and far between. And that's not always easy in the business world.

In sales, I never thought about how much I would make on a transaction. I rarely looked at the commission split (it varies in real estate). I did not want my personal motivations to potentially cause me to try to steer a customer to buying a house that would pay me more. I honestly can say I *always* put the needs of my customers first.

The same is true in my consulting career. I *always* do what I think is best for the client, even if that means I will make less money.

I am sure I would have been a lot more financially successful if I had a different viewpoint. If I did not pay my employees as much, or if I took advantage of customers, or talked bad about my competition, etc. But it just does not seem *right* to me. So, I won't do it. I think my parents raised me right.

OTHER

MASTER PERSUADER

I learned early on that I can be extremely persuasive. I can talk people into almost anything.

Part of this is because of my ability to change perspectives. It allows me to better understand the different sides of an argument, which makes me more effective in arguing a particular side. This skill was helpful in my short-lived debating career. But it also helped tremendously in both sales and consulting.

I am also very logical. (I was often called "Spock" in school, mostly because of my somewhat resemblance and the fact that I was a huge fan, but I also prided myself in my ability to use logical reasoning.) In sales, this can be handy as I can present logical reasons for buying.

But I think there is a lot more to it. Perhaps most important is that I can be extremely passionate. And when someone is passionate about something, they are much more persuasive. After all, if that person is so convinced about whatever it is, there must be a reason. And I am only passionate about what I believe in, and that shows.

I also think people naturally trust me. They always have as far as I can remember. I have always been a good confidant. Part of this is because I can be a good listener and part because they know I won't tell anyone. They know this because I never gossip. Ever.

I also rarely, rarely lie. I won't say never, because that would, in fact, be a lie. But I am pretty damn honest. Part of this is because I have strong ethics and morals that were passed down to me from my parents. And part is because I am usually a terrible liar. I hate lying, so it's hard for me to do it. Unless there is a really, really, good reason for doing it (like a white lie). In that case, I can be very convincing. (Because I am known to be honest, it has allowed me to pull a few good pranks in my life.)

Because I am so persuasive, I am good at sales. Not only am I persuasive, but I was also a student of sales techniques when I was younger. I absorbed Tom Hopkins and other sales trainers. I got so good, I even started to write my own sales book. I was fascinated because, to me, it was a matter of applied psychology.

My sales ability served me well after I sold my second business, IBS Mail Marketing. After discovering that Fortune 500 companies were NOT looking for bright entrepreneurs to situate in their corner offices, I had to do something to earn a living. I got both an insurance and a real estate license. But I was concerned the real estate market would tank (it did, this was 1991), so I chose selling insurance.

I started off selling health insurance, mostly to small businesses. Health insurance is something easy to believe in, so I was pretty darn effective and quickly rose up through the ranks. But then the company folded (another national company folding under me), and I joined John Hancock selling, among other things, life insurance.

Ok, I believe in life insurance. And I would do all the calculations to determine the proper amount of insurance, and that was what I would sell them. But then I began to realize that the definition of "proper amount of insurance" was being supplied by the insurance company. Was this really the amount they needed?

That's when I started to have problems with selling. I realized I could sell people *anything* but was I doing the *right* thing? It was right for me, but was it right for them? This was not an easy thing to answer.

This became a moral dilemma I could never quite solve. I not only was extremely persuasive in my own right, but I also knew all the techniques that were designed to get a person to say "yes." In other words, I could *manipulate* a person into buying whatever I'm selling. This caused me a lot of consternation in that even if I felt that what I was selling was good for them, I had a problem if the reason they bought it was because I manipulated them to do so. And I did not want to do that anymore.

As a result, I grew to hate sales. And I still do. I have had to do it, like when after declaring bankruptcy due to the Florida real estate crisis and the sudden downturn in golf led to a precipitous drop in consulting opportunities forced me to start selling residential real estate. The compromise I made with myself was that I would try as hard as possible *not* to be a salesman or a persuader. Instead, I would learn as best as possible what my client wanted and needed, then I would try and find it, and present it as objectively as possible, without ever considering the commission or any consequence to me. I would lose sales as a result, and not be as effective, but I could live with it. Yet, I still hated doing it – and still do. I just don't trust myself.

Of course, I still must sell myself when it comes to my main career as a golf course consultant. But I view this a bit differently. Mainly because I honestly feel I am the best choice for almost every job I go after (ok, make that *every* . . . I was just trying to be modest.) And I am naturally passionate about what I do, which comes through during the interview.

TAKING CRITICISM

One of my biggest faults (as Holly will tell you, the list is long) is that I do not take criticism well. I carry a massive brick on my shoulder and am extremely sensitive to criticism. This is especially true when I think I am being treated unfairly. In other words, if I perceived I was being attacked, not only would my defenses immediately flare up, but my impulse was to immediately attack back. With both Pat* and especially with Ann, these incidents became flash points. When I was being blamed unfairly, or unduly criticized, I would react with anger and more often than not, a fight would ensue.

It has also hampered me in both school and work. While I realize I'm not perfect and I will ask for help – especially in proofing a document that I've written, I will get upset with all the red marks I receive. My first instinct is to say they are being too critical, even though I realize they are *probably* right.

I have been determined to not let this happen with Holly. I have learned to ignore her when she makes harsh and sometimes hurtful statements. I am not going to rise to take the bait. I am finally learning these small battles are not worthwhile. Let them slide, you won't remember it the next day. But if I respond, it can escalate into a major row we both regret.

It may be the cancer, or may be just the result of getting older, but I find myself a lot less sensitive to criticism than I have ever been . . . Or maybe it's because I simply don't do things worth criticizing about anymore? Nope, my wife assures me that is not the case.

[Update August 2019 – I made the decision about six

months ago to become a full-time writer. Part of this was motivated by the downturn in the golf consulting world. But it is also fulfilling a life-long dream. I bring this up because as a novice writer (commercially), I suddenly found myself receiving lots of criticism. People picking apart my writing, noting all the seemingly endless amounts of mistakes I made. Here is what really surprised me. Not once did I get angry or upset, except perhaps at myself for being so careless. Needless to say, this was in contrast to most of my pre-writing life.

I believe the reason is twofold. First, the cancer has caused me to mature – in many ways. And one of them is the ability to withstand criticism and knowing the difference between someone trying to be helpful vs. someone just being mean. Second, I really, really want to be successful as a writer. Given that I am starting a new career at 65, I realize there is a lot I don't know. And I don't have the time to spend decades learning by trial and error. I look at each critique as a lesson and I am a sponge absorbing them. I am even non-plussed by all the hundreds (literally) of rejection slips I get from agents. It hurts, but it also tells me I have more to learn. It's a challenge, not an attack.]

SELF-CENTERED

As a child, I was both very self-centered and selfish. I know, what a revelation. Most children are. But I continued this as an adult. The problem was that I was not self-aware that I was being self-centered!

I always believed I was a thoughtful person. I certainly cared a lot about other people. And would do anything for someone – if they asked, or it was very, very obvious. But I was terrible at *anticipating* what someone may need, and then going out of my way to help. The truth is I found it very hard to look beyond my own needs and concerns.

In some ways, my "thoughtfulness" would follow the curves of my life's events. When things were going well for me, I was happy and a lot more thoughtful and generous. But when things were going poorly, as they often were, I found it hard to look beyond the dark cloud enshrouding my life.

It should be said that I am *extremely* good at *rationalizing* my actions. That voice in my head tends to be very self-centered, but intelligent enough to find a reasonable path that always ends up favorable to myself. And that voice assures me I am not doing others any harm in the process. I would never and have never deliberately hurt someone for my own gain. But that does *not* mean that I haven't unintentionally hurt others due to my actions that largely benefited me. It's just that in my clouded state I was not really aware of how my actions would impact others and my little voice assured me it considered those consequences.

I will give you a great example. One my wife frequently reminds me about. It goes back to when we decided to move to Texas. One of the big motivators for me, other than the desire to be closer to my family – especially my father, was the need to get away from my ex-fiancé – Pat*. Pat was still very much a part of my life and would come over frequently for one reason or another. Naturally, this did not go over very well with Holly, who had been living with me since Valentine's Day of '07. I knew if I wanted to preserve my relationship with Holly, which I very much did, I needed to get away from Pat.

But there was a significant problem. I had let Pat continue to use the car she had been driving when we lived together. But that car was in my name and I was still paying for it. It was obvious, even to me, that I could not continue to let her use a car that was in my name and under my insurance and that I was still paying for, especially if I was in another state!

Yet, even after what Pat had done to me (more on this later), I still cared for her, and especially her daughter Brianna*. I had no desire to hurt either. I also knew she could not afford to buy the car from me . . . or likely any car, because she had no money or credit.

So, it occurred to my little voice Holly had a much older car that was fully paid for. We could give Pat Holly's car and then Holly could drive Pat's car that was really mine. Remember how I could be persuasive? I managed to talk Holly not only to the exchange, but to also pay me for the difference in value of the cars so we could pay off what I owed on it and put it in her name. And it accomplished exactly what I wanted and needed to happen. One thing. I never stopped to think how it would affect Holly – or her emotional attachment to *her* car and her emotional hatred for anything associated with Pat.

There are many similar examples throughout my life. Probably many, many more that I don't even have a clue about. This is because I never realized I was hurting someone and unless they made me aware of it after the fact, I remain blissfully unaware I did anything wrong.

It is amazing, really, how much of a blind spot I have when it comes to viewing myself and my actions. Strangely, you would think facing death and suffering from cancer would make me even more selfish and self-centered. But I think it has had the opposite effect. Maybe because my situation has had such an obvious impact on others, it has forced me to realize just how much I have impacted them in other ways.

Like a lot of people, I have tried to minimize what I am going through when others ask. I try not to show my suffering out of a desire to not have others worry. Yes, I'm sure part of it is because I want to be "brave," but there is also a genuine concern for the feelings of others. As I have mentioned before, I honestly feel guilty about all the attention I have received. The very process of thinking of others in this situation may have made it easier for me to understand my impact in other ways as well.

Or maybe I simply want to improve my slate for the final judgement, even though I don't believe in such a thing. All I know is that I'm doing my best to be much more considerate of others and trying harder to view things that include me from their perspective. Well, no matter what the reason, at least I am making a strong effort in the right direction.

MORE FAULTS

I would like to think that one of my biggest problems is my modesty. But I can't find anyone that agrees with me.

I am sure I have only begun to scratch the surface of all my faults. But thinking about them just gets me more depressed. If you really want to know, just ask my wife. Or my ex-wife. Or my kids. Or my sisters. Any of them would be glad to give you a list. Just be prepared, because I'm sure the list is long.

Trust and Relation- ships

Business Partnerships

December 2017
I am an incurable optimist, which admittedly has been seriously challenged in the past year, both with my health and with the political situation in this country. Yet I remain optimistic. It's just my nature.

However, related to the incurable optimism is a trait that has proven to be both a positive and a negative. It is that I am a very trusting person. I tend to trust someone until absolutely proven I can't. Even then, I have trouble not trusting them.

I did learn early on, though, that I cannot put unearned trust in people I don't know. I am very alert about scams and cons. But when it involves people I know, well my blind faith in them has unfortunately hurt me badly several times.

Let me give you a few examples. There are two times when I took a friend on as a business partner. Both turned out badly for me. Encore and Golf Management.

Maybe because I had so few friends, I trusted them unconditionally. Or maybe it is because I have trouble reading people who are interacting with me. But either way it cost me. The first time was with one of my best friends, Greg, who partnered with me on my first business venture, Encore. I wound up doing most of the work before the business opened – including writing the business plan. Greg did help bring in some money, although I raised most of it. Then a few months after we opened, Greg left the business completely. This meant it was entirely up to me to run the business and made returning to graduate school impossible. But I never got upset at him. I knew he had to devote his time to his own thesis. But it still hurt. And it made my work that much harder.

In setting up the business, I signed for everything. That meant when the business went south, it took me with it. Greg, who never put any of his money into it (neither of us did, we were gradual students in debt over our ears), lost nothing. He did have a friend invest, who lost his investment, which I felt badly about. But my family invested a lot more. Plus, I would later get a loan from my Uncle's bank (that I also personally guaranteed). I also worked the last year and half without taking a penny in salary.

When the business folded (a story I will detail later), I

had to declare personal bankruptcy. But shortly after the bankruptcy was finalized, I got a big surprise in the mail. Xerox sent me a check for several thousand dollars! Apparently, we had built up equity in the equipment. But we had owed Xerox many times what they sent back, so I thought they would surely come and ask for it.

I told Greg about the check. He wanted me to distribute the check equally to all the stockholders. But I was convinced Xerox would come calling, so I held on to it. (I guess my ethics wasn't strong enough to return the check!) I would later use the money to pay back my uncle's bank as well as reimburse myself for all the legal fees I had to front for myself and the company.

Though Greg never confronted me about it, apparently, he resented my doing this and felt that I should have given the money to the stockholders. But the stockholder's loss was limited to their investment. I lost everything. And Greg lost nothing. So, I did not really feel that guilty about it. I really did not think Greg felt that strongly, either, as he never confronted me. But apparently, he held a grudge as he told our mutual friend Andy about it. And while Greg and I have met several times since and have had great times together, Andy refuses to talk to me. Even today, thirty odd years later.

More recently, my friend and business partner, Paul, let me down regarding our management contract, as I mentioned previously. An outside observer would likely conclude Paul was deliberately sabotaging me with the owner. He even sent an email to the owner supporting the contention I was a bit unbalanced, where he described an incident where I got a mad at a waiter when he kept interrupting me when I was having a serious conversation with Paul at Chilis. (I still have no idea why he sent that). Paul also told Howard my projections were unrealistic, even though I had sent them to

Paul previously asking him for his input, which he never gave. He did this again when I submitted the business plan at the end of February, which the owner rejected – in part because of Paul's input

What could be Paul's motivation? Well, after I was removed, Paul took over the management contract. Further, he has promised to pay me a referral fee for both the contract to do the renovations (a multi-million-dollar contract) that I worked hard to get for him, and later for the management contract. But to date, I haven't seen a dime from either. (Paul says he never was paid extra to manage the facility, which may well be true).

Nor was this the first time Paul has let me down. When I first got into the business, I won two management contracts. In both cases, I partnered with Paul's company. Although at that time, Paul had a partner, Barney, who was my main contact and who was their "operations" guy. In both cases, I lasted six months until the owner (with input from Barney) decided I was not effective and fired me but retained Signal. I never got a severance or any future reimbursement. I blamed Barney for both of those instances, even though obviously Paul was involved as his partner.

Further, I have brought Paul in as a consultant on several projects, including another one that led to him getting the contract for renovation. So, you would think that Paul would reciprocate? Well, I can think of only one time where Paul came to me with a suggestion that we partner on a project. We did not get the job.

Sounds bad, right? Yet, I still have a very hard time believing that Paul deliberately was trying to screw me. Instead, I chose to believe that Paul was being very loyal to Howard (the owner). They both knew I was very sick, and I think Paul believed I would not be able to complete the contract. He was also concerned that I was still charging the full fee, even though in December and January I was clearly not putting in the hours. (I kept trying to explain that I had factored in a slow December and January when I was calculating the flat fee.) And I still hold out hope for the payment, given that the project is still not complete. Hopefully, Paul will pay me when he gets paid the final amount. [Update: He didn't]

Thus, just a few months after Paul's impersonation of Brutus, I was bringing him onboard on my next project. My wife doesn't understand and thinks I'm crazy. I probably am. But I would much rather think a guilty man is innocent, than to believe an innocent man guilty. I will always give my friends the benefit of the doubt. Besides, he is damn good at what he does, and I want the best for my clients. [Update: I have much more on this relationship in the Epilogue, and its not good].

Misplaced Trust

I talked above how I misplaced trust in my business relationships and in a personal one with Pat. However, the worst example of misplaced trust nearly got me killed – and still might. And that was trusting my doctor, Dr. Freud. Having multiple doctors in my family (my sister and brother-in-law), perhaps I am more trusting of doctors than I should be. And he had been recommended. Further, he had a nice bedside manner. So, it never occurred to me to not trust him.

My sister, Juliette, though did warn me about in-house CT scans, noting that doctors who had their own CT scanners often used outdated equipment. So, I asked when I went in. The tech admitted it was an older machine but added that its guts had been replaced last year, so it was functionally new. (That turned out to not be true. The radiologists I consulted later said the image was of poor quality.) Now I know and now you do too. Don't trust doctor-office CTs or MRIs! Especially if they give you negative results. And always get a copy of the scan so you can have someone else review it if you are not comfortable with the reading.

First Marriage

December 2017

Trust must go both ways. And I have always tried to live up to the trust others give me. I'm sure this is one of the reasons behind what success I've had with my consulting practice. I've been doing this now for over twenty years, and I honestly cannot think of a single dissatisfied customer (except Howard, but I think that is due to extenuating circumstances). This is because when someone is trusting me with their multi-million-dollar project, I take it very seriously. They are always going to get my best effort, and I think they know that. And when I'm through and deliver my dissertation-length reports, they know it is thorough. Whether or not they agree with my conclusions, they know that I did my homework in reaching them.

Yet, I have not always held up that trust. I failed in the biggest trust relationship there is – my first marriage. I violated that sacred trust and it is something I will always regret and will forever be sorry for.

Ann and I met at my first business, Encore, when she and I struck up a casual conversation as she was using the self-copier. We hit it off instantly.

In some ways, Ann and I were opposite. We came from different backgrounds – not as different as my parents, but still different. She was raised in the Boston area. Both her parents were dedicated public servants – her father a fire captain and her mother a nurse. Her mother was of French-

Canadian decent and her father pure Italian. Ann's family were devout Catholics and were ecstatic when she went to Notre Dame for college. She had to look up Kansas on a map to see where it was located when she was accepted at KU for graduate school.

Yet Ann and I were similar in many ways too. And it was our similarities, not our differences that would create the difficulties.

We moved in together about a year after we started dating. Given her conservative background, we did not share this information with her family. And since they were halfway across the country, it was pretty easy to keep our living arrangements secret.

THE WEDDING

We got engaged in 1983. At the time, I had just started working for Scriptomatic, which kept me on the road most of the time. Naturally, Ann wanted us to get married back in Beverly Farms, where she was from, and in the church she had gone to all her life. One problem, she hated the priest, who was famous for his fifteen-minute masses (the normally last an hour). I had been going with her to services in Lawrence at the KU Catholic Center and we both loved the priest there, Father John. So, we decided to ask him to perform the service, which he was happy to do. But that did not endear her to the local priest, whose church we were using.

Because the service was half-way across the country, my constituency was small. Only my immediate family and my best man, Jeff Gordon and his wife and infant son. Given Ann has a large family and was very popular, we were outnumbered by about 200 to 8.

Perhaps the strangest thing, though, was that at the time of the wedding, we were no longer living together. In fact, we were separated by about 1,500 miles. A few months prior, I had been promoted to National Marketing Manager and moved to Philadelphia. Since Ann had to finish her doctorate, she remained in Lawrence. Worse, she had to do her internship, which was going to be in North Carolina. So, we knew we would be living apart for the first fifteen months of marriage.

At least Scriptomatic was generous in giving me the time off for our Honeymoon, which was in Puerto Vallarta. We had a wonderful time.

KIDS COMETH

Ann and I got along well, until the kids arrived. Then things started going south. But not at first.

Matt came along in 1988. By this time, I had my second business, IBS Mail Marketing in Cary, NC. Elizabeth came three years later.

The problems arose when the kids got to school age. You know the mother's curse – where they hope you have kids that were just like you? Well we both were victims.

Our kids got a lot of our good traits, as they were both very smart. But they also inherited our worst traits. The both had very bad ADHD (thanks to me) and horrible anxiety (thanks to Ann). As a result, they were difficult to manage, especially when they got into a school environment.

Ann and I are both Leos. And we both share the traits most often associated with Leos. Two, in particular, were bound to create a conflict – and they did. We both like to lead, and we were both very, very stubborn.

Our main disagreements occurred when discussing how to handle the kids. Ironically, Ann, the child psychologist, did not adhere to many of the modern principles. It wasn't that she did not believe in them, it's just when your kids are doing something bad, you tend to act instinctively – trying to get the behavior to stop immediately. But that is often not the best strategy.

Things got a lot worse when my business went south, and we started really struggling financially. That added an incredible amount of stress, which understandably, Ann abhorred. It also exhausted whatever emotional reserves either of us had. It did not take much to light the fuse.

Our marriage was in trouble. We both knew it. We were fighting almost every night, often in front of the kids. And these were not polite squabbles, but loud screaming matches.

We tried counseling. But that ended as soon as the therapist hinted part of the problem might be Ann's. She was very happy when she could blame me for all the problems but was not willing to share in the blame. (And, yes, I certainly bare my share of the blame.)

I knew this was a terrible situation for the kids. Children should not be raised in an environment where the parents were openly hostile to each other. (Although we were both united in our love for the kids). Especially since most of those fights were about them.

Yet, I just could not accept that our marriage was likely over. Instead, I think in the back of my head I thought that if I had someone else that could provide emotional (and yes sexual) fulfillment, perhaps that would give me the strength to cope with my wife. So, when the opportunity presented itself, I was ready to accept. Yes, this was an extremely selfish act that I was rationalizing as being healthy for my marriage.

I can never forgive myself for the hurt and harm it did to my family and especially to my children. I am so sorry. I was so weak.

PAT

I would pay for my violation of the sacred trust.

I met Pat online. One of the reasons I was attracted to her was her story. She had a very tough life, including being abused as a child by her adopted father and being kidnapped and used as a sex slave when she was in high school. She lived near Greenville, about two hours away.

The more we chatted, the more intrigued I became. I thought she had a great story to tell and I fancied myself a writer, so I volunteered to help her write a book. We arranged to meet for lunch. I made the hour and half drive, questioning my sanity and motivations with each mile.

When I first saw her, I became concerned I had been badly duped. It appeared she was a he. First, there was the name. "Pat" could be short for "Patrick" or "Patricia." Second, she was tall. Third, she was wearing a uniform that, shall we put it mildly, was not flattering. Fourth, there wasn't much to see that was flattering (i.e., no big bumps). Fifth, she had no make-up on. Sixth, while she had long hair, it was not brushed and was mostly under a cap. And lastly, she had a very husky voice.

I was still not fully convinced even after we sat down for lunch at Pizza Hut. But I did become very intrigued as our conversation wore on. She invited me back to see her small apartment, and I accepted. As they say, one thing led to another, which led to my discovering she was definitely a she.

Pat had a four-year-old daughter who was living with her in her one-bedroom apartment. I was honestly appalled at how she was raising her, like allowing her to stay up all hours of the night and also to watch R-rated films, full of both violence and sex. She also frequently left her alone. While that should have sent me running and screaming away, it had the opposite effect.

This is because I seem to have a hero complex. I want to be the shining knight in armor that rides into to rescue the damsel in distress.

I have always been a good and sympathetic listener. Perhaps this is why people have always seemed to bare their souls to me. They know I will listen, and they know they can trust me. But too often, I cannot resist the temptation to try and help. Because I lacked the wisdom to know that what they really needed was the sympathetic ear and not someone to try and solve their problems. It was much, much later in life that I learned the difference, although I still struggle with resisting the urge to interfere.

Pat had a thing about abusive boyfriends. And I mean the kind that did physical harm. The breaking point for me was when she started seeing one of her exes who I knew had been very abusive to her in the past.

All my protective instincts combined with my hero complex and I knew I had to intercede. And the only way I could do that effectively was to become much more active in her life. My need to be needed was extremely strong with both Pat and her daughter. Ann did not need me (at least she did not seem to). And while my kids did, they still had their mother, and I would always be a part of their life. Pat and her daughter had no one else.

I thought it was love. But in hindsight, I really believe it was more the fulfilling nature of that relationship as opposed to the constant conflict seen in my marriage. I left my wife and moved in with Pat. Actually, I had her move to Durham. This was both to get her out of a dangerous environment and so I could remain very close to my kids.

I honestly think one of the reasons why I was so willing to have an affair was I knew deep down that my marriage was not going to last. I also knew I didn't want to be alone. That really scared me.

Leaving my kids was the toughest thing I have ever done. I almost didn't go through with it, but I did.

We stayed in Durham a year, living less than a mile from my kids. On school nights, I went over there virtually every night to help them with their homework.

However, neither of the ladies was particularly happy with this situation, to say the least. After about a year, I knew I had to do something drastic. I also knew to preserve my relationship with Pat, I needed to get away from Ann.

Since I had done a lot of subcontracting with the National Golf Foundation, I called Richard to see if by any miracle they needed another consultant on staff. To my surprise, they did. They had just landed the largest consulting contract ever for them, a massive study for the state of West Virginia that would entail visiting every golf course in the state. They hired me and put me in charge of the study. So, Pat and I were headed to south Florida. NGF was headquartered in Jupiter. We found a house to rent in Hobe Sound, which was close to Jupiter. [These are two more examples of misplaced trust – both Pat and NGF ended up letting me down.]

The study took eight months to complete. I did all the research and almost all the writing. Naturally I went overboard. But the results were good. The purchasing director told us that it was not just the best golf study they had ever had; it was the best review of any industry he had seen. That certainly made me proud.

NGF promptly rewarded me by laying me off. They were downsizing and laying off a lot of people, about 20% of their workforce. Since I was the last one hired, I was among the first to go.

Pat and I stayed in South Florida for another six months, then moved to Jacksonville. We chose Jacksonville because we loved the town and Pat had a very close friend who lived there (her husband was in the Navy). Plus, it was a lot closer to the kids.

We were happy, I thought. In fact, Pat and I later got engaged. But then the roof fell in and it was me who was the victim of greatly misplaced trust.

With my father's help (he guaranteed the loan) we purchased a house in Jacksonville. It was new construction in a nice middle-class neighborhood, near Orange Park. Not long after we moved in, Pat befriended a neighborhood boy, who was about 13. He was a foster child of a neighbor at the end of the block. He told her about how they were mistreating him, so she took him under her wing and gave him a person to talk to.

About six months later, Jonathan* was kicked out of his foster home. Pat convinced me (it wasn't hard, I have a very soft heart) for us to become foster parents. We did (it took about a month as we had to take classes, etc.) and were able to get Jonathan as our foster child. He moved in. A few months later, we also were able to get his sister – who happened to be the same age as Pat's daughter. Both kids had been abused – physically and sexually – by their biological family.

About the time Pat and I got engaged, we adopted the two children. Well, Pat did. This was the first indicator to me that something was terribly wrong. Because when I returned home from a long trip, I was told by the three of them that they wanted Pat alone to adopt them. I was very hurt but went along with it. I loved them very much and figured that when Pat and I got married, I would end up adopting them anyway.

Tracy*, Jonathan's sister, and I always got along great. But Jonathan and I had a more difficult time. One of the issues I had was that I did not like how Jonathan interacted with Pat. He was not treating her like a mother, but more like a girlfriend. I saw it in how he looked at her, sat near her, and even putting his arm around her when we all went bowling. (Bowling became a family activity. We all joined leagues, with the kids bowling together and Pat and I bowling together.) When I brought up the issue with Pat, she completely dismissed it. I even mentioned it to the bowling coach of the kids' team, and he thought I was imagining it.

Jonathan had been living with us now for two years. He was fifteen, about to turn sixteen. And he started dating, which I thought was great. But Pat never liked any of his girlfriends. By this time, Pat had become a substitute teacher. One of her longer-term assignments happened to be teaching Jonathan's class. He was in a special education class for kids with emotional disorders.

Then came that fateful night when my world came

crashing down. We were in a hotel in Orlando. We were there because the three kids were participating in the state bowling tournament. Our team, as well as a lot of other kids from Jacksonville were staying at the motel.

After checking in, the kids decided to go swimming. Pat and I took a walk. We wound up by the pool, looking to supervise the kids. There we found Jonathan in the pool with his arm around one of the girls he had dated, and who Pat didn't like.

What happened next was a complete shock. Pat erupted. She started screaming at the girl, cussing her out and calling her a whore, among other things. In short, she was acting not like a mother, but like a *very* jealous teenager.

Jonathan disappeared. It was late at night before we were able to find him. We were extremely worried, as was the coach. When we finally got the kids settled, Jonathan insisted on talking to me, alone.

That's when he told me everything. You see, Pat and he had been sleeping together – from the very beginning. They would do it when I was out of town. He was thirteen the first time.

Suddenly, everything became clear. I realized he was telling the truth.

As you can imagine, the rest of that trip was an emotional haze for me. Pat denied it, saying Jonathan lied to get even. He also wanted to hurt me. Made sense. Only deep down, I knew he told me the truth. But I just did not want to accept it. I was a mess emotionally.

When we returned to Jacksonville, I decided to call Jonathan's social worker, who had been giving him therapy. I turned to her because I honestly didn't know what to do. I was hoping she could help me sort things out. Well, what I didn't realize is that she was compelled to call social services.

They came out that night. I was still an emotional wreck and now deeply conflicted. I knew if I told them what I thought, they would have no choice but to take the kids – all three of them. But I loved them, and I did not want to lose them. That would be punishing me as much as Pat as well as hurting the kids. At the same time, I couldn't lie. So, I simply refused to talk to them. Meanwhile, Jonathan, who knew what the consequences would be if he told the truth, told them he had lied to me. Pat backed him up and they left.

Complicating things was that my kids were coming that week to spend a couple of weeks with us! I felt I had to hold it together for their sake. And I was still in limbo. I so wanted to believe Pat. The concept of a 35-year old women (at the time) sleeping with a 13-year-old boy was just such so disparate from my own vanilla world, I had an extremely tough time accepting it as a possible reality.

Over the next several weeks, I learned from my neighbor Jonathan had basically told them the same thing he told me. They had dismissed it at the time as a boy exaggerating in order to make him seem bigger, etc. But now they realized it was true as well.

I also did a lot of reflecting on Pat's and my relationship, and all the stories she told me about her life. Certainly, she would fit the profile of a child abuser – having come from that environment, as had her victim. I also realized Pat would often act very differently from time to time. I knew she had psychological issues when we started dating. But I deceived myself into thinking that I had helped her recover from them. Certainly, most of her behaviors were conforming to what most people would consider normal and her parenting skills had markedly improved.

It was during one of these reflections I had a minor epiphany. What suddenly made sense was that Pat suffered from dissociated personality disorder – i.e. she had split personalities. And one of them was a teenage girl. It was this personality who was responding to Jonathan in a romantic way. It was even possible the adult Pat was not aware of this.

I confronted Pat with this theory. After talking it over for a long time, Pat finally admitted that it was likely true.

After the kids left, I finally got up the nerve to break up with her. (Her teenaged self immediately wanted to get even, and she called my daughter to tell her about it). One problem. She now had three children. Yet the house was mine. I was not about to give it up, but I couldn't in good conscious kick them out immediately, either. So, I agreed to let them stay until I could help Pat find another place to live (yep, I helped her.) This took nearly six weeks.

Sometime during all this, Pat ran into another one of her former students, Burt*. Burt was a couple of years older than Jonathan but had befriended him in school. They were in the same behavioral class Pat taught.

Burt had just suffered a devastating tragedy. One that is hard to comprehend.

Burt was nineteen when I met him. A year earlier, he had gotten a girl pregnant. But they loved each other and decided to keep the baby and were going to get married. Like Burt, she had come from a broken home. They found a cheap place where the three of them (including the baby) would live. And they planned their wedding.

One night, Burt was talking to her while she was driving home with their baby. He then heard her scream, followed by a loud bang.

A drunk driver had run a stop sign and slammed into them. Both his girlfriend and baby died, and Burt had been talking to them when it happened.

Naturally, this caused Burt, who was already emotionally unstable due to his abusive upbringing, to fall into a deep depression. This, in turn, caused him to lose his job and his truck. He had moved back in with his mother, who was abusive, and they fought all the time. It was a horrible situation.

When Pat ran into him, she brought Burt home and introduced us. Naturally, Jonathan was excited to see him. I liked him as well and felt incredibly sorry for him.

Pat would take him under her wing, spending a lot of time with him. When the situation at his home got to the boiling point (police were involved), Pat asked if he could stay with us for the short term. By this time Pat and I had officially broken up (although I never got the ring back). But I could not turn him away, either. So, he moved in. But he was not alone. He brought with him his very pregnant cat.

I love cats. I love dogs as well. In fact, I love most animals. And I am about as soft-hearted as they come.

When Pat and I first got together, we had a single cat, Cloe, who was Pat's cat that she had for nearly ten years or so. We got a second cat, Cleo, after we had been living in Hobe Sound for year. We got her from the humane society.

But things started to get out of hand when we moved to Jacksonville. It seemed like every stray cat found its way to our home and of course, we took them in. Once a women Pat met at the veterinarian gave her one. Later, when I bought a house to turn into a rental, we discovered the previous owners had abandoned a couple of kittens. Naturally, we took those in as well.

My daughter, Elizabeth didn't help. Pat would take her to a flea market and three different times, they would return with a furry creature. The first two times it was a kitten that someone was giving away. But then Pat surprised me with a puppy. Not just any dog, mind you, but a pure-bread Siberian Huskie, whose mother had been in some movie.

At the time, we did not have a fenced yard. We decided to try an invisible fence. This is basically a buried electrical cable. The dog wears a device around his collar that gives them an electrical shock if they get too close to this fence.

Well, apparently Siberian Huskies are notorious for ignoring invisible fences, as we soon discovered the hard way. This prompted me to build a wooden fence around our back yard, which I did with my neighbor's help.

We had Alliah for about a year when Pat convinced me raising Siberian Huskies could be very profitable. So, we bought a male purebred Siberian puppy, Damon. This was just a few months before the fateful bowling tournament.

Thus, when Burt moved in, we had eight cats, two dogs, three kids and two adults. Shortly after he moved in, Jonathan's cat had six kittens. Now we had fifteen cats, two dogs, three kids and three adults. In a three-bedroom house. Crazy. The kittens, though, would play a big role in my next relationship. But that's another chapter.

We were finally able to find a house for Pat to rent. It was not far from my house – about five miles. Pat took the kids, four of the cats and both dogs. (I knew I couldn't keep the dogs because I traveled too much). Burt also went with them. However, he left his cat and her six kittens. I just inherited seven more cats! Oh yeah, she also took our newest car, and a lot of the furniture. It was the car she had been driving, but it was also only in my name. I didn't argue about anything.

I can't remember why I had to go over to Pat's house that day. But it was something relatively important, like a paper she had to sign or something. It was mid-morning. Pat greeted me and we went into the kitchen to deal with the papers. But where I was sitting, I could look straight down the hall to her bedroom. That's when I saw a naked Burt in the bedroom, heading towards the bathroom. Yep, Pat was now sleeping with the 19-year old former friend of her adopted son and apparently former lover.

Seeing Burt that day was a bit of relief. For that removed any remaining doubt I had regarding Pat and Jonathan. The whole thing still sickens me.

HOLLY

As so often has happened in my life, my darkest days yield quickly to much brighter ones. After breaking up with Pat, I wanted to get right back on the saddle rather than wallow in self-pity. I started using Yahoo Personals (that was a thing back then), and found Holly, who would become the love of my life.

We communicated back and forth for nearly six weeks before our first date – first by email and then later by phone. But I did not want to go out until my house "guests" left.

Finally, the big date came – August 17th, 2007. We were to meet at the Carrabba's in Orange Park, about ten minutes from my house, but nearly thirty from hers. But she agreed! We picked a place close to my house because Holly was interested in the kittens I inherited. And while they were still weaning (they were born on the first of July, in Jonathan's bottom drawer, which, as was often the case, he had left open), she wanted to see them with the idea of adopting one when it was time.

Naturally, I was twenty minutes late. I did have a good excuse, though. I had an important business call come in just before I was to leave. (We still had land lines back then.) When the call ended, I immediate called Holly to apologize and tell her I was on my way. Fortunately for my sake, she decided to wait.

Holly, who was forty-six at the time, had never been married. She had been in a long-term relationship (seventeen years), but that had been several years previous.

Her mother had cancer. Holly moved back home (Waycross Georgia) to take care of her, fortunate that the local museum had an opening for a director. When her mother got worse, they moved to Jacksonville, where Holly became the first Executive Director of the Beaches Museum in Jacksonville Beach. This was a great opportunity as Holly became deeply involved in the planning and building of the museum. Meanwhile, her mother was in Hospice care, but living with Holly. She was given only a few months to live, but that turned into several years.

She had no interest in dating while she was taking care of her mother – or for a period after she passed. Finally, her good friend and coworker insisted she get back out there. She had been going out for about a year, without meeting anyone she really cared for. I imagine her expectations were equally low for me.

To my very pleasant surprise, we immediately hit it off. If there is such a thing as love at first sight, this was it. Throughout dinner, she entertained me with stories of her nephew's wedding she had just attended in Georgia. Her description of the Georgia wedding had me in stitches.

I could not believe just how comfortable I felt with her. I even commented after we finished dinner, that it was as though we had known each other for years. Or perhaps in a previous life. She agreed and told me she had the same feeling.

After we were married, Holly confessed to me that when she saw me walking across the parking lot at Carrabba's to meet her for the first time, a feeling came to her that "this was going to be the man I am going to marry." What makes that thought more interesting is that Holly was not looking to find someone to marry. She was quite happy living alone, as she had done all her adult life.

For my part, throughout dinner I could not help thinking just how wonderful she was and how lucky I was to be there with her. I never dated the real popular girls. I think I felt myself unworthy and was convinced they would not go out with me, so I never really put myself out there. But here I was with the most charming woman, who, no doubt, was very popular. (And it's true, to know Holly is to love her. And she has perhaps the most infectious and unique laugh that she employs all the time. That's how I will find her in a large store or mall. I just need to wait for that laugh, which I know will be coming soon. And it does. She is always meeting and befriending strangers and finding something to laugh about.)

After dinner, we went back to my place to introduce her to my kittens. As soon as she came in the door, one of them, Hiccup, who was the runt of the litter, immediately came up to her while she was standing at the door. Hickie then proceeded to rub against her leg, before laying on her foot and instantly falling asleep. Holly was in love. Not with me, but with Hickie. But more on this later.

Holly was my first date after a long-term relationship that ended under about as bad a circumstance as possible. I knew I was extremely vulnerable to a "rebound" relationship. And I did not want that. I wanted to make sure that my next relationship was genuine, and my love was true.

Much to Holly's dismay (and she continues to remind

me how awful it was for me to do this), I insisted on going out with others, while we dated. Yet there was no competition. After a few months, I completely lost any interest in dating others. There was no need. I knew my love for Holly was real.

PETS

June 2017

While I'm on the topic of Holly, I want to share a quick story. Animals have figured prominently in our relationship. Currently, we have eight cats and two dogs. Except for Cleo, who was purchased at an animal shelter, the rest were rescue animals where we were not looking for an additional pet.

WAXAHACHIE

As I mentioned previously, when we first moved to Texas, we rented a house in Ennis. We were hoping to buy it but were not able to due to the fact we had not sold our houses we had in Jacksonville. We had six months to sell our house and buy theirs according to our contract. When we couldn't do it, they sold the house from under us.

We looked at homes in Corsicana and Ennis, but could not find any we liked, or were able to rent first, then buy. Finally, we found a house we really liked in Waxahachie, another twenty miles up the road. We loved the house and we loved the town, but it meant a forty-five-minute commute for

Holly each way. It was a sacrifice I was willing to make. Fortunately, so was Holly. We rented it for six months. During this time, we were able to sell Holly's house in Jacksonville and then were able to purchase the one we were living in Waxahachie. (I had to declare Chapter 10 bankruptcy to get rid of the two houses I had in Jacksonville). We lived in that house for five years, before the commute just got too much for Holly. And we found a house we loved in Corsicana . . . but I'm getting ahead of myself.

PUMPKIN

Pumpkin, our now fat tabby, was found by a nurse who worked for my sister. She heard this kitten's meowing across a busy six-lane street in Dallas. Two problems. It was Thanksgiving (hence her name) and she was allergic to cats. Holly and I to the rescue. Pumpkin still has a very loud meow. ("The meowth of the south," we call her.)

LUCKY

Lucky, our big black male cat, was found when Holly and I happened to be walking through a house under construction in the Dallas area. It was on a Sunday and it was over 100 degrees out. We heard this meowing, which I was able to trace to the attic. Given the heat in that attic, that cat would not likely have survived the day, hence his name. We took him door to door in the neighborhood, but no one claimed him. So, we did.

PEANUT

One day, after we had been living in Waxahachie for about a year, I went into the garage and saw a black and grey mop head lying on the floor. Only we didn't own a black and grey mop. As I bent down to explore further, the mop head moved. Once I climbed down off the ceiling, I discovered the mop head was really a small dog with long, matted hair. The dog appeared emaciated and could hardly move.

I brought it some water and food. But it was terrified and hid under the cabinet. But eventually, it would come out. Because the dog moved so slowly and looked so bad, I assumed it was very old.

I was able to finally lure the dog out, who was scared, but friendly. I picked the dog up and carried her to the back yard, which was fenced. I then went to the store and bought a small bag of dog food, a collar and a leash. I went home and brought the dog in to introduce it to our cats. They did what cats do and ignored it and the dog just curled up and went to sleep.

When Holly got home, she instantly fell in love with the dog, who she promptly named "Peanut." But we knew we couldn't keep it. Not with all our cats. So, we put the leash on the dog and tried to take him for a walk, with the idea of trying to find out who's it was. We had identified it as a him, because when we picked him up there was a matted tough of hair that we assumed was surrounding its penis.

When we got outside and put Peanut down, the dog took a few steps, then stopped and would not go. We tugged and pulled, and he went a few steps, then refused to go any further. We ended up picking it up and carrying it around.

When no one claimed him, he became ours. Holly then trimmed his long-matted hair, and a puppy emerged. He wasn't this old dog, but rather a very young and obviously neglected one. That would not be our only surprise. We took him to the vet the next day to get him checked out and discovered he was a she. We also learned she was a shiatzu.

Prior to Peanut finding us, neither Holly nor I wanted a dog. I traveled a lot, so having a dog was impractical for me. Besides, we had a lot of cats and we both thought a dog would be disruptive.

Peanut, though, never realized she was a dog. After all, she was a young puppy when we got her, and she was surrounded by cats. Naturally, she thought she was a cat as well. Not only would she play with them, but she mimicked them . . . including purring. Yep, our dog purrs. Or at least she tries. When she is happy, such as when her belly is rubbed, she makes this sound that sounds like a cross between a purr and an asthma attack.

While we were in Waxahachie, we lived in a wonderful neighborhood with friendly neighbors and lots of kids. We would take Peanut for long walks and Peanut would run up to everyone she saw and immediately flop over so they could have the pleasure of rubbing her belly. Every kid in that neighborhood knew Peanut's name.

FERRIS

Ferris came into our lives after we moved to Corsicana. We found him in the country in a vacant house I was showing (I did some residential real estate on the side when we were living in Waxahachie and later Corsicana). He was a survivor as the family had moved away at least a month previous and Ferris was still a kitten when we found him.

BEAU

Peanut had a major hand in our getting our second dog. We were living in Corsicana at the time. We had a fairly large house (about 4,500 sf) on three acres, plus a detached workshop in back that I had converted into an office. One day I was working in my office and I heard Peanut, who was in a small fenced area that went from the workshop to the house, barking her head off. This kept up for quite a while, so I decided to investigate.

Peanut was barking at this tan dog who was lying down under a tree in our yard outside the fenced area. I could tell immediately there was something very wrong with this dog. For one thing, he was not reacting at all to Peanut. (The sex of this dog was never in doubt! He would make most human males jealous.) But it was also covered with flies and was doing nothing to shoo them away.

As I got closer, he continued to not react. He just looked up at me with these incredibly big, sad eyes. He was emaciated. You could just tell the dog had given up and came to lie under the tree to die.

I got my car and drove it around to the tree. The ground was hard, so I was not leaving big ruts in the yard to do so, not that it mattered. I then lifted him (despite his size, he did not weigh but about thirty-five pounds) and put him in the back seat. I tried to pat him on his head to reassure him, but when I did I, it moved! That's when I discovered the top of his head was covered completely with maggots! Gross.

I took him to our vet, Beau. He identified him as likely part pit-bull and part black-mouth cur. He strongly suspected he had been a "target dog." That is, a dog who was used to train pit bulls who were being used in dog fights. He was a mess. In addition to his open wounds, he apparently had been deliberately injured so that he could not move fast . . . basically, he was a cripple.

The vet did what he could to save him. He treated the wounds and nursed him back to health. He kept him seven days before turning him back over to us. During this time, we advertised to see if we could find an owner, or someone who might be interested in him. I named him "Beau de guarde dog" in honor of the vet and the fact he was part pit bull.

CHARLIE

The latest member of our pet family Charles Sanford Heathcliff Wait, came to us much more recently. In fact, only three months ago – September 2017 (around the first anniversary of my discovering I had cancer). I was taking Daisy to the vet because she was "thinking outside the box," so-to-speak. Holly was with me. Next to the counter was a kennel and inside the kennel was this very cute kitten.

When we asked about the kitten, they told us it was our next cat and then handed him to us. Apparently one of their good clients had found him. She could not take him in, so she brought him to the vet. Further, she paid not only for all his shots, but to also have him neutered when it was time. As he was four months old, that meant in two months.) The reason he has so many names? He had been given the name "Heathcliff" by the women who found him. Holly added Sanford, but we would end up calling him Heathy. Only one problem, he would not respond to any of those names – Sanford, Heathcliff or Heathy (or damn cat, or any of the other names we would call him when he would get into trouble – which was frequently. One morning, the name "Charlie" came to me with regards to him. So, we started calling him Charlie and he responded. We'll see how long it lasts.

His true name, though, is "Trouble." That cat is always getting into mischief. He is playful and loves house plants – as food. But his main trouble-making skill is that he loves carrying things around. And not necessarily tiny things, either.

One night, I put my watch on my nightstand on its charger like I normally do. The next morning, the watch was gone. We looked all over the bedroom and tore the bed apart, nothing. As the watch had a habit of falling off my wrist (horrible design), Holly suspected I had lost it somewhere outside the house. One problem. I did not leave the house that day.

We scoured the house, prompting a thorough cleaning. But the watch was not to be found.

Weeks passed. Then months. I planned on asking for a new watch for Christmas.

Holly had the exact same watch. She had her charging station on the floor next to my dresser. One morning she got up and exclaimed, "why are there two watches here?" Yep, my watch was right next to hers – oriented exactly like hers.

To be fair, we never saw Charlie with the watch. But who else? Unless we have ghosts.

The ghost / gremlin theory picked up a bit more merit when a couple of weeks later my entire key chain disappeared. The key chain is a lot heavier than the watch. And similar circumstances. I remembered putting them on my nightstand. And I know I had them as I got something out of my car earlier that day. But I never left the house other than going to the car. We searched everywhere, including tearing the car apart. Nothing. The keys have never turned up.

[Update: The keys still are missing and now a backscratcher is gone. The backscratcher is wooden, about eighteen inches long. I keep it in the drawer by my bed. It is always there or on the nightstand. But one night, it disappeared. That was six months ago. Still gone. Again, we can't prove it was Charlie. But he is definitely our leading suspect. Only where is he hiding them? I suspect when we move, whenever that is, we are going to find a treasure trove somewhere.]

THE THREE SISTERS

That leaves the other three cats – Daisy, Sunshine and Hiccup. They all played an integral role in my courtship of Holly.

As I mentioned, I inherited the mother, Sasha, and all six kittens from Pat's new boyfriend, when he was staying in my house. And I used the pretext of showing Holly the kittens to lure her to my house that first date.

Sasha was a very small cat herself. I was told later she was a dwarf cat. But she looked like she was barely a year old herself. She was about half the size of any of my other cats.

Two weeks after our first date, it was my bowling league night. I was leaving for a four-day business trip the following morning. I was sitting at my desk when I noticed Sasha laying under the desk. She looked sick. But as I was running late for bowling, I decided to wait till I got back to see what was wrong.

Two hours later, I came back to find Sasha dead. Now I had six kittens who were only eight weeks old and not yet weaned. It was 10 pm and I was leaving in ten hours for the airport.

I immediately called Pat and Burt and was shocked to learn two things. The first was that Sasha was not one year old, but, in fact eighteen. (The vet later told me she probably died of malnutrition – feeding the kittens literally starved her to death as she just was not big enough or young enough to handle them). But what was worse, they were not going to raise a finger to help me. Not only were they not going to take care of the kittens, but he was not even going to come over to bury Sasha – a cat he had since he was an infant.

It was late in the evening by this time. So, I trudged out

in the darkness and dug a hole to bury Sasha. But I had a bigger problem. What was I going to do about the kittens? I had to leave in the morning, and they could not survive on their own. Hello, Holly.

Amazingly, she agreed to help. She could not stand the thought of the kittens being left alone. So here we were, having only dated a couple of weeks and she was coming over in the middle of the night to take the six kittens home with her.

She kept the kittens, hand feeding them until they were old enough to eat on their own. Eventually, she would give three of them away. But we kept the other three – Daisy, Sunshine and Hiccup. All three share their mother's petite stature, although not to the same degree. They are all under eight pounds, with Hickie barely over six. Both Cleo and Lucky weigh over sixteen, and Pumpkin fourteen.

GOD AND ME

FEELING PHILOSOPHY

A consequence of being faced with my eminent demise is. I instantly became a lot more philosophical. Naturally, I started thinking about death. What it means and what happens next . . . if anything.

I have always loved Philosophy. It was one of my favorite topics in High School and College (before the real-world interrupted).

WESTERN CIV

This leads me to a sidebar about taking Western Civilization in College. Western Civ at KU was a required course. It was split into two two-hour courses to be taken over two semesters. And it had a lot to do with philosophy, so I felt I would enjoy it.

I took Western Civ I the first semester of my Sophomore year. I really enjoyed the subject matter. And I worked hard in that class. I read every assignment and I was probably the biggest participant in class discussions, which was supposed to count as a major part of the grade.

But there was a problem. My teacher was, at least to my way of thinking, a fascist. Certainly, his viewpoints were diametrically opposite of mine in almost every area. This was not a big problem for me as I love a good debate!

I have always loved debating, well before I ever learned what that term meant. And it didn't matter what side of an argument I took. I always felt that you learned the most about a subject by thoroughly examining both sides of an argument, which is most economically accomplished with a good debate (not argument, debate. You need to leave emotions out of the equation in order to be open to learning). I have also had the ability to see both sides of an issue – to be able to change my perspective. This enables me to be able to argue proficiently either side of an issue. Thus, I can start a debate even when I'm with people I would normally agree. And, to my friends' non-delight, I often did.

But in the case of my Western Civ teacher, I genuinely disagreed with him. And I was not shy about providing my arguments. I felt I did an excellent job stating my case, and I was enjoying the debate. But I forgot one little fact. He was the teacher and therefore responsible for giving me my grade.

Even though I had disagreed with the teacher on almost every issue, I still felt I deserved an "A" for the course. I did the work and knew I did a good job on it. So, when I received a "C+" for the course, I was very upset. But there was nothing I could do about it. Except vow it would not happen again.

The next semester I really loaded myself up. I was taking twenty-six hours. And it included some heavy classes like chemistry, physics and abnormal psychology. [Yes, I was a masochist with no social life, but technically not insane. I just really loved learning. If I had thought I could get away with it, I would have loved to become a professional student.] So, I was not about to repeat my mistake from the first semester. I decided to take Western Civ as a "pass-fail" course. This means you get either a "pass" or "fail" for your grade – no A, B, or C to worry about. An A, B or C gives you a "Pass". A "D" or "F" merits a "Fail."

Now if you're going to take a course pass/fail, the objective is to obviously get as low a C as possible. In which case, you win. But if you end up with an "A", you lose – because that could have helped you with your GPA.

In order to help ensure a "C", I decided I would not read *any* of the assignments, which usually took the form of a book. I started the semester reading the Cliff Notes on the books, but later, I didn't even do that. After mid-year, I did absolutely NO homework for the class.

But I couldn't help myself. It became a game to me. How good a grade could I get if I did absolutely no work, or at least as little as possible?

The one thing I did fastidiously was attend class. (It was easy as it was between two other classes). And I was a very active participant in the class discussions, even though I often knew absolutely nothing about the subject. This was easier than it sounds as the material (book) was usually about a famous philosopher, not about history. So, I just had to figure out what the subject's philosophy was.

Class participation was important as it counted for 25%

of the grade. Here was my strategy. I listened for the first ten to fifteen minutes (it was a ninety-minute class) or so of the class discussion. This would give me an outline on what the subject matter was and in what direction the discussion was heading. I then made logical conclusions as to what it meant, which allowed me to add my two cents worth. And I was a pretty good guesser and a great b.s.'er. It also helped that the discussions usually started on-topic, but quickly degenerated into more general philosophical or current issues.

It further helped that my teacher this semester was the exact opposite of the first semester teacher. I liked her. [It didn't hurt that she qualified as being "hot." But she was also a very good teacher.] And, she seemed to like me. So much so that I knew I had her snowed.

There was only one written assignment for the year. It was our mid-term project that we were supposed to have been working on since the beginning of the semester. It also counted for 25% of our final grade.

The project was for us to be clipping articles from the newspaper and then relating them to what we were studying in Western Civ. Now it was the night before the project was due and I had not clipped a single article. It would have been way too much work to try and dig up some articles now (remember, there was no internet back then. We didn't even have personal computers) – and then write about them!

But I had a creative alternative. I was a big Bob Dylan fan and somehow, I suspected my teacher was as well. One of my frat brothers was a good musician and Dylan fan. He had a Dylan song book, with the lyrics to his most popular songs. I borrowed his book, then wrote an essay relating *his* lyrics to our Western Civ discussions. It was all b.s. since I hadn't read any of the books. But it was very good b.s.

The teacher naturally loved it. At mid-semester, I now

had a high "A" in a class I was hoping to get a low C. That's when I gave up reading the Cliff Notes.

Fast forward to finals. I was very confident I still had a strong A going into finals. Our Western Civ final was divided into two parts, a written essay test, accounting for 30% of our final grade, and an oral exam that would account for the remaining 20%.

I did not study a minute for the final. I had several other finals that week that were important, including one in Abnormal Psychology immediately after the one in Western Civ.

For the essay test, we were to write one essay. We were given our choice of about ten topics. The one I chose was "'Money is the Root of All Evil,' would Marx agree or disagree with this statement." I thought about it for a minute, then began chuckling.

Let me paint the picture. Here was a test accounting for 30% for the final grade of a required class for graduation. Everyone in the class was dead serious, except for one idiot in the back of the class who was chuckling.

I was thinking that you cannot talk about the 'Root of all evil', without talking about the entire *tree* of evil. So, I spent about 90% of the essay describing the tree of evil, and how the people were the sap. My tongue was so far in my cheek, I'm surprised it didn't pop out.

It was without question, the funniest thing I had ever written. I was extremely proud of it. In the entire essay, which filled the notebook given us for the test, I devoted maybe two paragraphs to answering the actual question.

When I was finished and left the class, I laughed out loud, and continued to laugh all the way to my next class, the psych final, which was across campus. (I had refrained from doing so during the class, although I know a chuckle or two escaped). The Abnormal Psychology final was very important to me as Psychology was my major.

There were six of us in my Frat house (AKL) taking that test. (It was a huge class of about 300). The night before we gathered together to study and quiz each other. Of the six, I probably was third or fourth in terms of knowing the material.

Heading into that final, though, nothing was going to get me down. I was still very much on a "high" from the Western Civ final. Indeed, throughout the Abnormal final, I was still giggling – so proud I was of that essay! I had really achieved what most students dream of – just totally and deliberately trashing a final. And getting away with it.

When the Abnormal final results were posted, I was surprised to learn not only did I get an "A", but I had the highest score in the class! This taught me a lesson on taking tests. Like most people, I suffered from test anxiety. I would do ok, but it was always a struggle. But here I was getting the highest score in a class of 300, when I knew the night before I was at best third out of six in my frat house. What happened?

The answer was that I was incredibly relaxed for the test. Nothing was going to get me down after that Western Civ test. So, from that moment on, I would always do something to make sure I was relaxed right before a big test – like read a comic book, etc. I also made sure I was well-rested. Any midnight oil burning needed to be done two nights before a final, not the night before. I successfully applied that strategy to my other finals that semester and for the rest of my college career. It worked. I got straight "As" from that point on. (And graduated in three years with honors in two different schools).

But back to Western Civ. Even though I had factually blown off the written final, I knew my writing alone was extremely clever and my teacher may have liked it. Since my goal was a C, that meant I had to make sure I blew the oral exam (get your mind out of the gutter).

The oral exam was a one on one affair held in her office. I did not do any prep work for it. I was ready to go down in flames. But, again, I could not help myself. I had to test my bs skills (they would come in handy during my sales career!)

A very popular TV show on at the time was Columbo, starring Paul Falk. I loved it. Columbo was a detective who solved cases by asking key questions in a very humble manner. He also had a habit of restating a suspect's statements as a question that would reveal even more.

I decided to play Columbo during the exam. (I at least showed enough restraint not to mimic his voice, although I think I might have slipped once). The professor would ask me a question. I wouldn't have a clue as to what the answer was. But I felt if I knew a little bit more, I could figure out what answer she was wanting. So, I restated the question, changing it just slightly to give me a clue as to what direction the answer should be. She would then affirm the restatement. All the time, I was watching her reactions very carefully. I continued to watch her body language and facial mannerism as I framed my answer. If I saw a positive reaction, I continued the path I was on. If I detected a negative reaction, I said something like, "of course that was not what was happening in this case," and head off in the opposite direction. In a very real sense, the teacher was taking the test for me!

In the end, I would fail. No, not the class. I ended up with a high "A" and thus failed to achieve the goal of getting a C-.

There was one other footnote to that semester. About a third of the way into the semester, I came down with a real bad case of mono. I was quickly sent home by the KU doctors. My own doctor wanted to hospitalize me and would have, but there were no beds available at his hospital. He let me stay home also because my sister was in medical school at the time and assured him, she would look after me.

I got very sick. I also developed a lot of side effects, like jaundice, liver swelling and other things. I remember for two solid weeks I could not breath out of my nose. It hurt so much to swallow that even soup was painful. I was told by several that I had to drop out of school.

I was back in class in three weeks, although still very weakened. I never dropped a class. And I ended the semester with straight A's for the first time in my college career. All thanks to learning how to take finals.

WHY ARE WE HERE?

But back to philosophy. Philosophy largely deals with the big question of "why are we here?" It is a question that has fascinated me all my life. And now that question is a lot more "real" to me.

There are only two ways you can go with this question. Either there is a purpose or there isn't. And if there is a purpose, then that directly leads to a higher power choosing that purpose. Which leads to a discussion of the existence and nature of God.

IS THERE A GOD?

Before suddenly entering the business world, I thought of myself as a scientist. As such, I always harbored doubt about God's existence because it was unable to be proven. And a scientist has a natural disdain for things that cannot be proven. It is their mission to push the limits of knowledge, not justify faith.

Philosophers, though, argue with reasoning rather than solid evidence. They will point out, for example, that even if the Big Bang (the one that started the universe, not the TV show) happened, there had to be *something* that created the original particle in the first place. And there had to be a trigger for the explosion.

I take a similar, though much more personal, perspective now. And I combine my appreciation of philosophy with my passion for science to form my personal belief, no faith, in God. For example, in science *probability* is often used to prove or disprove scientific theories. If the probability of something happening by chance is less than 1 in 20, or being more conservative, 1 in 100, science will say that the result is "statistically significant" and that it was unlikely due to chance. If the experiment is repeated with similar results, it is usually taken as solid proof.

I look back at the events in my life and ask, "what are the chances these were just random." Well, let me describe a few and let you decide.

My Relationship with God

October 2016 (from videos) and May 2017
I have a deep faith in God. I know this will surprise most of the people who know me, because I never talk about religion. I am not one to proselytize. (Although, in the back of my mind I have often wondered if I should become a preacher). And I don't go to church, except to accompany family. (When I was married to Ann, I would go with her to church as she was a devout Catholic, and I knew it was important to her that I go. When we had kids, I went every week because I felt it was important for them to have a structured religious upbringing. My compromise with Ann was that when they got older, I would share with them my non-Catholic views.)

The truth is, I have issues with organized religion. A lot of issues. The biggest problem I have is that most churches seem to espouse the doctrine they and only they have the right answers. If you do not follow their doctrine, you were condemned or otherwise disdained. I also have a huge problem with preachers who get very rich from preaching. (Recently one Texas preacher was pleading with his congregation how important it was for him to have his *fifth* private plane.) How is that following Jesus? Talk about rampant hypocrisy . . .

This never made sense to me, even as a child. As I mentioned, I am a very logical person. And logically, it never made sense that one and only one religion had the "true path to God" and *everyone else was wrong*. It was the latter part of that statement that bothered me the most. No matter what faith you practiced, it meant that *most* of the world's population was wrong and thus condemned. And yet, each one of them truly believed they had the answer and could support their conclusions in similar fashions. Why, I wondered, couldn't they all be right – at least to a degree. Perhaps they all have piece of the truth, but that truth is much bigger than any one vision – just like a window only gives you a limited perspective of the outside world.

Almost all religions rely on doctrine handed down through the ages, often in written form like the bible and the Koran. These are supposed to be holy works, written straight from God. Yet God, himself, did not physically write any of them. They were all written by man. (Ok, a word about pronouns. I will often use "he" when referring to God, but I certainly do not believe that God is a "He" or a "she". After all, why would God need a sex organ. Nor do I believe he is an old man with a beard sitting on a throne. I have no doubt that God has no physical form we can identify. But more on that later. I will also use the word "man" to mean "mankind," which includes women. English is an imperfect and inherently sexist language!). Because of the human mediation (even if they have a divine inspiration), these works are thus subject to human interpretation, limitations and failings. Indeed, we know the actual construction of the bible today was determined by a council of humans (the Vatican), who chose what to include and what to exclude. And there were definite political influences at play when they did so. In fact, the only thing that anyone has claimed was written directly by God were the ten commandments. Yet, the Bible gives two different accounts of them (Exodus 20: 1-17 and Deuteronomy 5: 4-21.)

It was also clear to me the bible could not possibly be literally true as Genesis violated almost everything we know from science (and I have always considered myself a scientist). And if one chapter could be filled with so many inaccuracies, how can one believe the other chapters are somehow sacrosanct and true word for word? Especially since the bible we read in English is the result of numerous translations from the original Hebrew and Aramaic? And each translation provides a different interpretation.

I also have trouble with the concept of "worship" with "God." Does God really want to be *worshipped?* Worship is defined as expressing adoration and reverence to a deity. Is God so vain that he requires our adoration and reverence? That, to me, sounds like a human emotion, not a divine one. Indeed, it seems to make God guilty of one of the "deadly sins" -- pride. It is something a massive ego, like a certain President of ours, would desire. I just don't think the supreme being has such a fragile ego. (I do understand the need for us humans to be *humble*, recognizing that there are powers that are greater than ourselves and have great respect for its power and wisdom. But I believe it is possible to be humble, without having to *worship* that greater power).

At the time our major religions were established, the leaders of the world relished in adoration and reverence, so it was natural to assume God, too, wanted this. But, to me, it never made sense. I would like to think that God is well above these petty human emotions and has a much stronger ego than that. This seems more like humans projecting their imperfections on God, rather than God demanding it. Certainly, I would expect God wants our *respect*, both for what he has done and for the power he possesses.

However, I do think worshipping God serves a *human* need. That is, I think it is important for us to acknowledge there is something far greater than ourselves. That we are just a part of a much larger story, much as a single letter is to *War and Peace*. This is very humbling, of course, and I think that is the whole point. There is a reason why *pride* is one of the "deadly sins." It also reinforces the need to follow His commandments (as interpreted by humans).

Nor do I believe *God* requires us to go through *rituals*, which, after all, are tied to worshipping him. Rituals are a mainstay of religions. And they make sense as a tool of both education and self-depreciation. To the degree they help people, they are worthwhile. But I do not think <u>God</u> *requires* them. Their main purpose is through repetition they are reinforcing the particular doctrine of that religion. Which is consistent with my idea that no religion has a monopoly on God. So why would any given ritual be more valuable to God than any other?

I do see the benefit of rituals for some people. It can help them focus and reaffirm their faith. By going through a ritual, it is making a *sacrifice* – which is another tool to reinforce your belief system. If you are making sacrifices and going through ritualistic behavior, it *reinforces* your belief in the underlying cause, otherwise why are you doing it? And repetition is definitely an effective tool for learning. It is also highly effective for brain washing. That's why every cult practice them in one form or another.

Again, like church, I feel rituals are good for some people, but they are not right for me. I do not need them to improve my faith in God. It's already strong. And I don't need them to depreciate myself, I do a pretty good job of that myself. And I have my wife to help!

Churches have great power over people. And by extension, the people overseeing the church (at all levels) have power. With great power comes great responsibility (says that great religious leader, Spiderman's uncle . . . It also comes with great temptation. Too many times this power has and continues to be misused. Too often those that crow the most about righteousness have the most to hide. (We see this often in politics as well.) The leaders will preach fervently against what they themselves practice.

Be assured I do not think all those in the church are hypocrites or in it for any reason other than faith and altruistic principles. But churches are very powerful and often very rich with much of their income in the form of (untraceable) cash. This naturally attracts people with nefarious intentions as well as those of genuine faith. Indeed, I believe most involved with churches are there because of their faith and not because of a desire to manipulate people. But those few who see it as a means of power or corruption can do almost as much harm as the rest do good. More people have died in the name of God than for any other reason. More wars have been fought over religion than any other reason. Is that truly what God wants?

We can never forget that much evil has been done in the name of God. So many political leaders have claimed to be divinely inspired if not divine themselves. Then use this proclaimed righteousness to justify horrendous acts such as genocide, repression, theft, rape, you name it. The problem is too many people are willing to accept it. We inherently want answers, even if they are wrong.

God and church make too convenient an excuse by those in power, or seek to be in power, to justify abusing that power for their own sake, or to put down others because of their faith. This notion that *my* religion is the only *true* religion and thus all others must be wrong, has created more problems generated more hate and justified more wars than all other reasons combined. And yet most people do not *choose* their religion. They are indoctrinated into it from birth or early childhood, so they really know no other faith. And when they do learn about other faiths, these religions are seen through the prism glass of their own faith, rather than as a possible alternative truth. Our perception of God and our faith is shaped mostly by where we are born and raised than any insight or revelation we have had personally.

The irony is that most faiths teach tolerance of others, not forced conversion. That part is all man made.

MY HERITAGE

Like everyone else, I am a product of my upbringing and heritage. One of the few things my parents had in common was that neither was very religious. In most other ways, my parents were about as opposite as you can get.

My dad was born and raised literally (and, yes, I do mean "literally" in the true sense of the word) in a three-room house he shared with four other siblings (really six, but two died in infancy) and his parents. The house was located one mile outside of Protection, Kansas, a town of about 1,000 people located 142 miles from the nearest city – Wichita. It had no electricity nor indoor plumbing, nor did it even have an outhouse – just convenient woods. He was raised as a farmer and brought up as a Southern Baptist. [The house still exists, although my uncle moved it and converted it into a storage building. It's tiny and hard to imagine how a family of seven could live together in it . . . without killing each other!]

Mom, on the other hand, grew up in what was one of the largest cities in the world – London, England. Her family was well-to-do, and she had a full-time nanny growing up. Her father owned a rather famous restaurant in London, Selby's, that was frequented by royalty. Her family was Jewish. Her parents were children of immigrants who had come to England to escape the Pogroms going on in Europe in the late 1800's. Her father's family was from Russia and her mother is from Prussia. (Ironically, my father's family was originally English, but most have been in America since the 1600s.)

The differences between my mother and father extended beyond cultural and genealogical, they were also opposite in personalities. My mother being extremely outgoing and my dad very reserved. In fact, my sister's and I did not even realize my father could talk, let alone have such a wonderful personality, until mom died . . . because he always deferred to her and let her shine.

They met during World War II. My father was in the Army Air Force. When they met, my dad was serving as the flight officer at Heathrow. At the time, Heathrow was two air bases – one British and one American, separated by a major road. After the war, the bases were combined into one large airport, becoming the Heathrow we know today. (My dad's experiences growing up in the Dust Bowl and Great Depression along with his exploits during World War II were fascinating, and the topic of a book that I helped him write: *From Dusty Plains to Wartime Planes.*)

One night, dad was looking for something to do, so he treated himself to an ice show. After he bought his ticket, he was invited by this middle-aged woman to join her and her 13-year-old son in a private box to watch the show. (Londoners loved the Americans and treated them well.) Dad agreed. He was soon to learn she had two daughters in the show (chorus, not the stars). During a break, the two young women came to the booth, where they were introduced to my father. One of them was wearing a dress with card suits on it. She would become my mother, with the card suits foretelling her future as a duplicate bridge master . . . (I will have more to say about my parents later as it is a fascinating story). They were married on May 10th, 1945 – two days after VE day.

The older I get, the more I appreciate what my mother did. She gave up everything she ever knew for my dad. Remember, in the 1940s, getting back and forth from the US to England was not easy and certainly not cheap. There were no jet airlines. Flying was an all-day affair and involve multiple stops and was very expensive. Ocean liners took a long time to get there (although not nearly as long as back in the colonial days!). So, she knew she would not see her family or friends very often. And calling overseas was also very expensive, so she knew that even communicating with her family was hard. She was giving up the only home she ever knew, as well as her family, and all her friends. She was also sacrificing her way of life – to move to Kansas.

At least she was not going to be living on a farm. That was not the plan. His end of the deal with my mother was that he would not pursue farming (which he wasn't really wanting to do anyway), and they would live in a city. His dream was to become a pilot for the airlines. Unfortunately, that was the dream of most of the pilots from the war. As a result, the airlines were very fussy. One of the things they insisted on was that the pilots be at least 5'9" tall. Dad is 5'8". He stayed in the Air Force until 1947. Then, when mom got pregnant with Cheryl, dad got a job with Sears and they moved to Kansas City. Dad remained with Sears until he retired.

I must tell a quick story about how mom got to the US after the war. Because of the number of war brides, the US military commissioned a passenger ship to bring them to the US after the war. But that ship wasn't leaving until December and mom did not want to wait that long as Dad was being sent home in August. So, her father bribed a freighter captain to take her on his ship. Her trip took about a week.

In the meantime, Dad was flying his plane back to the US. The path back had them stopping in Iceland for refueling. But when they got there, an early fall storm snowed them in. He was stuck. He was there for three weeks. He then flew to Goose Bay on the southern tip of Greenland at the end of September but was once again snowed in for another week. Still, he was not worried as mother was not due in the US until December. He had no idea her father had bribed the Captain to get her there early.

As a result, Mom got to the US (New York) well before Dad. But there was no one there to greet her. Not only did she not know anyone in America, she also arrived with little money. They were only allowed to bring $20 in cash. There were no credit cards back then. Nor could she get ahold of Dad. But she did have dad's parent's address. So, she telegraphed them and told them of her problem. They immediately wired her money for a train ticket, and off she went on a cross-country adventure on a train full of returning military men. (I'm sure she was very popular on board!)

A couple of days later, she arrived in Wichita for the last leg of the trip. Upon arriving at the station, she immediately made her way to the restroom (naturally). There she saw someone she had recognized from a photograph my father had showed her. It was dad's sister-in-law, Velmarie Riner, whose brother, GT, had married dad's youngest sister, Doris. Velmarie also happened to have a sister who used to date my father. Naturally, they sat together on the train to Protection, with Velmarie happily telling mom stories of dad's past, including his past romantic adventures!

Dad's family made mom feel welcome. [His father had

become a successful farmer, in fact prospering during the dust bowl years as he developed innovative techniques of farming. So, they had a much larger, though still modest, home than when dad was young. It even had electricity, which they did not have before the war.] But you can imagine the cultural shock she must have had! A couple of days later, my Dad called his parents to tell them he had finally arrived in New York. After talking to him for several minutes, my grandmother asked him, "well do you want to say 'hello' to your wife?" Dad was flabbergasted! He had no idea mom was in America!

The marriage worked because both of them were willing (to a degree, at least) to compromise. Mom did not want to give up the City life and could not see herself on a farm. Which was fine with dad. That's how they ended up in Kansas City.

While neither were religious, they both agreed church was important for the kids when we came along. But what church? Mom was Jewish (which, by the way, makes me Jewish according to Jewish tradition), while Dad was Southern Baptist. The compromise? They took us to the Unitarian Church, which is one church that acknowledges the validity of other faiths. We went to the All Souls Unitarian Church in Kansas City until I was about thirteen. At that point, I guess they decided I had enough religion and we stopped going. Either that, or they realized I was a lost cause.

Really, I think they just got tired of trying to get us to go. The girls did not want to go, and both had stopped a few years previous. And I was not exactly enthusiastic about it either.

According to Wikipedia (that "infallible" source of all knowledge):

John S. Wait

Unitarianism *is historically a Christian theological movement named for its belief that God is one entity, as opposed to the Trinity which defines God as three persons in one being; the Father, Son, and Holy Spirit. Unitarians believe that Jesus was inspired by God in his moral teachings and is a savior but a human being rather than a deity. Unitarianism is also known for the rejection of several other Western Christian doctrines, including the doctrines of original sin, predestination, and the infallibility of the Bible. Unitarians in previous centuries accepted the doctrine of punishment in an eternal hell, but few do today.*

Notably, one of our founding fathers and later President, John Adams along with his son and another President, John Quincy Adams were Unitarians.

In our church anyway, we were also very accepting of other religions, believing that all faiths had something to offer. Which I still believe today. We even studied them in church school.

However, as I grew older, so did my disdain for organized religion. I noted the number of wars predicated on religious belief – even though, ironically, all major religions are against killing. And I certainly saw all the hypocrisy often seen within churches. (Look under the definition of hypocrisy and you will see a picture of a church parking lot after service has let out. Watch people cutting off other church goers, so they can get home thirty seconds sooner.) One also observed great hypocrisy on TV with the self-serving ministries (Jimmy Baker comes to mind) whose sole purpose seemed to be to get money out of the listener to be used for their own personal benefit. It was sickening to me then, and still is, how often people will use religion, the church, or the bible to justify whatever they want.

I will quickly point out that not all churches are bad, not all ministers, hypocrites. Indeed, churches do a lot of good. And they can be extremely comforting to those in need. It is because I recognize the good in churches that I strongly supported sending my kids (and even accompanying them each week) to church. But by the same token, I do not need someone else telling me how to have faith or practice my beliefs.

I also grew up in the 1960s, a period where church membership was at historical lows and even the media publicly questioned whether God existed or was still alive. (Time ran its famous cover story: "Is God Dead" on April 6, 1966, when I was 11 1/2). Remember, we were mired in a very unpopular war (Vietnam), our leaders were being assassinated (John and Robert Kennedy, Martin Luther King), riots were a regular occurrence, we were still recovering from the atrocities of WWII, especially the Holocaust, other atrocities were occurring around the globe, our environment was a mess, we were mired in a bitter cold war making nuclear war not only a very real threat, but it seemed inevitable. People naturally wondered, "why would God allow all this evil to continue?"

In my late teens, I was, at best, an agnostic. And there were times I was probably an outright atheist. I certainly did not believe there was a God watching over us and guiding our lives. Supporting this attitude was the fact I was a strong believer in science. And it seemed much of what organized religions were teaching was against (at worst) or not at all supported (at best) by science. If there was an all-powerful God out there, I reasoned, it was less likely to be a "being" as we understand it, and more likely to be a combination of pure energy and the collective conscious of all beings.

Kansas City

May 2017

I know for most people who are not from Kansas, it is a bit confusing there are two Kansas Citys. And while "Kansas" is its first name, the biggest Kansas City is on the Missouri side of the river. That's where the skyscrapers are, the sports complexes, the airport, and now, the casinos.

Casinos in Kansas City. That still takes some getting used to. They weren't there when I was growing up, or when I left the area for good in 1984. Indeed, Kansas and Missouri were both extremely conservative. Especially Kansas. It was one of the last states to repeal prohibition. Even in 1984, you could not get anything but 3.2 beer in a bar or restaurant ("3.2" stands for the percentage of alcohol allowed – 3.2% by volume). Only in private clubs could you be served "hard" liquor. The thought of a casino in Kansas back then was as silly a notion as a TV show host, with no political experience, becoming President. Now, Kansas has four casinos that are *owned* by the state . . . plus, five more owned by Native American nations.

OF PRIDE AND PREJUDICE

Back to Kansas City. Kansas City, Kansas is on the other side of the Missouri River from Kansas City, Missouri. It is home to the Kansas Motor Speedway (which was not there when I was). It is also located in Wyandotte County. We lived in Johnson County, which is south of Wyandotte County. Johnson County was a prototypical suburban area. It was mostly affluent and almost exclusively white at the time I was growing up. Indeed, the only school I attended that had a black student was my high school, Shawnee Mission North. In a school of over 2,000 students, I doubt we had more than a dozen black students. And none were in any of my classes. In fact, the first time I ever interacted with a black person was when I worked at Sears, starting my Junior year in High School. (I continued to work at Sears, at least in the summers, through my Sophomore year in college.) At Sears, though, there were many black employees I got to meet. Two really stood out. Karl (I am not sure that was his name, now, it's been so many years ago) was the head of security. No one would dare mess with him. For one thing, he was built like a linebacker – big, husky, muscular, yet obviously agile. But here's the thing that was not fair. While he looked like he could tear you from limb to limb, he was also a nationally prominent karate black belt. He even had competed against Chuck Norris. He was also a teddy-bear (thank goodness). One of the nicest and gentlest people I ever had the privilege of meeting.

The other was Rod. Rod was my age and we quickly became close friends. He and I both loved air hockey and we played at an arcade in the mall during our breaks. (We both became really good. Although I never entered any tournaments, I did beat someone who claimed to have been the KC champion.)

Sadly, it was with Rod I got to experience racial prejudice first-hand. And it came from a most unlikely source . . . my father. I invited Rod over to our house after work. He was still there when my dad got home from work. Dad's face, when he met Rod, blazed for a second before recovering to smile and shake his hand. But after Rod left, I was told, in no uncertain terms, that Rod was not welcome in our house . . . ever.

Up until that moment, it never occurred to me my father was prejudiced. He certainly never showed it, at least in a way that I saw. He never disparaged blacks at home or complained about them like you see with most bigots. Besides, my father married a Jew! And I had several Jewish friends, including my best friend. But there it was, right in front of me. My father was a closet bigot.

The only other time in my life where I saw my dad's prejudice involved Juliette. When she was in med school (KU Med), she started dating a fellow whose name happened to be Wilt Chamberlain. No, not *that* Wilt Chamberlain. But nonetheless, when Dad heard she was dating *a* Wilt Chamberlain, he threw an absolute fit and forbade her to ever see him again.

I never met Wilt (either of them), and I never asked my sister, but I doubt strongly if her Wilt was even black. And I know, if anything, if he was black, dad's pronouncement probably would have made her want to see him more, not less. But alas, that relationship was short-lived anyway. (I do know she participated in the civil rights demonstrations at KU, which were many at the time – and made sure not to tell our parents).

I was always pro civil rights (for all people, regardless of race, gender, religion, sexual orientation, etc.) While I, personally, have never been subject to racial persecution, it is a part of who I am. (Few people even know I am Jewish – until now that is. I don't look Jewish and do not have a Jewish name). Both of my mother's parents fled eastern Europe due to Pogrom in the late 1800's. The Jewish people historically have been the most discriminated against people in the world, predating Christ, and probably remain so even today. It would be completely hypocritical for me (or for that matter, anyone) who has been subject to prejudice to turn around and exert that same prejudice on others. I can honestly say that I have never assumed anyone to be "inferior" due to the color of their skin, their sex, their religion, or any other demographic. But if they drive slow in the left lane, that's another matter.

Because I was pro civil-rights and it was the 60s then 70s, I became anti-south. Because, at that time, the south was synonymous with bigotry and civil rights abuses. But God is mischievous. Where have I spent the last thirty-five years of my life? In the South. First North Carolina, then Florida, Texas and now Georgia. Fortunately, things are a lot better in the south than they were in the 60s!

EARLY DRIVING LESSON

Back to Kansas City. One more story before I get to the real point I want to make about Kansas and what it means to me. This story, though, is relevant as I think it demonstrates just how mischievous God can be.

As I mentioned, Kansas City, Kansas is in Wyandotte County. I think historically, KCK has always had a bit of chip on its shoulder. One way it has shown its "independence" from the other Kansas City (and, indeed, the rest of the metropolitan area) is in how it names its streets.

In Kansas City, Kansas, the numbered streets go north

and south. Everywhere else in the metropolitan area, including where I lived, the numbered streets go east and west. This little fact gives you some interesting intersections like 32nd street and 32nd street, etc.

It would have been nice if they had told you this little fact in driver's ed. But they didn't. And since we never went to Kansas City Kansas, I had no real knowledge of it growing up. I certainly had never been there when I turned 16. And I was blissfully ignorant of its nonconforming street names.

It was two weeks after I got my driver's license. It was still summer, so I was not in school. At 7am the phone rang, and my mother answered. It was dad. His car had broken down and he wanted us to pick him up as he was having to have his car towed.

First mistake. Dad never talked to me. He gave the directions to my mom.

I love my mother dearly. She was a wonderful, wonderful person who everyone loved. She had so many endearing qualities. Driving was not one of them.

This was 1970. Mom absolutely hated freeways. (I-35 had not been open that long in Kansas at the time.) Whenever she drove on a freeway, her instinct was to immediately exit. She famously ended up in the Kansas City stockyards during one of her premature exits.

And my mom, bless her, had absolutely no sense of direction whatsoever. (My father was the opposite; he had an unerring sense. Fortunately, I am more like my father and have a pretty good sense of direction.) As a result, my mother would habitually get lost whenever she tried to go somewhere the first time. I'll give two quick examples.

The first was in the early 1960s when her mother came to visit. (It was her last visit as she died before she was sixty, ironically of cancer). Mom wanted to take her shopping in

St. Joseph, which is about forty miles north of Kansas City. Well mom and her mother took off. Soon they were in the countryside. After about an hour (and no doubt, unending conversations), they started coming into the city. Then mom noticed the skyscrapers and remarked to her mother that she did not realize St. Joseph had skyscrapers. It doesn't. Mom had managed to drive in a complete circle.

I also remember riding with her after they moved to Dallas. I can't remember where we were going, but sure enough Mom got us lost. But soon her face brightened as she turned to me and said, "don't worry, I've been lost here before."

Back to that early August morning in 1970. The plan mom and dad had was for mom to drive her car to the scene and I would follow her in mine. Then mom would give dad her car and she would ride back with me. Simple.

The problem was I had absolutely no idea where we were going. Mom never told me. I was just to follow her. The other problem was mom didn't really know where she was going either.

Naturally, she got lost. That goes without saying. However, this was way before the days of cell phones. So, I had absolutely no idea she was lost, especially since I had no idea where we were supposed to be going. Nor did I have any idea where we were as I had never been there before.

What I did know was that it was rush hour.

Mother was bad enough as a driver when you were riding *with* her. She turned out to be impossible when you were driving behind her.

The traffic was very heavy. We were driving down a busy street and came upon a stop light. The light turned red. Mom turned right. (This was before it was legal to turn right on red after stop). Cars were already coming the other way into the intersection. There was no way I could follow.

But that was not the only problem. The bigger issue was that the right turn takes you over a long bridge. By the time the light turned green (and it was a *long* light) and I made my way over the bridge, mom's car was nowhere to be seen.

There was no such thing as "GPS" back then. And I had no map. (Remember, I only had my driver's license for two weeks. But since that episode, I made sure to always have a map in the car). I had absolutely NO idea where I was, let alone how to find mom . . . or dad . . . or home. And while I could probably have found my way home by retracing my steps, the mission was to pick up Dad.

I first drove up and down the street I was on, in hopes of finding my mother. I figured sooner or later she would notice I was missing and turn around, or park in an obvious spot and wave me down. Wrong on both parts.

Now my logic kicked in. Assuming (wrongly as it turned out) that my mother had known where she was going, then my father's car was somewhere between where I was and his office. My father worked at the Sears and Roebuck catalog plant, which I knew was at 16th and Cleveland. I saw a street sign indicating that I was on 18th. So, I turned right, went two blocks and got on 16th. I figured if I drove long enough on 16th, I would eventually hit Cleveland. And dad's car had to be somewhere along the way.

Unfortunately, I did not know I was now in Kansas City, *Kansas*. And even if I had known that, I certainly did not know that 16th street in KCK ran north and south, not east and west. In other words, I was never going to find Cleveland Avenue on this 16th street.

I turned left onto 16th and proceeded cautiously, looking for my mother's car, my father's car, or the Sear's plant. Now 16th street was wide, but other than the center line, there were no other lines indicating separate lanes going in each direction. So, I assumed it was just one lane, which was what other cars were doing. (It turns out to be what is called "a lane and a half"). I had gone a few miles, when I realized that this cannot be right. It seemed I was heading away from the business district, instead of into it. Further, I never saw a freeway. Sears was just off I-70. And I was wondering why Dad would not have taken the freeway to get there. Clearly, he would never have taken this road. I began to realize what happened. My mother had gotten us both lost.

I decided it was time to go home. I saw a convenience store to my left, and I figured I could get a map and find my way home (I was very good at reading maps). Here is where my driving inexperience betrayed me. I swerved *slightly* to the right in order to make the left turn.

Oh, one other thing. My turn signal did not work, and it was raining. Dutifully, I cranked down the window (no power windows in those days unless you had a very expensive car) and stuck my arm out as I started my left turn.

That's when I ran into the police. Or rather they ran into me. More specifically, an off-duty police officer in his personal car crashed into my car.

He passed me because I was driving so slowly and assumed, I was turning right when I swerved slightly in that direction. If it had been anyone else, I'm sure that driver would have been given a ticket and been declared at fault as he trying to pass me on the left and hit me from behind. But he was a policeman. A Kansas City Kansas policeman. And we were in Kansas City Kansas. So, like the Chiefs on the road, I was not going to get that call.

Mom never found dad. He ended up hitching a ride with the tow-truck driver. After dealing with the not-so-nice policeman and learning the hard way what you do in a car accident, I bought my map and made my way home.

AD ASTRA PER ASPERA

While I was born in Missouri (the "show me State,"), it was only because that was where the closest hospitals were located to where my parents lived in suburban Johnson County – on the Kansas side of the Kansas City area. Despite my "accidental" birth across the state line, I consider myself a native "Kansan." And I am very proud of that fact.

I love Kansas City. I love Shawnee Mission, where I grew up. I deeply love Lawrence and KU. But mostly, I love Kansas.

I come by the love honestly. Not only did I grow up in Kansas, my father is from Kansas and most of his family still lived there when I was growing up. He grew up in Comanche County, which is just over half-way across the state on the Oklahoma border. He also had family and two farms up near Scott City, which is in far western Kansas, not far from the time zone line.

I always loved going to western Kansas and seeing our family and our "farms." (Dad did not have a lot of land, by Kansas standards. He had a total of less than a section of land (640 acres). Two-thirds of this was in Logan County, between Scott City and Oakley, and the other third, which I would eventually inherit, was in Comanche County, just a few miles from the Oklahoma border and about ten miles from where he was born and raised.

As a teenager, I spent three summers in Western Kansas, staying with one of my Aunts and Uncles, while working with them on their farms. (They had lots of land). I certainly learned the meaning of hard work, but I really enjoyed my time there. Before I went the first time, I took an extension course in Lawrence that taught me how to drive and work on a tractor. I was thirteen.

While I learned how to operate a tractor, that did not mean I knew what I was doing, as my uncle would unfortunately find out. Uncle GT gave me a simple task, to plow a field. The field was square in shape. I was on a good sized-tractor, dragging a 20' wide (or so) plow implement behind me.

Things started out fine. I made several successful laps around the field. I was very proud of myself. Sadly, no one explained to me how you handle it when the field starts to shrink. I was making tighter and tighter turns. The tractor was able to make these turns, no problem, thanks to power steering. But I forgot I was dragging a 20' wide implement that does not make tight turns. Well, I turned so sharply, the implement ran up the back wheel. (No real damage was done, and the lesson learned.)

As I grew older, though, I began to realize not everyone shared my profound love of Kansas. Indeed, Kansas is often mocked. "Flat Kansas," my wife still chides. They complain there is nothing to see as they are driving along the seeming endlessly long I-70 on their way to Colorado. I happen to find it beautiful. I love seeing the farms and the land. There is nothing like seeing the waves of golden wheat flowing in the breeze near harvest time. I also love being able to see for miles and miles in all directions. (It's very hard to sneak up on someone in Kansas!). Kansas is referred to frequently as a "fly-over" state. It just happens to be in the way while you're flying to Colorado or to one of the coasts.

But I appreciate what Kansas means. I understand the value of those farms and the seas of wheat. But mostly I love the people. I love that strangers wave at you when you pass on a country road. And they use the whole hand, not just a single finger like in some places I've been. And I love the work ethic. (Admittedly, I am not as fond of the politics.) But the people are wonderful there.

People will often say that New York and Los Angeles are great places to visit, but you wouldn't want to live there. Kansas City is like the opposite, it's a great place to live, but maybe not the most exciting place to visit --- unless you love BBQ or steaks.

But one thing I really love about Kansas, is its motto. *Ad Astra per Aspera. To the stars, through difficulties.* We learned the motto in grade school. And I loved it then and adopted it as my own. Back then, I wanted to be an astronaut. I took the motto literally. I wanted to go to the stars, and I knew there would be plenty of difficulties along the way.

But I think that motto is a good one for life, in general. No matter what our goal, there are difficulties we must overcome to achieve it. That is what life is about. Keeping our eyes on the stars as we wade through what life throws at us.

Along with a great motto, Kansas, along with my family, gave me most of the values I still hold dear today. It also gave me a great education, and a fantastic basketball team.

JAN

May 2017

As I am writing this our nation is going through difficult times. But this is not the first time, nor will it be the last. And as bad as it seems right now, it is nothing compared to what we went through in the 60s and 70s. Those were times when a lot of people, me included, had grave concerns about whether there was going to *be* a future. And, perhaps more than any time previous, people were abandoning God. Or rather, their faith in the existence of a benevolent being watching over the world was seriously challenged. How could there be? With all the problems we had. The riots. The wars. The injustice. The cruelty. Surely, if there was a God, he was either dead or uncaring. I certainly did not believe there was a sentient living, caring being watching over us.

My doubts about a "living, caring" God came to a climax when Jan left me. Jan was my first true love. We met while I was in gradual school at KU, working on my master's in Experimental Psychology (that's a misnomer, it should be called "research" psychology as experimental seems like we were toying with people's minds) and Jan was a senior working on an Honors project. My mentor had her work with me on my thesis project, which dealt with the effects of alcohol on visual perception (yep, I got to get college kids drunk. Although, only half of them received alcohol while the other half got a placebo. Yet even the Placebo group showed effects of drinking! Such is the power of suggestion.)

We dated seriously for a couple of years. She was from Kansas City as well, but her family moved to Hawaii. (Boy, did I want to go visit! But, alas never got the chance). One summer, I drove her to the airport for her trip home. Only the airport was in Los Angeles (we left from Lawrence, KS). The airfare was so much cheaper from LA, the savings more than paid for our drive to LA. What a fun trip!

I was so serious about her; I was ready to propose. But I never got the opportunity. One evening, we met up with her older sister, right before Jan was to leave for Hawaii. We were at some bar, having a good time when the subject of Kansas, specifically western Kansas, somehow came up. Apparently, her sister spent some time there for some reason (I think it was with a boyfriend). Anyhow, she started really dissing on Kansas in general, and Western Kansas in particular. I took exception to this. I lost my temper. (I just could not stop that little voice from egging me on and defending my state.)

Anyway, back to Jan. Seeing me lose control like I did, I think, really scared her. She basically broke up with me right afterwards. She would confirm the breakup by dating someone else while in Hawaii.

During this time, I was desperate. I so wanted her back! So, I turned to an unusual source for me – God. I prayed and prayed for her to return to me. But these prayers went unheeded. She was gone for good. So much for prayer and for God, I thought.

John S. Wait

Encore

It was a few years later when my faith would turn around for good . . . when God made his presence known to me in a very real and personal way. When I needed a miracle . . . and got one. Let me set the stage.

It was summer of 1979 when my good friend Greg and I were having lunch where all big decisions are made – at Burger King. At the time, I was working on my dissertation and he was working on his master's thesis. We were both complaining about the process of generating the finished reports. Not the research and work that went into it, but the actual production. While it may be hard for today's generation to understand, but back then we did not have personal computers. The most sophisticated thing we had for writing was the IBM Selectric – an electric typewriter that had a correction ribbon on it, so you could "erase" mistakes. In reality, it did not "erase" the mistake. It simply typed over it with a white powder that made the mistake *mostly* disappear. And, no, it would not point them out for you – you had to see the mistake as soon as you typed it – or at least while the page was still in the typewriter. Otherwise, it was too late, and you had to resort to "white-out" (applying a quick drying "paint" over the type) and then try to carefully realign the type –

which you could never get exactly right. In short, it was a painful process. And if you had a major change – like wanting to insert a paragraph or remove a paragraph on an earlier page – you had to *retype all the pages following* as the pagination, spacing and page numbers would be off. This process was especially hard on guys as back in those days, girls often took typing classes, so they could be prepared to take secretarial jobs, while guys avoided them like the plague. It simply wasn't manly. (Boy were we sexist back then! Although my mother made me take typing in summer school one year – and am I glad she did). As a result, you usually resorted to hiring a typist. And even if you could type somewhat decently, you *always* hired a professional typist for the final draft as it had to be perfect.

After the thesis or dissertation was typed, you then had to take it to a copy store and get several copies made. Finally, you had to find a binder who would bind the copies into nice hardback editions, with embossed lettering on the covers and spine.

As we were complaining about the process, the thought occurred to us that someone should create a company that would do all those things for you . . . the typing, copying and binding. The more we thought about it, the more we loved the idea. Let's do it, we said. (Honestly, I can't remember if the initial idea was Greg's or mine.)

We quickly learned there are three things you should have when starting a business. First, you should have a good business background. Ok, between Greg and I, the best we could come up with is that once I cut through Summerfield Hall (the business school) on my way to class. Check.

Second, you should have experience in the field you are going into. Well both Greg and I had stood in line at Kinkos (a copy store chain that later sold out to Fed-Ex). Did that count? Check.

And most importantly, you must have money. Lots of it. Well, we were both graduate students, so not only did we NOT have money, we were both deeply in debt. So, check, check and check. Of the three things essential to starting a business – between Greg and myself – we had exactly none of them. But two things we did have, stupidity (for trying to open a business without any of the above) and persistence (to continue to prove the stupidity).

The timing was critical for me as well. For the previous several years, I had been supporting myself through a teaching fellowship at KU (in addition to waiting tables). I was an Associate Instructor and taught my own class that I created – *"Parapsychology: The Scientific Study of ESP."* I was the first to teach the subject at KU, at least as an accredited course. But that summer, the head of the Experimental Psychology Department came to me and practically begged me to take their research fellowship, which meant giving up the teaching. The reason was they had no one else who could take the fellowship and if no one took it, the government would take it away permanently. That's how government worked. So, being a team player, I relented and took the position. The problem was I *loved* teaching. And now I really missed it. So much so that after a couple of months, I applied to teach Psychology at Johnson County Community College.

Knowing what we didn't know (which is an important step), I sought to get advice. I was able to find a business professor who was highly recommended to us who specialized in small businesses. He told us if we wanted to raise money, we needed to create a *business plan*. What the hell was that? We asked. And he told us. And then he gave me some samples.

What I quickly discovered was that this was real work! I had to do actual research. Who knew you had to do research in *business*? This was not a negative to me. As a scientist, I loved research. Somehow, the fact business required research made it *more* appealing to me.

To cut a long story shorter, I wrote a very thorough business plan, including the necessary research on the industry and the competition, as well as my first attempts at cash flow projections (something I now get paid to do for others). Armed with a business plan, we set out to raise the money.

One problem. How do you find investors? No idea. Naturally, we hit up family first. But we were also able to get a few outside investors as well. Actually, I think we got two, including a friend of Greg's. In total, we raised about $14,000. To us, this was a freaking fortune! (Back then, you could buy a new car for a few thousand dollars). But I would soon learn, it was not nearly enough. Ideally, you should have enough not only to capitalize the venture initially but be able to fund six months of operation without any revenue. Nonsense! We would make an instant profit, I was convinced.

My mother came up with the name – Encore Copy Corps. I loved it (the double entendre). And so, Encore was born. It was December 1979. Now we had the money, and the name, the next task was to find a location.

Lawrence, at the time, had about 35,000 people in it. Most of whom were associated one way or another with the University of Kansas. (KU, back then, had about 18,000 students). There were currently two copy stores in town – House of Usher and Kinkos. Both were strictly copy stores and both were located downtown (about four doors from each other). Back then, no one had personal printers or digital cameras that would do convenience copying for you. Only the biggest companies had their own copier. Nope, if you wanted a copy of something, you had to go to a copy store to get it.

We were smart enough to realize if our main competitors were downtown, maybe we should be on the opposite side of town. We found a perfect spot in a shopping center owned by John Kiefer, whose store, Kief's records, anchored the strip. Kief's was the most popular record store in town by far. (That's right millennials. Records. As in vinyl. As in 45s and albums. That's how you listened to music in those days. You either turned on the radio, went to a live show, or bought records – or sung in the shower. There was no streaming service or digital media. And certainly no cell phones.) The storefront we moved into was previously an art gallery. As a result, it was fixed up nicely, complete with a loft and a fireplace. High class!

Next job was to get the equipment. Hello Xerox. The equipment was incredibly expensive. The Xerox 9200, which was to be our main copier, cost over $100,000 – and this was in 1980! But they had this wonderful thing called a lease-purchase. Never mind we were paying 30% (yes!) interest. In addition to the 9200 (which we replaced a year later with the 9500 when it came out), we had two smaller black and white copiers (one for self-service – an innovation back then) and a color copier (the second in the town) plus two word-processors (also Xerox) – the first of their kind! And the only ones in town, at least that we knew of. It still amazes me they leased us all that equipment, after all, the business only had $14,000 with a nice business plan but no experience and our personal net worth was negative. They did require my personal guarantee on the papers, which I signed. I was able to keep Greg from having to sign. If it went south, I didn't want it to take both of us with it.

FIRST DATE

That Xerox 9200 would also figure into my first marriage. I met my first wife, Ann, while she was doing self-service copies at Encore. I was sitting on the couch in our lounge area next to it. (Yep, we had a lounge area around the fireplace. First class.) We struck up a conversation, which became more interesting when I learned she was a graduate student in Clinical Psychology. Naturally, I knew a lot of the students in the program.

I finally got brave enough to ask her out. The excuse I used was there was a new movie out that happened to feature a Xerox 9200, which I had recognized in a preview. The movie was *9 to 5* starring Jane Fonda, Dolly Parton and Lily Tomlin. Surprisingly, she said "yes."

Honestly, it is absolutely amazing there was a second date, given how that first date went. First, I had forgotten when I asked her that I had agreed to let Greg borrow my car that night. That meant Ann had to drive, which was kind of a no-no back in the sexist 70s.

Ann's car was something else. It was a hand-me-down from her Aunt Rose, who lived next to her parents and who just adored her. Well, Aunt Rose had that car for about twenty years before giving it to Ann. It wasn't exactly sexy as it was an old station wagon. Ann's family lived in Beverly Farms, Massachusetts – on the North Shore in the Boston area. This meant every winter the roads were frequently salted to melt the ice. Well this salt is not kind to cars as it eventually corrodes the underside.

So, Ann picked me up in this battle wagon and I got to watch the road as she drove, by just looking straight down at my feet. There were holes in the bottom of the floorboard! (The car would last another two years, before Aunt Rose got a new car and gifted her the other car. Ann sold the battle wagon to someone who drove it in a demolition derby!).

We got to the theater and I went to buy the tickets. But then I discovered I had forgotten my wallet! So, Ann not only had to drive, but she had to pay for the movie – and a couple of drinks afterward. I guess after doing all that she felt she had a vested interest in me, which is why she would agree to a second date.

But I'm getting way ahead of myself. I would not meet Ann until December 1980, after the store had been open about nine months. Getting back to how it started – and don't worry, there is a point to this story.

TIMING

The next task was to find a manager. Again, we knew we knew nothing about running a copy store. Because of this, we knew we wanted to hire someone who had experience, given we had absolutely none. We first approached the manager of Kinkos. She was very nice, but politely declined. However, she strongly recommended her assistant manager, Joni, for the position. We were extremely grateful for the recommendation. We talked with Joni and loved her instantly. She was perfect! (And she did a wonderful job for us).

So now we were set.

Then something unexpected happened. Johnson County Community College called. They wanted me to teach Psychology for them – starting the next semester which was in a few weeks. Now I had a real dilemma on my hands. I could return to teaching, which I loved and would be very happy. But I had just spent the past several months raising money for this business. Do I just abandon my stockholders and Greg? I had made a lot of commitments, not just to Greg and the stockholders, but to my family, to Xerox, to the new landlord, to Joni, etc. Do I just turn my back on them?

This became a major turning point in my life. I chose

Encore. Naively, I thought I could work part-time at the store and still be able to finish my dissertation. Boy was I wrong! I was soon working literally (yes, literally) 100 hours a week at the store . . . and loving it. I took a leave of absence from the Department, suspending my dissertation. (I was ABD – "all but dissertation." I had completed all my work for my PhD except for the dissertation.) I never returned.

In addition to not raising nearly enough money, we happened to be opening a business in our country's worst year in to open a business in its history. We were in the middle of the worst inflation our country had seen. Prime rate was near 20%, meaning any money we borrowed was at interest rates approaching 25-30%! (Today, the prime lending rate for most banks is below 4%).

By the time we opened, technology was just starting to take off. Xerox introduced the first *word processor*. This was essentially a computer that was dedicated to word processing. This was revolutionary at the time as neither Apple nor the IBM PC had been invented (Apple would "borrow" some of the Xerox technology for its MacIntosh computer). The Xerox word processor had an extraordinary improvement – a pad that allowed you to move the cursor around on the page . . . which they called a CAT. I can't remember what the initials stood for. Before this, the only way to control the cursor was with keystrokes. (Apple then came out with a "mouse" . . . coincidence?) So, we had the first word processors in Lawrence and would revolutionize thesis writing! We also had the latest in copy machine technology.

I found an outstanding typist, Nancy, who could type some 110 words a minute without a mistake! And that was on a typewriter. She took to the word processors like a duck to water. The keys blurred into a symphony when she typed.

You could not distinguish individual keystrokes.

As I mentioned, I was having a blast! Previously, I always thought I was lazy. Really. I always put in the minimal amount of work needed to get what I wanted. Even when I was taking twenty-six hours of classes, I don't think I put in a full forty-hour work week studying. I was always able to get by without doing a lot of work (remember, short-cuts). But this was different. Suddenly, I was working around the clock. I often slept at the store (upstairs in the loft). And I honestly felt I learnt more in the preparation for starting the business and in the first three months of operating it, than I had in the previous two years of school. I felt I earned an MBA in the school of hard knocks. (I would end up with a PhD in this field).

Ironically, it was while I was at Encore that I saw Jan for the first time since our breakup several years previous. She and her *husband* had just bought a bar a few stores down from us. It hurt so much seeing her again, I would never go to her bar for fear of seeing her. I just could not stand it. Nor did she ever drop by the store to see me.

Greg

I am going to interrupt the story to talk a bit more about Greg. When I was young, Greg helped fill a huge void in my life – when Jeff left. He and I became very close. The friendship carried on to college, where Greg (and two other friends of mine from grade school, Don and Brian) joined me at AKL.

Greg and I also became travel buddies. Our first three big trips together were planned. The first, which occurred while we were undergraduates, was a car trip to the East Coast. It was a lot of fun. On our way east, we visited various college campuses. Where possible, we snuck into the football stadium and kicked field goals. I remember doing this at Purdue and Ohio State, but we visited other campuses as well. (Note: neither of us was that good at kicking field goals, mind you, but it was fun. However, another friend of ours from way back, Robert Swift, tried out for the football team and became KU's main kicker.)

The next trip occurred in 1974. Greg and I were both sophomores at KU. It was in March and KU had made it to the NCAA Regionals, which were being held in Tulsa. There was a lottery for the students to be able to buy tickets to the game. I can't remember if it was me or Greg that won, but we had agreed to go together if either had won.

God decided to play a little trick on me, though. Right before the tournament, I developed a very painful pilonidal cyst in my rear end. It required surgery, which occurred the day before we were to leave for Tulsa. I want to say Greg picked me up at the hospital, but I may have gotten to go home first. But if so, it was only briefly.

As you can imagine, my tush was extremely sore. I was given a "doughnut" to sit on, which was both funny and awkward. But it also meant I could not drive. So, we made the trip in Greg's VW Bug. (The original bug, not the horrible redo).

The games were held at Oral Roberts in the Maybe Center. It was a tremendous experience . . . made all the better by the fact that KU won the regional. We had an awesome time, even if I was the "butt" of the jokes. (Keeping our tradition alive, we kicked field goals at both OU and Oklahoma State during side trips).

That was not the only road trip Greg and I would take to watch KU play. We also went to both Hilton auditorium (Iowa State) and Hearn's Center (MU), the two of the most hostile arenas for KU to play in. They were fantastic experiences. I think we won both games, but that may be revisionist history.

In gradual school, Greg and I drove out to the San Francisco Bay area (stopping in Colorado to visit my Aunt), where Don was working as an appraiser. That trip, which was great fun in many ways, had a notable side adventure, and another example of God's mischievous sense of humor. Don took us to meet a girl he was dating, who happened to live on the other side of the bay. She shared her house with several other girls . . . hello set-up. Well, I wound up hooking up with one of her roommates, which was a bit out of character for me. I was not usually into one-night stands, but this was a special circumstance. (After all, Don drove. How were we to get home if we did not stay?)

Anyway, while we were in bed, she happened to mention her boyfriend was a hitman with the mob (a story Don later confirmed). That might have been a bit of knowledge I would have wanted to have before I wound up naked in her bed. But wait, there's more. About 2 am, the doorbell rings. Yep, it's her gangster boyfriend coming over for a bit of late-night tail. Fortunately, she was able to send him away without incident – as she was rightfully upset with his very late and unexpected booty call. (Again, this is before cell phones and texting!). I would hate to think what would have happened if he had been more persistent, or suspicious, that night . . .

Greg, who is aptly named as he is without a doubt the most gregarious person I have ever met, with an infectious grin that almost always is on his face, could be impulsive, as well. Which happened to fit in well with my own impulsiveness.

Our first impulsive trip was as undergraduates. We were talking about some of our high school friends (including a former girlfriend of his . . . one of many) who happened to be at K-State, about an hour and half away from Lawrence, where we were. He lamented how much he missed her. We decided it was a good idea if we dropped everything and drove to Manhattan (Kansas). And we did.

It was my first visit to Manhattan and K-State. And we did it right, visiting Aggieville and seeing his ex and having a blast. We crashed that night at the K-State branch of AKL.

The second trip was the most bizarre, and it firmly established to me God has a very nasty sense of humor and loves to play practical jokes. It occurred when we were both working at Encore . . . where we were the two owners. We were driving back from Ottawa, about thirty miles south of Lawrence, after delivering an order to a customer. We were on US 59, driving north, when one of us (I can't remember now which one, but I think it was me) stated, "I wonder where this highway goes . . ." After a bit of discussion and guessing, I suggested "we should find out!" And by that, I did not mean stop and buy a map, but to continue on the highway to see where it would lead.

To my surprise, Greg agreed. But he had a stipulation. We had to first stop back at Lawrence and get some clothes . . . and he had to call his girlfriend du jour, Heidi. (He and Heidi were quite an item for several years, and the reason for another spur-of-the-moment trip to Colorado, but that was later.) Before leaving, we called the store to tell Joni we would be gone for the rest of the day and next. The excuse? I told her we were visiting my uncle in western Kansas who had invested in the store.

Heidi was not home, so Greg was not able to get her blessing, but he decided we should go anyway. He would continue to call her along the way. (This was not as easy as it sounds today. Remember, there were no cell phones then. So, calling meant finding a pay phone and then shoving lots of quarters in it because it was a long-distance call. I realize these are two concepts foreign to those under thirty in that sentence – "pay phone" and "long-distance." Google them.)

Off we went! Heading north on US 59. As we crossed a state line, we pulled over and celebrated by tossing a football back and forth. By the way, US 59 merges into I-29 in Omaha, and then ends up in Winnipeg. Sadly, though, we never made it that far.

Greg continued to call Heidi every few hours. Finally, when we arrived in Sioux Falls, South Dakota (about 420 miles north), Heidi answered. Well Heidi lacked the sense of adventure Greg and I had. She promptly scolded him and admonished him to return home immediately. Well, by this time it was late at night, so we decided to stay at a cheap motel for the night. But not before making a twenty-minute side trip to the Minnesota border so we could say we had visited that state.

We made it back to Lawrence about 3 pm the next day. Upon arriving, I immediately called the store to check in. That's when God no doubt chuckled. For visiting the store *at that exact moment* was the very uncle from Western Kansas I had told Joni we were visiting! Now, to my knowledge, Uncle Merle *never* before went to Lawrence. In fact, in my entire life to that point, I had never known Merle to come this way, because he would have visited us if he had. And I can't remember why he was there this particular time, except that I know he had some business reason (he owned a bank in Protection, and I think it had something to do with that and not farming).

I immediately headed down to the store. Naturally, Merle was curious as to why we were visiting him in Protection while he was here in Lawrence and I had to quickly explain that Joni misheard. We were visiting *Greg's* uncle, not mine. I think he bought it . . .

GOD'S SENSE OF HUMOR

While I'm on the tangent of God's sense of humor, my first wife was another example. No, she's not that funny. It's her background at the time we met. As you might have guessed, I am a huge KU basketball fan. I never missed a home game when I was in Lawrence . . . even after I left school and could not afford a ticket. That's because I figured out a fool proof way to sneak into the games. This was after trying several methods that did NOT work, including posing as a reporter. I actually "interviewed" the Athletic Director. After the interview, I tried to hide in the restroom, hoping to sneak into the field house, which was attached to the offices. But I think they suspected a scam and a guard made sure I could find my way out.

I now found myself outside the field house in the throng of students waiting for the doors to open. I saw some friends and started talking to them, thinking fast. Then the doors opened, and a mass of students mashed towards the doors, I got my inspiration.

At each door, there were two ticket takers, one on each side of the door. As the mass of student humanity made its way towards the doors, I moved along with it, chatting with my friends. When we reached the door, I went to the ticket taker on the right. I then mumbled an apology about not having my ticket ready and reached in my pocket and pulled out my wallet – but not moving all that fast. After a few seconds, the ticket taker moved on to the person behind me. As soon as he did, I pivoted to the ticket taker on the left. But now I was already in the door. As I looked at him in the eye, I put my wallet away. The ticket taker on the right assumed the one on my left took my ticket and the one on the left assumed I had given it to the one on the right! This proved to be an outstanding trick. I would use successfully for the next three years. It never failed. But back to Ann.

Back in the last 1970s and including 1980, when I met Ann, if you were a KU fan you "hated" two schools passionately. Missouri naturally was one. That is a blood rivalry dating back to the Civil War days when the thugs from Missouri, led by Quantrill, came to Lawrence and burned the town down. We have never quite forgiven them, or the state for that.

The other school, perhaps surprisingly, is NOT K-State. No, K-State has always been more of a friendly rivalry, like one you would have with a close friend or brother. Competitive, yes. Hatred, no. One school might be a bit jealous of the other (like KU of K-State's football success over the past twenty years or K-State of KU's 110 years of basketball success . . .) but we tend to root for the other school when they are playing someone else.

No, back in the late 70's, the other school you hated was Notre Dame. This hatred dated back to a NCAA Regional game in 1975 -- the year after Greg and I went to the Regionals. We had perhaps an even better team in 1975 than the year before. Notre Dame, coached by Digger Phelps, had a strong program as well. That year Notre Dame was led by a phenomenal player named Adrian Dantley.

This should have been a great game . . . but the referees absolutely ruined it. There is no doubt in my mind they were horribly biased. I know, you always think that about the refs, but in all my life, no other game came close to matching this one for obvious bias. Even the network announcers could not believe the calls. You see, we kept fouling Dantley by constantly hitting our faces against his elbows. Every time we started to make a move, the whistle would blow, and blow, and blow. Amazingly, by the end of the game *seven* KU players fouled out of the game, including ALL FIVE starters! Yet, we still only lost by six points. (Look it up, if you don't believe me.)

As fortune (read: God's sick sense of humor) would have it, the following several years, KU and Notre Dame would play each other on a home and home basis. (I think we did for four straight years.) And in each game, the refereeing was particularly horrendous. Now I realize that to every fan, the refs always seem to favor the other team. But these games *really* stood out by the sheer volume of seemingly bad calls. So much so that KU fans grew to absolutely hate Notre Dame.

So naturally, where did my first wife go to school? Yep, Notre Dame.

THE MIRACLE

Back to the story already in progress . . .

The Euphoria of opening did not last long. We turned out to be *too* much of a success. We attracted the attention of another student who was the opposite of Greg and me. He had lots of money and no brains. He saw how successful we were and decided he could do it as well. So, Lawrence went from having two copy stores to four in the space of a few months.

But while Greg and I were smart enough to locate in a different part of town, he wasn't as wise. Instead, he opened his copy store two doors down from Kinko's and on the same block as House of Usher! What an idiot!

Naturally, Kinkos and House of Usher did not take too kindly to this intrusion, and immediately started a copy war. They would drive the price of copying literally (yes) below cost. (You had to pay a "click" charge to Xerox for each copy made on the machine as part of the service contract. They were charging less than the service charge, and that did not account for the toner and paper costs. They were losing money on every copy they made). I quickly realized that if you were losing money each time you made a copy, you were not going to make it up with volume! On the other hand, I would lose all my business if I was charging double their price. As a result, I felt I had to drop my prices considerably (but not below cost). Making things worse, the idiot opened right after school let out for the summer. Meaning this was the slowest time of the year, when it would be hard to be profitable without the added competition and certainly without charging below cost.

This was when I discovered I had a flare for marketing. It was right after the second *Star Wars* movie came out. I took the *Star Wars* theme and created "Copy Wars" ads, with my competitors filling the roles of the villains. The ads were a big hit. (The ads were on this thing called "newspapers." Gore had not invented the internet yet.)

I quickly learned, though, I could not survive charging as little as I was. So, I gradually raised my prices. In the meantime, the strategy of my competitors proved effective. The idiot was out of business in less than six months. While we survived, it was only barely. And we did so by running up a lot of debt. Which, at 25% interest and higher, proved impossible to pay back. Encore ended up folding after three years, even though it was always *operationally* profitable – meaning we generated more revenue than our operating costs – but we could never pay down the debt.

Back to 1980. When the idiot opened his store, it hurt us. Suddenly cash flow became extremely tight. One day, I didn't have enough money to make payroll, so I told everyone it would be delayed a day. I really did not think that would be a big issue. One day. Boy was I wrong! The employees were VERY upset (I think I learned a few new words that day.) I also learned an extremely valuable lesson. NEVER mess with payroll! I vowed never to be late again. (And I never have.) But it got close.

A couple of weeks later, I was in the same predicament. Payday was the next day and I was exactly $200 short in the bank account. What the hell was I going to do? If I missed another pay day, I would surely lose some very good people. It was too late to go to family for more money – even if they had agreed, which was dubious. And I had no money to contribute. Neither did Greg, although by this time, he had stopped working at the store to concentrate on his thesis.

I would like to say I prayed again that day. It certainly would make a great story. But the truth is I don't remember. I could have. But then again, I had not forgiven God for the Jan thing. So, if God existed, we certainly weren't on good terms. Anyway, that night my own personal miracle happened.

I was back at my apartment doing laundry – which I did every month or so whether it needed it or not. I had my own washer and dryer I had bought used a couple of years previous. They worked fine.

I was putting the clothes into the washing machine when I noticed the cap on top of the washer drum was loose. I started tightening it when I realized there was something underneath. So, I took it completely off. And there, under the cap, was a gold ring.

Who knows how that ring got there. It wasn't mine. And I had that washing machine for at least two years and was the only person who used it. I lived alone. So why did the cap suddenly come loose then, at the *exact* time I would need it the most?

I told Greg about the ring and he agreed we should take it to the pawn shop the next morning. Guess how much the ring was worth? That's right. Exactly $200. The exact amount I needed to make payroll. I am not making any of this up or exaggerating.

At this point I recognized this was just too much of a coincidence. It was just too unbelievable. Perhaps it was no coincidence as well that Greg's master's degree was to be in Theology.

At this point, even I, who was still very skeptical of God's existence, had to admit that this certainly *appeared* to be a case of divine intervention. What other *logical* explanation could there be? But I still was not totally convinced.

Let's review what happened, then ask yourself (as I did) what are the odds this all happened at random.

1. The need: It was a critical time. If I missed payroll again, I was in grave danger of losing my employees, which would likely be the end of Encore.

2. It was the *night before* the payroll.

3. I was doing laundry that night. That alone was a rare enough occurrence. Let's put the odds at somewhere between one in seven (not realistic) and one in thirty (more likely) . . . i.e., how often I actually did laundry.

4. The top cap came lose. I had the washing machine for years without any issues with the top. Why did it choose that night?

5. There was a ring under the cap. How many people lose a gold ring in a washing machine? And then never find it? How the heck did it make its way *under* the cap that had been screwed on tight? (The space certainly did not seem large enough for that to happen.) And the ring was not mine. Given I was the only one to use the washer and I had owned it several years, that ring had been in there a long time.

6. The ring was worth *exactly* the amount I needed to make payroll. Not a dollar more, or a dollar less. (And, no, I never suggested the amount to the pawn broker).

Taken together, I would conservatively put the odds at somewhere near 1 in a bazillion.

Later that weekend, I was driving to Kansas City for some reason, I can't remember exactly why now. My parents had moved to Dallas two years previous. But I was gazing up at the little puffy clouds dotting the sky. Staring at those clouds through the windshield gave me an idea of how I could possibly prove to myself that God, indeed, exists. I would put him to a test. But one that no one else would notice and that would not result in a personal gain for myself (which I felt was unethical.) I realized putting God to the test was taking a big chance. Maybe the big fellow would not take too kindly to it.

I decided to pick *one* of the dozens of small puffy clouds at random. If I could make that one cloud disappear without the other clouds disappearing, then it would mean either God intervened, or I had psychic powers. [I certainly did not dismiss the latter as I do believe in ESP, etc. as I will discuss more later]. But, in my mind, even that explanation would indicate the presence of God. I kept a close watch on that cloud as I drove. The cloud disappeared. *None* of the others did.

I recognized the fact that while I tried to pick the cloud at random, perhaps I subconsciously picked a cloud that was already disappearing. So, I repeated the experiment, picking another equally ambiguous cloud, only this time I picked a cloud that was larger than the others and did not appear to be changing. It was also surrounded by other clouds, so it was hard to imagine it disappearing by itself. But the result was the same. The target cloud disappeared while the ones around it did not change. I did not dare try again. I figured God might not take too kindly to being challenged repeatedly! (I repeated the experiment twenty years later and had the same result. I don't need to prove it anymore).

While the "miracle" and the "experiments" did not absolutely prove the existence of God to me, it certainly made me much more willing to consider the possibility. And the more I considered it, the more I realized it was true.

IT ADDS UP

Since that time, I have had many other occasions where similar "miracles" have occurred . . . where an unbelievable set of circumstances would come together at just the right time. These unexplainable events have occurred on both sides of the ledger. I have had equally unbelievable bad luck as often as I have had good luck.

I will give a somewhat humorous example of the latter as an illustration. It happened before my "revelation" and was responsible for ending my career as an astronomer before it got a chance to start. It all had to do with math. It is also another example of God's mischievous nature.

I have always been good at math. And, unlike most normal people, I really loved math. But when my senior year in high school came around, I developed a *severe* case of senioritis. I mean it lasted all year long. I honestly do not recall *ever* bringing homework home. Any homework I had, I would complete in study hall or not at all. Reading? Studying? Nope. The only reading I would do was science fiction – and it had nothing to do with school.

John S. Wait

During my senior year in high school, I took calculus, which was the highest math class offered. In my class were some true geniuses – the smartest kids in the school (I was decidedly not among that select group). The class was taught by one of our assistant football coaches, Mr. Hicks. Let's just say as a math teacher, he was an outstanding football coach. Indeed, we won the state championship all three years I was in high school. He did not believe in assigning a lot of homework. Not only was he bad at teaching, he had absolutely no control over the class. In fact, during tests he made the mistake of physically leaving the room. BIG mistake. So, what happened was one of the geniuses in the front row took the test, completing it in about ten minutes. The test paper would then make its way around the room. We all shamelessly copied. If Mr. Hicks caught on, he certainly did not show it. I don't think he would care even if he found out. This went on for the entire year.

But this created a dilemma for me when I started my Freshman year in college. I had tested out of math, so I did not need it to graduate. (Back then, you could test out of a requirement, but you did not get college credit for it. Man, I wish we had the opportunity of earning college credit in high school like you can today). But I knew I needed it for my scientific career. The problem was – what math class should I take? I realized I did not really learn much from my senior year calculus class, so I would probably be lost in Calculus II. Yet, if I took Calculus I again, I risked being bored out of my mind. Then I saw the answer. KU offered an honors class for Calculus I. Perfect. Sign me up. I thought this would still be an easy course as I had *some* retention from the year before. Yet I should learn more since it was an honors class, and it would look good on my transcript. Boy was I wrong.

To further prove how dumb I was, I enrolled in twenty hours of classes my *first* semester in college. I loved to learn and was thrilled with all the choices I had! (Twenty hours, by the way, was not my record. One semester I enrolled in twenty-six hours). I also learned once you got to fulltime status (thirteen hours), there was no additional charge for extra classes. Fantastic! Again, I was thinking that Calculus would be one of my "easy" classes . . .

By the way, registering for classes back then (1972) was an entirely different experience than today. Remember, no computers, no internet. We had a printed catalog of classes about an inch thick that was mailed to each student a couple of weeks prior to registration. Each class had about a paragraph description and its prerequisites . . . that was it. That's all you had to go by.

The physical registration occurred in the field house and was done by class. The seniors went the first day, followed by juniors, etc. Inside the fieldhouse (the famous Allen Field House) and other buildings, each department had a number of tables set up. On the table were boxes labeled for each class. Inside the box were punch cards. If you wanted to take a class, you would take a punch card, which you would turn in at the end of registration. There were only enough punch cards for the allotted number of students for that class. If you got there too late and there were no punch cards left, you were SOL. This resulted in a mad rush upon the opening of the doors as students scrambled to get in the most popular classes, or those classes required for graduation but were limited in number.

Two things about taking an honors class. First, the class is usually a lot smaller. And second, the class is taught by an actual professor, not a graduate student (unlike many Freshman courses). It was the latter that proved problematic, surprisingly.

I started to realize I may have made a big mistake the instant the professor walked into the room for the first time. He did so accompanied by a cane . . . a white cane he was tapping repeatedly on the floor, while wearing Stevie Wonder sunglasses. Yep, my *math* teacher was completely blind.

Now you might think being blind might pose some problems in teaching *math*, especially calculus, after all, it requires writing a lot of complex equations on the black board (or the projector). You would be right! Dr. Salinas was a brilliant man. He could solve complex calculus problems completely in his head. And I'm sure he *thought* he was doing a great job writing these equations on the board. But, then again, who had the nerve to correct him? The fact the equations that should run horizontally on the board more closely resembled a ski slope? So what? But the fact you could not *read* the symbols he scribbled, that was a bit of an issue.

What may be especially surprising, however, was that being blind was NOT his biggest handicap in teaching the class. The biggest? He was from Brazil. Ok, there is absolutely nothing wrong with being from Brazil. It was not his point of origin that was the problem. The issue was that he had an extremely thick accent. So thick, in fact, that you (or at least I) could not understand a single word he said. Because apparently, he thought he spoke perfect English as he did so at a very rapid clip. And there obviously were no visual clues – like the panicked look on our faces – to tell him otherwise.

So, here I am taking calculus from a teacher I could not understand and whose writing I could not read. Kind of made going to class useless. But still, I had taken calculus a year before, so it should not be a problem simply reading the book and doing the work, right?

Wrong again. Much to my shock, it turns out calculus can be approached (and taught) two different ways. You can start with integration or you can start with differentiation. (At least I think those were the terms). We did it one way in high school. But, unfortunately, this class was being taught from the completely opposite way. In other words, what little bit I had retained from high school *was completely useless for this class.*

Given that I had already discovered twenty hours of credit might have been a bit overzealous for my first semester of college, I was greatly pleased to make a new discovery – you could drop a class you did not like, without any penalty! Thus, I made the not-so-tough decision to drop Honors Calculus. I realize that I could have gone back a semester later and started over, but my pride had been hurt. Besides there were other sciences I could study where math would not be as rigorous as it is in astronomy or physics.

To be fair, math and I have always had a love-hate relationship. I love math and was always very good at it. But I did not always get good grades. It was not because I didn't know what to do . . . I did, always. The problem is that I have mild dyslexia. I flip 9s and 6s. This is problematic in math. I would do the work, but because the 9s and 6s flip, I would get the answer wrong. This still plagues me to this day. I have to always double check my work, and even then, I won't catch it all the time as it will flip again.

College calculus is just one of many examples of where a set of bizarre circumstances came together at just the right moment to cause a life-changing event for me. After a while, you start to think there must be a reason.

Career Track

May 2017

Before going any further, I think it might be helpful to provide a bit more relevant background information. As a lot of my fortunes (pun intended) dealt with my professional career, let me fill you in on what happened.

After a year at Encore, it was obvious the debt mountain was going to be tough to overcome. I decided the best solution was to shed its biggest paycheck . . . and that was mine. I fired myself, leaving Joni in charge. I was still intimately involved, but I would no longer work there, nor draw a paycheck. Instead, I took a job selling this new technology that had just come out − personal computers. I was approached by my Xerox rep, who was quitting Xerox to start selling Xerox personal computers (they were one of the first to sell them). David was a great salesman, with outstanding training from Xerox.

I was starting to get the hang of it, when IBM decided to get into the personal computer market. And that killed our sales. (Xerox had just introduced its first hard drive . . . which had an amazing 5MB of storage! Previously, we were working with eight-inch floppy discs. If you don't know what a floppy disc is, google it. Just be sure to spell it correctly . . .

I left the exciting field of personal computers and took a job as a district manager for Scriptomatic, which was the leading manufacturer of addressing machines. Again, pre-computer, churches and other organizations would use a Scriptomatic machine to address their bulk mail. They would type the addresses on these cards, which would feed into the Scriptomatic and using a process like a mimeograph, would transfer the address onto the envelope or mailing piece. When I joined the company, they had just started selling a labeler, which would take computer generated mailing labels and transfer them onto the mailing pieces.

As a district manager, my job was to sell to the dealers. I took over the lowest performing (by a considerable margin) district in the country. It was also the largest (by far) in area. It included North and South Dakota, Nebraska, Kansas, Missouri, Iowa and parts of Illinois, Kentucky and Arkansas. I was able to turn the district around, more than doubling sales, and making it one of the best in the country . . . in just under two years. This earned me a promotion to Philadelphia to become national marketing manager.

I was just settling into this job and gaining a life-long appreciation of cheese steaks, when the company was sold (ironically to Xerox), and a new President was brought in. We loved the old president, who was a father figure and very sharp. This was not the case with the new President, Harry. Not only did he have a horrible personality, but it was clear he wasn't there to build the business, but to tear it down. (Xerox was more interested in our technology and our customer list). And one of his first acts was to get rid of the position I was now occupying. I had been there less than three months.

This led to one of the most bizarre sequence of events in

my life. They were going to put me back in the field as a district manager. However, the only open territory was one centered out of Indianapolis. Meanwhile, I had become engaged to Ann, who was going to be doing her internship at the University of North Carolina. At the same time, the district manager in North Carolina was interested in transferring to Indianapolis. So, it would seem like an easy fix. Move him to Indianapolis and me to Chapel Hill. Only to this new President, nothing so simple could be easy.

All this was happening at the same time as Ann's lease was about to expire in Lawrence and she was needing to move to North Carolina. So, I flew back to Lawrence to help her pack. We packed, cleaned and loaded up the car and U-Haul trailer, still awaiting word on where we were going. Nothing.

Now it was June 30th, moving day. We had to vacate the apartment, but we still had no idea where we were going. All we knew was that it was east. So, we departed, heading east on I-70. We made it to Carbondale, Illinois, where we stayed the night. Still no word. We were treated to the "honeymoon suite," which, given there were only about twenty rooms in the motel, was not what you might think. Indeed, think of the world's most tacky hotel room, made out in an "Elvis" theme, complete with the requisite velvet Elvis, and you have an idea of where we slept.

The next morning, we took off east again. But we soon came to the crossroads where we either had to stay on I-70 to go to Indianapolis or turn south toward North Carolina.

I pulled over and found a pay phone. (Dark ages before cell phones!) I called the office, hoping for an answer. Finally, good news. They had a decision. My career was heading south. Wait, that sounds bad. The trade had been approved!

We found a townhome to rent on the southside of

Durham, off highway 54, in a neighborhood called Parkwood. Parkwood was one of, if not the first, PUD (planed urban development) in the country. It was close to Chapel Hill, as well as the airport, and right next to the Research Triangle Park (RTP). In short, it was at the very heart of the area known as the Triangle (Raleigh, Durham, Chapel Hill). When we moved there, we had no idea of what RTP was, or its significance. Well it's one of, maybe *the*, most successful industrial parks in the country. It is centrally located, right in the middle of the Triangle. It is huge. It also had two unique requirements of its tenants. One, a large percentage of their land (I think 60%) must remain greenspace, and two, only 40% (or some such number) of their building space can be devoted to manufacturing – and no smokestack industries!

As a result, you can be driving right through the area and never realize you are in the middle of a major industrial park, one that is home to several major pharmaceutical companies and had a huge IBM plant, where they made the IBC PCs. The area is also the major employment center in the metropolitan area, surpassing all the downtown areas – including Raleigh, the State Capital!

The Triangle is also home to three major universities – UNC (Chapel Hill), Duke (Durham) and NC State (Raleigh). They all would play a role in my family's future. But I'm getting ahead of myself.

I was miserable being back in the field. While my ego had been dinged by the downgrade (through no fault of mine), the major problem was dealing with the company's President. He was a real slime ball who had absolutely no problem lying to your face, or to your customers. (He could have gone into politics.) This really upset me. I could not stand the fact that I would tell my customers one thing, then discover the opposite was true.

But if I left, what was I going to do? Well, I had been happy running my own company, I thought, maybe I could do that again. So, I contacted a business broker who happened to know of a mailing service that was for sale at a price low enough, we could afford it. Mailing service? Here I was selling mailing equipment! This seemed like too good to be true.

I could not quite give up selling the equipment, though. I decided to set myself up as a Scriptomatic dealer . . . though that quickly faded as I became more fed up with the company as well as becoming enamored with my new business. But at the time, I thought the equipment sales would be the main part of my business. Because of this, I named the company "Independent Business Systems." The mailing service then became "IBS Mail Marketing." (I know, appropriate for a bs'er.)

The company I bought was strictly a mailing service. They would handle bulk mailings for companies – doing the folding, inserting, addressing, sorting and mailing. It was a very small operation, with just two employees plus me.

But I was aggressive and built up the business. We quickly doubled in size, requiring us to move into a much larger building after a year. A year later, we were again doubling in size and moving to yet another new (and much nicer) location. I was adding services, like design, printing (which we subbed out), first class presorting, and later fulfillment services. We eventually became a full-service mail marketing firm. We could take a project from inception through completion. We also grew to over twenty employees.

But again, I learned a hard lesson about *cash flow*. The problem was we were growing *too* rapidly. We had to lay out our expenses before we got the money to pay for them. So again, while we were profitable on paper, it was not translating into the bank account.

After five years, it became too much, and I had to sell it. And while the value might have been impressive, so was the debt I had to pay off, so I did not walk away with much money.

John S. Wait

INTO INSURANCE

Upon selling IBS, I had visions of getting a job with a nice corner office with a Fortune 500 company. After all, I had an impressive resume with what I did at Scriptomatic and later with IBS Mail Marketing. Sadly, I was to discover that Fortune 500 companies did not *like* entrepreneurs. They did not appreciate independent thinkers (this was 1991).

Frustrated, I got both my real estate and my insurance licenses. In looking at the two markets, I decided the real estate market was about to tank, so I chose insurance. (I was right, the market did tank). I chose to sell health insurance to small businesses, as I was very familiar with the target market. I went to work for the American Health Care Association/Keith Woods Agency – which sold a quasi-group coverage. This was a national company headquartered in Ft. Worth.

Again, I met with success. I was able to choose where I worked, and because I loved to play golf, I chose the Pinehurst market as well as Brunswick County (the NC side of Myrtle Beach), in addition to locally. After a couple of years, I earned a promotion, first to district manager and then to Regional Manager and had offices in both Raleigh and Wilmington.

I am obviously allergic to success, though, because the company went broke. Not mine, the insurance company, and without any warning. I was suddenly out of a job and more money (to pay for the leases of the offices I had rented).

Let's pause for a moment and review my career history up to this point:

Astronomer: Killed before it started when I took a calculus class taught by a blind professor who has such a strong accent, we could not understand him.

Psychologist: Killed when I was asked by the department to give up teaching in order to take a research position. This directly led to be getting into the business world.

Encore: Encore started off with flying colors and was immediately profitable. So much so, that we were in talks to franchise. Then an idiot decides to open a fourth copy story, only he does it practically next door to the other two competitors. It may have taken a bit for us to die, but the death blow had been struck.

Xerox PC sales: Kabooshed with release of IBM PC.

Scriptomatic: I was a rising star, newly promoted to the home office and given a great job and title, national marketing manager. Only to have the company sold three months later and a hatchet-man hired to take over, immediately eliminating my position.

IBS: Victim of our own success. Grew from three people to twenty and from $100,000 in revenue to well over a million in just three years. Profitable, but could never overcome the cash flow issues. This is really the only career change I could have prevented with better management.

AHCA: Started as an agent, and rapidly worked my way up to district manager then regional manager, with offices in Raleigh and Wilmington, only to have the insurance company go belly-up.

I was beginning to feel like I was jinxed. You will also note another trend. Except for the first two careers, which never really started, and for the three months while I was national marketing manager, I never had a steady income. The sales positions were all straight commission. And with my companies, I may have paid myself a salary, but it was variable. In tough times, I would skip my paycheck to meet payroll for the others. In short, no job security, no stable income. Sadly, this situation would plague me the rest of my life with one brief exception.

Money now being very tight again, I had to do something. Since I had been selling insurance, I took a job with John Hancock. Fortunately, the agency I worked for also allowed us to sell group insurance, so I continued to sell group health insurance, while learning to sell life insurance – mostly for buy-sell agreements and for charitable trusts, as I concentrated on the business market.

GETTING INTO GOLF

As Pinehurst was one of my markets, I eventually gained a golf course as a client. This was where I first met Paul, who was the superintendent there. But I really did not have much to do with him as I worked with his boss, Mike, and the business manager, Barney (who would later partner with Paul to form their own company, Signal). (Paul and Barney both later became insurance clients of mine).

It was when I was working with them that I had an epiphany. The golf course was very successful. But, in my opinion having run two businesses of my own, it was horribly run (as a business, not as a golf course). This got me to look more carefully at the industry. As I did, I began to realize several things.

> The golf business was **BOOMING** (this was 1994). You could open a golf course about anywhere and it would

be successful. You never heard of a golf course failing, as a result—

Banks were throwing money at the industry, making ridiculous loans;

Golf courses, as a rule, were horribly managed; and

Golf courses were horrendous at marketing. But they did not need to market. Because of the high demand, customers would beat a path to them.

This was all very interesting. I researched more and learned that there were well over 500 new golf courses under construction, and the trend was increasing. At the time, we only had about 12,000 golf courses total. This meant we were adding about 4% or so to the supply every year.

Most of these courses were being built as part of residential real estate developments as golf courses added great appeal, increasing both demand and prices.

Doing the math, I realized it would not be long before golf would likely reach a saturation point. But because of the poor business practices being employed and a total lack of knowledge about marketing, these courses, and their owners, would be completely unprepared for it when it happened.

The problem was made worse by the real estate development courses, which made up the vast majority of the new construction. The developers did not care whether or not the course was successful. They only needed it to *look* successful long enough to sell their houses or lots. Thus, courses were being built in areas that simply could not support them.

Since I knew how to run a small business and had a great appreciation of marketing, I felt that this could present a great opportunity for me. So, I made the fateful decision to get into the industry, with the hopes of being established by the time the saturation point came. (My vision was prophetic, but what I did not realize was that golf course owners are like doctors, you can't teach them anything. They refuse to accept someone else may know better than them. As a result, even though the need was there, few independent operators would hire a consultant. That's how I wound up working mostly with municipalities, who really needed and appreciated the help.)

I was very fortunate. I was able to make Legacy, the course Paul worked at, my first golf course consulting customer as I helped them with a marketing plan. Then an insurance client of mine in the Pinehurst area was building a golf course. I was able to hook him up with Barney and Paul to help him. This would become my first management client as I became the General Manager. This did not last more than about six months, however. While we were doing well, the head pro, who was in place before I came aboard, resented my presence. Further, the owner did not like some of the decisions we made, which were all either made by Barney or approved by him. However, Barney apparently convinced him I was to blame, and I was given the ax, while Barney remained.

By this time Barney and Paul had formed Signal as a golf course management company. Meanwhile, I was trying to build a consulting practice. I can't remember now who referred me, but I was able to get my first big consulting job, which was a feasibility study for a golf course as part of a proposed real estate development. As I was a novice, I brought in an experienced consultant to help me, Doug. He was referred to me by Barney, if I remember correctly.

This project turned into an eye-opening experience as I quickly learned Doug was not my kind of consultant. His goal was to do everything as easily as possible, while playing as much free golf as he could. He had me gather information and then he put it into a boiler plate he already had written. He then asked the developer what he wanted to show and manipulated the data to show the desired results. This is not my idea of consulting!

It was the last time I would work with Doug and the only time I would ever use a "boiler plate." Nor have I ever asked my client what they wanted the results to show. My feeling was that I would rather deliver bad news (the project is not feasible) and save them millions of dollars, then to sign off on a project I did not believe would work and have them fail. Indeed, I was one of the few consultants during this period (late 1990s) to recommend *against* golf course projects. Although most of my studies were positive.

Signal also came across consulting projects, which they would bring me on to help (defined as doing most of the work and most of the writing). We did several feasibility projects together, many of them for the same client. But that golden goose died, and I got burned as I did not get paid for the last project.

I also sold a management contract to another client, this one in Kentucky. Again, I brought Barney and Paul in to help. But six months later, the same thing occurred as with the first management contract. This time the pro was upset because we put in a policy about him doing lessons on his own time rather than on the company's time. The policy was Barney's, but I was the one to implement it. He complained to the owner, and Barney decided it was all my fault. So, I was let go and Barney retained. It should be noted that in both these cases, Barney did not make it more than another six months before the owner realized Barney was the problem, not the solution.

While I was trying to get established, I embarked on my only real marketing campaign for myself. Dallas was a hotspot for golf course consultants. This was largely due to the presence of the largest golf course management company, ClubCorp. At this time, ClubCorp was privately owned and very successful. But many of its executives left to form their own enterprises. Because they did not want to move, these companies remained in Dallas.

So, on one of my trips to visit my parents, I decided to do some cold calling. I went around and visited as many golf course management and consulting companies as I could, including attorneys who specialized in golf courses, etc. Sadly, no one jumped at the chance to hire me.

Then about nine months later, one of the people I visited, Lynn Fry, called out of the blue. Lynn, a former ClubCorp Vice President, had a company called American ClubServ. (While at ClubCorp, Lynn accumulated a lot of ClubCorp stock as he would always take his bonuses in stock. As a result, he became the largest non-family stockholder in ClubCorp, which paid off handsomely years later for him when ClubCorp went public.) Lynn's company did both management and consulting. He specialized in private clubs, which was an area I had little experience. He proved to be a tremendous teacher and resource. He also became a good friend.

That first call, though, was for a feasibility study in Arizona, not far from Las Vegas, Nevada. For this first project, we worked closely together as he was getting a feel for my expertise. He must have liked what he saw, because he brought me in on several of his projects. And, unlike with Barney and Doug where my education was more in the way of learning what *not* to do, Lynn was a fountain of knowledge. This was especially true with private clubs and with food and beverage. And I was a sponge soaking it up.

Lynn was responsible for hooking me up with the National Golf Foundation's (NGF) golf course consulting division. They had contacted him about doing some subcontract work and he did not want to do it, so he referred them on to me. That began what has been a long (18 years and counting) and very successful relationship for me.

Lynn also brought me in to help him manage a private club in the Tampa area. He had fired the previous GM and had me, and another person alternate as intermediate GM's until a permanent one could be found. This really helped me with my knowledge and understanding of private clubs.

While I started Sirius Golf Advisors in 1995, I continued selling insurance as I knew it would take time to build up the consulting practice. I set up my own office near my house. I rented an office in a building right in Parkwood, from a realtor, Sol Ellis, who owned the building and ran his real estate practice from it.

Sol was a wonderful gentleman. He also had a passion for UNC basketball, which I shared. But he was able to take his one step beyond. He worked as a security guard for the team at home games, escorting Dean Smith on and off the court, and standing near the bench during the games. He had been doing this for over twenty-five years when I met him. Oh, the stories he was able to share!

I was very fortunate to be able to get to see a lot of Carolina's home games, thanks to Ann's best friend, colleague and mentor, Mary Beth. Mary Beth had two season tickets. Ann was not exactly a sport's fan, so Mary Beth took me to several games a year – including the Duke game every year. She always took me, she claimed, because she knew I was a very vocal supporter of the home team! (By this time, Ann was now working on the faculty at Duke. But that did not stop me from rooting vociferously for UNC when they played Duke!).

REALLY? REAL ESTATE

My business grew to the point where I hired a part-time administrative assistant. That proved to be a fortuitous decision. One day, she mentioned to me she was thinking of buying a house. Well, I still held my real estate license, even though I never had used it. So, I approached Sol, who was willing to take me on part-time and mentor me.

I helped my assistant with her house. And then later helped her sister. I discovered I had a talent for real estate and enjoyed it a lot more than insurance. From that point on, I focused on real estate as my secondary occupation while I continued to build up the golf business.

Selling residential real estate also helped my golf career. This is because at the time (late 1990's), real estate was the primary driver for new golf course construction. Thus, the more I learned about the real estate side, the more I would be able to help my developer clients.

Notably, I continued to sell residential real estate part-time until we moved to Georgia in 2015. Initially, I intended to get my Georgia and Alabama license, which was relatively easy as I was a Florida broker and there was mutual recognition (I just needed to pass the Georgia state test). But, after twenty years, I was just tired of selling it.

BECOMING A BROKER

When I moved to Florida, I discovered that my NC experience counted, and I was able to get my broker's license without having to get a salesman's license first. This meant I did not have to work under someone else. This opened an intriguing possibility for me. I could combine the real estate with the golf and sell golf courses, which was a pretty strong market, at the time. Thus, in January 2004 Sirius Real Estate LLC was born – as a golf course brokerage (that also sold residential real estate in Jacksonville).

Four years later, my new wife, Holly, and I would move to the Dallas area. While I continued to operate Sirius Real Estate as a golf course brokerage, I felt it was better for me to work under a broker for whatever residential real estate I would do as I was not at all familiar with the south Dallas market. We were living in Waxahachie at the time. Fortunately, Texas real estate law allowed me to do this. I ended up working for another great guy, Bill Stivers, at Century 21 in Waxahachie. He not only was very helpful for what little residential I was going to do, but he was a passionate golfer as well. He remains a good friend.

LIFE CYCLES

May 2017

Contributing significantly to my conviction of God's existence are the extreme cycles that represent my life. My entire adult life has been like one giant sine wave. There have been few, if any, plateaus, but lots and lots of peaks and valleys. The sine wave periods are highly variable in length, though. They can last anywhere from a few months to two years, before changing direction.

    I realize everyone has ups and downs, that's to be expected. But most people get to enjoy at least some plateaus. Not me. And what is particularly notable, and often very frustrating, is that both the peaks and valleys would approach a threshold value, but never cross it. That is, I would get so close to achieving great success, only to have it taken away at the last moment. Fortunately, the same was true on the opposite end. I would get very close to absolute bottom, where things seemed hopeless and I was full of despair. But again, only to be saved right before it became pitch black. What's also remarkable is that these turns of fortune almost always came out of nowhere and involved things I had absolutely no control over . . . like the ring in the washing machine. Further, the peaks and valleys tend to be of the similar magnitude. If I had a really good year, it was followed by a really bad one, etc.

As I mentioned previously, I always thought as a youth that I was destined for "greatness". Yet it seems every time I was on the threshold of tremendous success, something totally unforeseen or unexpected happened that turned the curve around and sent me crashing. I mentioned some of the career changes in the previous chapter. I have also been close to realizing my dream of *owning* a golf course – even having it under contract – then losing the financial backer at the last moment. And most recently, I had finally achieved a dream by winning a management contract with a project that I had essentially created, so I could manage its transformation . . . only to develop cancer and losing it. And there are many, many more examples.

On the other hand, I experienced unexpected good fortune when things got bleakest . . . when things got so bad, you could not see a way out and just wanted to give up. I never did though, and something good always intervened. Like finding the ring. Such as winning a contract out of the blue or getting a call from someone you never heard of that wants to hire you for a big project that you had no knowledge of beforehand. Or being in deep financial distress, with no way of paying your mortgage and no prospects in sight, then going to a casino and winning $9,500 on a 50-cent bet. Or to be once again weeks away from financial ruin, only to get a contract on your albatross home and win a lucrative management deal within days of each other. Or most recently, to be faced with both the termination of my career and, more importantly, my life due to my cancer tumors growing again, then suddenly have the new treatment, which was just approved by the FDA weeks earlier, start working and the tumors starting to disappear, and then winning a major new contract, all within a few weeks.

Admittedly, sometimes the change in fortune – good or bad – was predictable. A lot of the good fortune changes were the result of hard work and not giving up. Some of the bad swings were triggered from poor decision making. But, in at least as many cases, the pendulum changes came out of nowhere. And before you can say "self-fulfilling prophecy", keep in mind the changes were often from completely unknown and unpredictable sources.

I will also admit my family rescued me a couple of times during extreme financial duress early in my career – my parents did it a couple of times and my sister Juliette really came through when I had nowhere else to turn. But these sources quickly dried up as you can imagine. They did not want to "enable" me in my "misadventures". And while my sisters helped me when I was down, they would not help when they easily could have when things were not so dire. Both easily could have helped me significantly by referring clients to me when I was selling residential real estate in the Dallas area, or when I was doing estate planning, which my sisters needed. I think neither of them ever trusted I knew what I was talking about, even though I was successful in both areas. They could only remember the failures and the fact that I am and always will be the "little" (and *much* younger) brother.

So, I never have been able to achieve that great success I dreamed about. But I also have not seen the very bottom (although I've been close enough, I could touch it). I never experienced a "real" tragedy like losing a child or a spouse, or, until recently, having a serious disease or physical handicap. I've never been homeless. But I have been through four bankruptcies. I've lost two businesses I put everything I had into, which, believe me, is a significant emotional loss. I left my wife and family for a woman who, six years later, turned out to be a pedophile, having an affair with a 13-year-old she then convinced me to bring into our family as a foster child when he was 14. And, oh yeah, that terminal cancer thing.

While I have never had a "plateau" last more than a few months, I can say some of the peaks and valleys were not as big as others. But in most cases, things would always go in the same direction. In other words, either all good things happen, or all bad things. Rarely do I have the good and the bad "balance" out at the same time. (A case could be made of my experiences last summer when I experienced the highs of finally selling our house in Corsicana, getting the management contract and finding the house of our dreams all while suffering from cancer. However, I did not *know* I had cancer at the time. In fact, the doctors were telling me it was nothing serious, just an infection, which was good news at the time. And physically, I was not feeling bad – until September, which is when the cycle began to really change directions.)

One difference between my life cycles and the sine wave analogy. As noted above, the changes in direction often are very sharp turns and completely unexpected, instead of a gradual transition as a sine wave would predict. My life more resembles the peaks and valleys of an EKG, spread out over decades rather than minutes.

I have also found that my luck in little things seems to come in waves, both good and bad. For example, I love playing casino games on my phone. (No, I have never paid for any of them.) What I have found is this – if I am lucky on one, I tend to have good luck on all of them. If I have a bad streak on one, I will have a bad streak on all of them. It is extremely rare for me to do really good on one machine but badly on the others. These games are not from the same manufacturer. So why does it seem they are coordinating? I have learned to take advantage, though. I bet small when I know I'm in a losing cycle and bet larger when on a winning streak. The problem is learning whether a random win or loss is indicating a change in direction or not.

Strangely, though, with each life cycle my faith in God has only gotten stronger, even when the swings were not in my favor. The sources of those swings were often so unpredictable that you start to realize that maybe its destiny . . . that there is a *reason* behind the turn. Perhaps I am not meant to achieve great success or suffer ultimate tragedy, but instead, learn to experience enough of both and deal with sudden changes of fortune and the emotional swings they bring . . . especially the incredible frustration. It's like constantly being teased, with the goal just barely, but forever, out of reach.

Certainly, I have learned from these cycles. When things are going great, I realize they are not going to last. So, I no longer "bet the farm" on the success continuing. Instead, I plan on it not. But I also know I must keep trying to find that ultimate success.

On the other hand, when I am in the depths of depression, I take comfort in *knowing* it will not last long. That somehow, someway, things would change. I believe strongly in the saying "it's always darkest before dawn" (hence the title of my book). I have learned to be patient in waiting for the light to break through And, it always has. There have been many times in my life that I've felt dawn must be coming soon because it sure the hell is dark out there. Now I know just be patient.

I am certain that this is one of the reasons I have not fallen to pieces with the cancer, and why I always remain calm when disasters strike, and why I tend to be a "rock" when things are really going bad.

That works for me. However, these cycles affect more than just me. They are devastating on my family. There is no doubt in my mind these cycles contributed heavily to the failure of my first marriage. Ann is extremely risk adverse and likes consistency . . . the exact opposite of my life. And while Holly is not affected as badly as Ann, it is still extremely hard on her. As it has been on my kids. For this, I am extremely sorry. It is not something I wanted. And it's not like I haven't sought stability. There have been several times over the past twenty-five years I have sent out numerous resumes, trying to find a stable job. But without success.

When you're going through these extreme cycles, it is reasonable to ask, "am I being punished?" when things suddenly turn bad, or "what did I do to earn a reward" when things turn around. And I will admit I am not immune to this speculation. Indeed, it has been a source of a lot of soul searching throughout my life.

But I can never come up with a real answer. I can't find anything I am doing or did differently right before the change in direction occurs. This only adds to my frustration.

Adding to the uncertainty, and resulting anxiety, that is constantly present is that these cycles, as mentioned previously, are of variable lengths. A good cycle may last only a few months before changing directions, with the down cycle lasting a couple of years. This makes it much more difficult to anticipate when the cycle is going to change. Although if a cycle has lasted a couple of years, I know it is overdue for a change.

So, if I am not alternately being punished and rewarded for my actions, then why are these things happening to me?

THE NATURE OF GOD

WHAT DOES HE LOOK LIKE?

May 2017
Now we have established God exists, it is logical to wonder: what does he look like? Is God a *being*, an *essence*, an *energy*, or something else? In fact, can we be so sure God is a single entity, or could Greeks, Romans, and various other religions have it right –there are multiple Gods? Perhaps, what we consider as "God" is really a super-advanced *civilization*, not an all-powerful being. After all, there is no doubt if we went back to ancient times with our modern technology – includ-

ing flying machines, the ability to communicate long distances, etc. – we would have been worshipped as gods. (There have been many science fiction books and movies with similar themes). Or perhaps, as speculated above, God is a collective, made up of trillions of individual "souls," much like our body is made up of billions of cells.

One thing I'm certain of, is that God does not look like an Old Man with a long beard sitting on a throne. I can understand the need for people to "humanize" God as it may help them relate. But the whole idea makes no sense. Think about it. Why would God need a nose? Does he breathe? He's immortal. It would not make sense he must breathe in order to live, so why have a nose? It serves no purpose. Nor would I think he needs to eat. So why would he need a mouth? God supposedly knows all and sees all, so would he really need human eyes and ears? They are too limiting. The eyes can only see in one direction, after all. Would God need hands and arms? His power is unlimited. Do you really see him molding Earth or the Universe by manipulating his fingers? Why would he have legs? That implies he has something to walk on. What would that be? Is it material? If so, *where* would that be? If it's not material, then why would he need legs to move? Isn't that too limiting for a being of God's power?

EXPANDING OUR PERSPECTIVE

Now it makes sense God could *present* himself to beings in any form he chooses, in order to make his message more understandable. But I certainly do not think any physical representation of God bears any semblance to reality. Indeed, I do not think we, as humans, even have the *capacity* to understand the nature of God, any more than a being living in a 2-dimensional world can truly grasp a 3D world. They may be able to theorize about it, but to be able to envision the shape of an apple would likely be beyond their capacity – just like it is beyond ours to imagine what a 4-dimensional object would "look" like. If a 2D being encountered a 3-D object, they would only see a 2-d image of that part of the object that intersects their two-D world. Something as simple as a banana would appear to be anything from a circle to a pointed object to two different and separated oval objects, depending on how that banana intersected his world.

In the same vein, as 3D beings, we cannot truly envision what a four-dimensional entity would look like. We could only see a 3D surface that intersects with our universe. And that shape would constantly change as the object changes its orientation to us.

When I was teaching parapsychology at KU, I used a similar illustration to explain how ESP may be working through the fourth dimension. I used the 2D to 3D analogy. I took a sheet of paper, which has a two-dimensional surface. I would then put two dots on it and ask, what is the shortest distance between these two points? Naturally, everyone would say a straight line. But then I folded the paper, so the two dots touched. Now what is the shortest distance? Well if you're a 2D man, it's still that straight line that goes the length of the paper. For him, the world has not changed. It still has only the two dimensions represented by the surface of the paper.

But for a 3D person, the shortest distance is going across where the two dots touch. Now imagine that paper folded into a tight ball. For a 3D person, they can access the paper at any point. But that 2-D person still sees a flat surface and still must trudge the length of the page to go from one dot to another. While that piece of paper is a wadded-up mess to us in three dimensions, it is still a flat piece of paper to Mr. 2D, because the fold is in a dimension he cannot perceive.

We have a great real-life example of this. Madrid and New York are approximately the same Latitude. So, one might logically think that the shortest distance between the two would be to follow the 40-degree North latitude line from one to the other. You certainly would not think looking at a two-dimensional map the shortest route involves going over part of Canada! But that's because we are used to thinking about maps in two-dimensions, rather than a globe, which is three dimensions. That's why a lot of airline routes are not the "straight lines" when viewed on a two-dimensional map but are the shortest 3D line that goes along the surface of a globe, and thus appear to be a curved line on our 2D map.

But God may exist in a lot more than four dimensions. One could argue "he" exists in all of them. So how can we, who are used to thinking at best in three dimensions, ever hope to envision what God really looks like? (And by using multiple dimensions, it can explain how God can be everywhere – or at least at multiple places at one time in our 3-D universe, if one simply assumes that this 3D universe is simply folded multiple times in each succeeding dimension. Just like we, as 3D beings can intersect the 2D universe of a sheet of a paper, at all points simultaneously, or at multiple points that would appear to be greatly distant from each other in the 2D world but are connected in ours.

When I was very young, probably seven or so, I read a book called "*A Wrinkle in Time*." This book had a profound effect on me and began a life-long obsession with science-fiction. I was thrilled to find recently it is being made into a movie.

In the book, they talk about a Tesseract, which is a cube that has been cubed again in the 4th dimension and represents the progression of line to square to cube to tesseract. I spent hours as a child trying to visualize this, with all the angles being right angles. I would come close, but then my brain would "hurt."

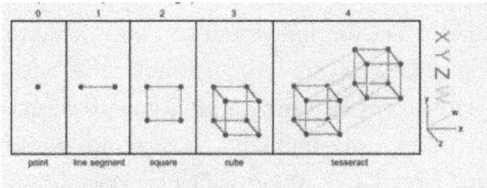

From a point to a tesseract. A one-dimensional cube is two "parallel" points connected by a line segment. A square is formed by connecting two parallel line segments, a cube by connecting two parallel squares. A tesseract, then, is simply two parallel cubes.

Below is a 2D representation of a tesseract. Keep in mind *every angle is a right angle and all lines are equal in length* and no square cuts out another.

Concept of a Tesseract from: http://lightscalar.com/articles/17/how-much-water-can-you-store-in-a-tesseract.

When I was in college, I came up with the theory that perhaps God was more-or-less like a combination of "the force" as described in Star Wars, and pure intelligence. I thought perhaps God was a part of us all. Or rather, more accurately, we are all a part of God. In other words, God represented a collective consciousness that binds us all. When we are alive, our senses and our own thoughts obscure our connection to this collective consciousness. But when we die, these restrictions release and we once again become aware of the collective consciousness.

There are several ways to think about this. 1) We could be deliberate creations of the larger entity, much like appendages, that are used for a specific purpose. In this case, once that purpose is fulfilled, the appendage could be discarded. 2)

We are like cells that are part of a much larger brain. As you know, our individual cells have a sort of brain (the nucleus). Cells act like independent organisms in that they take in food, discharge waste and reproduce. But they are not only dependent on the larger organism but are a part of it -- Helping it process information. Yet the individual cell may have no idea of the larger picture. It only knows about the information it receives and processes. One might argue a cell may be aware of those other cells immediately around it, but would a cell in your liver know about a cell in your brain? Yet they are dependent on one another to survive. Or 3) we may be like a network of computers. Each computer has its own brain and functions independently. But it is also part of a much larger entity – the network. And with today's technology, that network no longer has to be physically connected. Combined with the other computers on the network, it is capable of so much greater things than it can as an individual computer. (Think "internet.") And, like a computer on a network, much of the network processing could be done "in the background" such that it does not interfere with its regular functions. In this case, our "conscious" is not normally aware of the "network" processing. However we do sometimes become aware of it – perhaps as our "conscious" or as an "inspiration" or even a "psychic event". And, like the individual cell, the individual computer on a network may have no idea about the larger picture.

What would these theories state about the afterlife? Unfortunately, the first idea would not require an afterlife at all. We would be merely useful tools. Once we have served our purpose, we can be discarded. But the other two theories provide for the possibility, perhaps probability of an afterlife. Upon our death, we would simply be plugged into a different network connection or have different sensory inputs (cell).

However, the cell theory also allows for a much different afterlife. It is possible once we die, under this notion, our individual identity gets "swallowed" by the collective. We no longer have individual functioning or processing but essentially dissolve into the collective. Not very attractive. However, the cell theory also allows for the cell to "mature" or "evolve" and become something else . . .

The network concept appears more consistent with our notion of individual souls. We are both independent *and* part of a larger entity. Only in this case, our relationship to the entirety would be far smaller than an individual grain of sand is to all the sand on earth.

The analogy of a grain of sand can also illustrate our relationship to the universe. As a grain of sand (if it were a living thing) would be aware of the other sand around it, it would have no idea that there are other beaches in other parts of the world, or that there are other grains of sand buried beneath the earth and its oceans.

In the network theory, our physical body is like I/O devices on a computer, providing input and output to the processor. When we die, the nature of our "input" and "output" changes. But we are still part of the network, only our role within it has evolved.

If the collective conscious exists, our relationship to it may be very different than the three possibilities described above. Or it could be some hybrid of the three. But, to me, the most useful analogy is to think of God as an infinitely large network into which all living things are plugged. It is, in short, the "essence" of life. Our connection to the network is then some unknown "life force".

It is also notable that neither the cell nor the network theory precludes the possibility of a central processor controlling everything. In other words, we may be connected to

God, but there is still an independent intelligence running the show.

A DARK GOD

December 2018

Scientists estimate that at least 67% of the universe is made up of "dark energy" and 27% is made up of "dark matter." We know this because the known matter and energy cannot account for the movements and energy forces we observe. For example, known matter does not account for the effects of gravity we observe both within our galaxy and in the universe at large, as seen in the movement of the stars and galaxies. Something, other than matter we can see and that does not block known energies or particles and has no apparent mass, is generating gravity. This also means all matter we can observe and measure accounts for just 5% of the actual universe. Might God, in whatever form, account for some of this "dark" energy or matter? And, as mentioned previously, our souls?

The existence of a collective consciousness, especially when combined with the idea the collective exists in multiple dimensions, can also explain concepts like ESP and other paranormal activity such as spirits and ghosts. It can also resolve issues separating most of our religions, such as: is Jesus the "son of God." Under the collective conscious theory, we are *all* essentially the sons and daughters of God – or rather all a part of God.

As mentioned above, the collective conscious is much bigger than just humanity. It is made up of all life – both here on earth and elsewhere.

Moreover, if we are a part of God in some form, we

must also recognize that God must have existed before humans came around because "God created them" as well as the rest of the universe. Were our souls there as well?

One might ask, if we are a part of God in some way, why is there evil? Why do people act so selfishly? I could point out the concept of cancer cells . . . But the truth may be something completely different. We will talk about it more below.

BEYOND COMPREHENSION

I honestly don't think we can truly grasp what God is. How can we? If we are to assume our "God" is also *the* God that created the universe . . . well the power that implies is simply unimaginable. It is hard enough to consider the entire universe was once contained in a space less than the size of a pinhead, as modern cosmologists (scientists who study the origin of the universe, not, as our President may allege, the study of hair and makeup) speculate it was just prior to the "big bang", let alone to consider what kind of entity would have that much power to be able to create such a thing. Notably, cosmologists mostly stay away from the thorny issue of how that pinhead universe came into existence in the first place and what caused it to explode. Although some speculate the universe continually goes through cycles of where it expands to its limit, then gravitational energies force it to collapse it once again into the pinhead, before exploding out once more in a never-ending cycle.

Good vs. Evil: The Devil Made Me Do It

December 2018

If there is a God, is there also a devil? Personally, I have just as much of a problem imaging an anthropomorphic ("humanized") devil as I do an anthropomorphic God. I do not believe there is a red entity with horns running around under the earth's surface, or in Los Angeles. But that does not mean there is not a devil in some other form.

There is no question evil exists in the world.

The issue is whether the "evil" we see is being directed by an intelligence other than God. The key words here are "other than God." Could God also be behind the evil as well as the good in the world?

I believe this to be a real possibility. Why?

First, let's go back to a previous question – why are we here? If we are here to learn (or even if we are here to be punished), then it makes sense that there *must* be a destructive force in opposition to the constructive force in order to create the best learning environment.

YIN AND YANG

I have always believed the Chinese concept of Yin and Yang made sense. While they recognize there are two forces at play in the world, they do not construe them as "good" and "evil" but rather as "constructive" and "destructive." Further, they argue *both* forces are necessary and must be in balance.

Think about it. Every act of construction involves an act of destruction. When we build a house of wood, we must first destroy a tree. When we eat to survive, we must destroy other living organisms in the process. Etc. Etc. It works in the opposite direction as well. When we destroy one thing, we are creating something new. Even a force that appears destructive – like a forest fire, plays a critical role in the long-term survival of the forest as it makes way for new growth.

Some of our greatest "evils," like war, often lead to our greatest accomplishments, such as major advancements in science, bringing together differing cultures and civilizations, etc.

One can also argue that the internal struggle we have as individuals, between "good" and "evil" or doing the right thing as opposed to doing the easiest or most convenient thing, etc., helps "temper" our souls. It is often said the struggles and suffering we go through "builds character" and makes us stronger. In that case, I guess I'm pretty strong now.

But then you look around and see examples of pure evil – people who get their jollies from hurting others. You see Hitler and other dictators who actively engage in genocide and wonder how could this be a part of God's plan? You see Charlie Manson and all the other psychopaths . . . There must be another force at work – a negative force – a devil.

I'm sure we all have also experienced our own internal arguments with our "conscience". It does sometimes seem like there is an angel on one shoulder and the devil on the other. And too often the angel loses the argument.

I cannot argue against the notion there are two competing "life" forces. Whether we call them "good" and "evil" or "constructive" and "destructive", or "republican" and "democrat," it does not diminish the argument. The question, though, is whether the two forces are really manifestations of the same life-force or God, or do they originate from different places and with different objectives?

Whether or not they originate from different sources, I think it is clear we owe a lot to the fact that there *are* two different forces that appear to be equal and that work to shape our lives and the environment around us. I think we need this conflict to grow – both as individuals and as a species. But I also think it is quite clear the two forces must be kept in balance.

While it may seem obvious we don't want the "evil" force to win, why wouldn't we want the "good" force to dominate?

First, I object to the idea of assigning values to these opposite forces by labeling them "good" and "evil." That is like assigning the positive pole of a battery, or the north pole on earth, as the "good" pole and the negative pole of a battery, or the south pole on earth as the "negative" pole. They must both exist for the battery to work or the world to survive.

Again, I will go back to the example of a forest fire. On the surface, you might call it an "evil" act. But it is necessary for the long-term survival of the forest and, in fact, does a lot of good. Now certainly from the perspective of the squirrel who may have lost its home or its life, the fire was pure evil. But from the forest's perspective, it is not.

How can genocide be anything but evil? Certainly, from our perspective, it is. But we do not have God's perspective. Maybe from his perspective, it is necessary to introduce such horrendous acts in order to stimulate positive actions in response. Further, if we are to believe in the eternal soul, and further, if we believe that these souls are, in fact, a part of God, then the worst evil being done is to the survivors, not the ones who were killed. That is bad enough from my way of thinking. But then again, if the memory of such massive deaths and agony remains fresh on our minds, perhaps it helps keep our leaders from pushing that big red button that would send us to nuclear war and ensure even more massive death and destruction.

In no way am I trying to justify acts of evil. I think those that commit such acts do so because they have lost their own personal battles. But I also think we need this constant struggle between "good" and "evil" in order to advance, both personally and as a species. I choose to fight for "good" but recognize my concept of good can mean application of both constructive and destructive principles. I want to survive, so I must eat. Doing so means doing harm (or endorsing harm) to other living entities (be they animal or vegetable). For that living entity's perspective, I am, no doubt, part of the "evil" force that destroys their species.

It is also true that it is often not a simple question of "good" vs. "evil." Nor is the distinction always clear. There is the concept of the "greater good." Countries (and churches) will use this term to justify acts, when taken independently, would appear to be "evil" in nature, but when looked at from a wider perspective appears to do a lot of "good". A recent example may be the killing of Osama Bin Laden. Independent of other consideration, this would appear to be an act of murder, which most would consider "evil." But in the context of "Justice" and "what's best for the US" it is considered a "good" act. Indeed, any war or government sanctioned assassination falls into this category. Politicians will argue that cuts to social programs like Medicare and Medicaid fall into this category. The people being affected by these cuts and many others will consider them "evil" acts, but others justify them because they feel it helps strengthen the overall financial health of the country – the greater good. Evangelicals may help elect morally corrupt politicians because they feel these politicians will advance a cause they feel justifies the means.

It is also the case leaders will use the construct of "greater good" to justify acts that are more about personal victory or benefits than one benefitting the members of that group. We are constantly bombarded with cases of "evil" masquerading as "good," which only makes it more difficult to do the right thing.

A POLITICAL PERSPECTIVE

We see this in politics, in religion, in charities, in scams, and in many, many other forms. We must always be on guard for this possibility. But we must also guard against overreacting and dismissing legitimate "good" people, acts, and organizations simply because we fear they are a con. It is up to us to do our own due diligence.

This is why I think our forefathers were so wise in how the set up the government, with a balance of power between the congress, executive branch and the justice branch; and within congress between the House of Representatives, which reflect population, and the Senate, where each state is treated equally. It is also why I fall mostly in the middle, when it comes to politics. I can see where if either side, (let's call it conservative vs. liberal as the parties themselves are no longer clearly one or the other), dominates, it can be bad. In fact, I think we tend to progress the most when there is a balance of power (like the President being of one party and congress another, or the two Houses controlled by different parties) as it forces each side to work with the other to find common ground.

However, as clever as our forefathers may have been, it has not prevented our country from participating in what many today would consider "atrocities" or major acts of evil. We can easily look at some major examples like slavery, the horrible prejudice that has existed against black, Latinos, gays, etc. throughout our history, the unequal treatment of women, the Trail of Tears and other atrocities committed against native Americans, the Chinese Exclusion Act in 1882 and the Geary Act of 1892 which is the only US law to prevent immigration or naturalization based on race, the internment of Japanese Americans during World War II, etc., etc.

We can also look at our political world – in how we will work with dictators who commit atrocities against their own people or have horrible human rights records – because doing so is considered in our "best" interests, either politically or economically. As citizens, we may shake our heads or wag our fingers, but often we do so because we don't understand all the circumstances or consequences of the decision. There often is no clear "right" thing to do. Sometimes it is a matter of determining the lesser of two evils. It's also why it takes a special type of person to be able to make these tough decisions. And this is why these people are rarely all "good" or all "evil." Nor should we expect them to be.

Jimmy Carter is a great example. He is likely the most pious person we have ever elected to the White House, at least in modern times, and, to most, a truly "good" person.

After all, he still teaches Sunday School into his 90s and he has worked on humanitarian causes ever since leaving office. (Jewish people would argue the "good" label, though, as he had an atrocious record when it comes to Jewish people in general and Israel, in particular). But most would also consider him a terrible President. Did his strong moral and ethical codes prevent him from making difficult decisions that might have been for the better of the country? Who can say?

On the other hand, we have Richard Nixon. Most would probably consider him an "evil" person, certainly one who had a very low moral and ethical standard. Yet, he was also responsible for some of our best foreign policy advances. He ended the very unpopular Vietnam war, and greatly improved our relations with both China and Russia, taking us much farther away from the brink of nuclear war that seemed so eminent when he took office. We also made major strides towards improvements in Civil Rights under his Presidency.

Many of our best Presidents had a shaky moral compass when it came to personal matters. There are numerous cases of philandering Presidents. But we tend to overlook these personal flaws if they achieved the "greater good" (especially if it agrees with our own political beliefs). Indeed, today we see Evangelicals largely support a President who most see as being morally corrupt. But because they agree with some of his policies, they are willing to overlook the obvious flaws. And it may be the case that these moral flaws — and perhaps their struggle to control them — are part of the mindset needed for a person to be willing to expose themselves to public scrutiny and more importantly, have the will to make extremely difficult decisions that affect the lives of millions of people. After all, a President, for example, may have to decide to send soldiers into harm's way, meaning lives will be lost because of his or her actions. Would a person who is pure good be able to do something they know will bring others harm? Perhaps a person of strong moral character would not be able to make a decision that could mean the loss of a few lives in order to save many more . . . in other words, to overlook the harm to the individual or to the few in order to pursue the "greater good".

Perspective gives us a better way to judge. But it also can make the distinction between "good" and "evil" even harder to determine. For example, I think most of us, if we had the opportunity to go back into time and be able to kill Hitler before he rose to power, would do it because we know of all the evil he inflicted. But the act of killing him *before* he did all the evil, would, *at the time*, have been considered an evil act. The people of the time would not have the benefit of knowing the future to be able to judge the act in any other fashion.

This is one of the reasons why I feel history is so important for us to understand. There are periods of time in our past as a species or as a country, where one side dominates over the other. We only need to look at what happened as a result to understand the importance of balance. History also teaches us that in the long run, things tend to balance out.

You can see why I struggle labeling these forces as "good" and "evil." An act that may from one perspective, be a "good" act or an "evil" act, from a different perspective (especially over time), may in fact be the opposite. Even the terms "constructive" and "destructive" fail to truly represent these forces, though, as an act of one also becomes the act of the other. Perhaps the terms "Yin" and "Yang" may be the best descriptors after all. Or perhaps we call one "devil" and one "God", even if they both end up emanating from the same source.

PURE EVIL

On the hand, there are some people and some events, that appear to be "pure evil." Destruction or chaos for its own sake, without any intended construction. For example, a sadist torturing his victim for no other reason than his own pleasure or a pedophile abusing a young child before murdering them.

This is different from the evil we assign to those that simply act in a very self-serving way (like certain political, business and religious figures). Is there then a true "evil" that is more than just a destructive force? Which would imply that there is also a pure "good" that rises in opposition.

I'm sure you've had the experience as I have, where you look someone in the eye and just know they are either pure "evil" or pure "good." Where does this come from?

It would seem, then, that "evil" and "good" may be more than just a theoretical construct, but actually represent a "force" of nature, just like gravity. Perhaps some of us are prewired to receive or be influenced by one force more than the other.

Do these forces also exist in the afterlife? Or are they constructs from the same entity that gives us life? And if they do exist in the afterlife, are our souls fighting an eternal struggle, on one side or the other? We may not know in our lifetime, nor are we meant to. And personally, I am not that eager to find out.

ANGELS AND DEMONS

Closely aligned to our discussion of "good" vs. "evil" is the concept of these forces being manifested in physical creatures called angels and demons. Do angels and demons exist?

The concepts of angels and demons, or similar nonhuman entities that influence our life, predates Christianity and appears in a number of our religions. Given its prevalence, one must wonder if there is any truth behind the myth.

Of course, ancient astronaut theorists speculate that aliens could have been responsible for these concepts as their non-human appearance could be described in no other way to ancient peoples.

But we also have people in modern times swear they have seen angels. Exorcisms to remove demonic possessions still occur.

Are these angels and demons a separate entity from God? Are they non-human beings with special powers? Are they immortal? Or could they be a manifestation from our souls after we depart from the corporal world?

I honestly have no idea. I really have not studied the subject (perhaps for my next book?). So, I am open to all of the above possibilities. However, if they are a non-human beings doing the work of God or the Devil, it is difficult to understand why we seem to have such few interactions with them. It seems more likely that humans act more like an angel or demon because they become more sensitive or are more influenced by one of the primary forces of good or evil.

INNER VOICE

January 2018
This brings me to the topic of that inner voice we all have. Where does it come from?

I am going to assume you have a continuous stream of conscious like I do. A "voice" inside your head that talks in your native language and provides a running commentary on your life. It is that "thing" that perhaps we most closely identify with ourselves.

But we really don't talk a lot about its nature. Or how it interacts with our bodies. Or whether it is part of our "soul" that may survive our body's existence.

Let me share some of my own observations.

First, while that inner voice directs what we say and do, it does not seem to actually control anything. By that I mean, it acts like a supervisor rather than a technician. It issues the orders, but those orders are not always followed. Nor is it always involved in what we do. For example, our inner voice does not shout "move your arm," you just do it, while perhaps your stream of conscious narrates.

We are all aware of our reflexes and that this inner voice has no control over them. Ok, clearly reflexes are biological in nature. But what about our other muscular activities? Does your inner voice really control them? Does your voice tell your legs to move when you walk? Or direct the muscles in our hands to close when we grasp?

Really, about the only thing I can think of that the inner voice *may* directly control is what we are saying. I say this because the inner voice is rarely speaking to us at the same time we are talking. This suggests the inner voice originates in the same part of our brain that controls language, which makes sense as the voice is talking in words.

But is the inner voice the only "intelligence" working inside our brain?

We are all aware our brain is divided into two hemispheres. One hemisphere typically controls language, while the other controls non-verbal thought like creativity. Perhaps our inner voice originates from the language center, but we are also influenced by the other hemisphere in non-verbal ways.

Evidence of this comes from when our inner voice may be rambling on about something, but then a new thought or insight emerges from nowhere. Perhaps that "nowhere" is the other hemisphere.

The next question then becomes, who is in control? The inner voice or the creative side? Or somewhere else?

The inner voice does not seem to control our memories. We have all experienced "mind-farts" where we cannot think of a word, or a specific memory, when we want to. If the inner voice controlled the memory, wouldn't it be able to call up these memories on demand? But it doesn't. The memories seem to be triggered elsewhere and then appear in a place where our inner voice can give these memories "a voice." (Scientists tell us our "oldest" sense, olfactory, can trigger memories we otherwise cannot recall.) Sometimes we will get pictures or impressions long before our inner voice can interpret them for us. Yet our body will react to them before our inner voice has even recognized them.

While that voice may be originating from the language center, is it speaking only for that hemisphere of the brain? I would say "no." What I have found is that I can sometimes change the perspective of that voice. If I'm lying on my left side, for example, I may start pursuing one line of thought. If I find that direction objectionable, I will turn over to my right side and a new line will often develop. Or I might generate a different insight into whatever I had been thinking about while laying on my left side.

We also know the inner voice does not always speak in our native language. Those of us (and I'm not one of them) who are fluent in a foreign language find their inner voice will speak in the language they are using at the time.

Nor is it necessarily limited to spoken languages. I believe mathematicians and other scientists can sometimes have their inner voice speak in symbols and equations, while artists see visions.

Let me ask a different question. We already discussed that, except possibly for talking, the inner voice does not seem to control our actual actions, other than to "strongly suggest" what we do. Does the inner voice even make decisions? We know it helps filter data and "think" about things. But does it really make the decisions we follow? Or is it just narrating the process?

I would argue it doesn't. Yes, we will tend to follow the *recommendations* of that voice. But there seems to be many times when we don't. For example, when I get angry, that inner voice may be "egging" me on by recalling all the times the person, who I am angry with, has "wronged" me in the past – in other words, it will seem to be provoking me to get angrier, or to not listen to the other person. Yet, I will often ignore that voice and *not* get angrier, but instead start recalling "good" images. Where does that come from? The decision I make does not appear to be made by the inner voice, but rather by a "higher" conscious that is considering not only what the voice is telling me, but also what the other side of my brain may be saying.

Historically, we have labeled our inner voice as our "conscious," while everything else is our "subconscious." But I do not believe that is accurate. It implies we are not aware of the non-verbal side. But I believe we are constantly getting input from that side and that it directly influences what we do, perhaps as much as our inner voice. The confusion comes from our inner voice sometimes verbalizes the non-verbal input, and other times this input goes directly to the control center causing us to react before we can give it "voice."

Another issue is speed. The process of verbalization is relatively slow. We seem to "think" much faster than we can verbalize. Therefore, we will find ourselves reacting to stimuli before we have the chance to properly verbalize it, even in our "conscious". It often seems like our inner voice is more of a commentator than the actual player. Or perhaps more accurately, a coach, as it provides input and analysis, but we often must react before we can verbalize the thoughts of that action. And I am not talking about reflexes here. Often these actions are clearly the result of intelligence and not rote memory. Yet the inner voice played no role in their being.

The question becomes, "who controls this inner voice?" I'm sure you've had the same experience as I've had, where my inner voice may be pursuing a line of thought, when suddenly it changes direction in mid-stream. Where did that change originate? How does the inner voice even know what to think and report about?

And what about the times it is silent? Is that voice still

talking to you when you are concentrating on something else? Such as watching TV or a movie? Obviously, our verbal center is busy when we are reading or listening to dialogue, but what about the action sequences? Do you verbalize what you are seeing or simply absorb it? We are certainly conscious of what we are seeing, but the inner voice is silent. This alone argues strongly the inner voice is not the same as our consciousness.

If we think of our thought process in visual terms, we may picture the viewpoint straight ahead is being directed by the inner voice, but we are still aware of the things happening on the periphery. But again, I think this is giving the inner voice too much credit. I am not sure it controls the main screen, but rather is responding to it.

I also find it interesting the inner voice sometimes appears in my dreams and sometimes does not. I will have very realistic dreams where I find myself "thinking" i.e. "verbalizing my thoughts" throughout the dream. Yet, in others, I seem to be just an observer, watching what is happening without any verbalization. In yet others, I seem to be the director, able to change how the scene plays out.

So how much of our actual behavior is our "inner voice" responsible? That is a very good question. We already know reflexive behavior is not controlled by the inner voice. There is not enough time for it to respond. But Behavioral psychologists have demonstrated that a lot of our behavior is a conditioned response. This behavior can be shaped through positive and negative reinforcement. Sports coaches, in fact, try to ingrain behaviors in the athletes so they are instantly reacting to stimuli, without having to "think" about it. I would argue these behaviors are not being controlled by the inner voice, although the inner voice may *follow* the behavior – much like the commentator. But its dialogue occurs *after* the behavior has already been initiated, and it may attempt to *rationalize* that behavior by coming up with various reasons why it occurred. In this way, it is self-reinforcing the behavior.

Some behaviors appear to be directly controlled by our emotions, as well. Certainly, how we feel about something we are observing will be influenced by emotions . . . and even *what* we are perceiving is influenced by them. Body language is an obvious example. We don't tell ourselves to smile when we see or hear something pleasant. Nor do we tell ourselves to cry when something is sad. Fear can trigger an escape response or cause us to be paralyzed. We often find ourselves attracted to or repelled by others, without a verbalized thought.

And anyone who has a teenager, or for that matter, was a teenager, knows the power of hormones. Certainly, hormones play a large role in our behavior. While the hormones can manifest themselves as urges that we do feel, often we are not aware of how much they are influencing our actions.

For that matter, there are a lot of biological origins to our behavior. Pain, physical and emotional, certainly changes our behavior as we both try to avoid it and to minimize it when it is present. And, again, we are often not aware of these influences. We may unconsciously walk with a limp, or hold our body in a certain way, unaware we are doing so.

What about schizophrenics, who seem to hear multiple voices in their heads? One might think that if *both* hemispheres of our brain develop language centers that perhaps *both* might generate inner voices, causing massive confusion as to which to follow. Yet some schizophrenics hear multiple voices, not just two. It has been suggested that some of them may be "hearing" the inner voices of other people – i.e. via ESP. Or perhaps "hearing" the voices of spirits. Or maybe they are just crazy.

I may not have competing voices inside my head, but I will often have competing thoughts. However, I can only verbalize one at a time. But I may *act* on the competing thought before I have had a chance to verbalize it.

Where am I going with all this, you may ask. Well, for one thing sometimes I find my inner voice verbalizing things I would normally find distasteful or contrary to my ethical or moral being. It may be arguing for me to do something I would later find to be very bad. Admittedly, sometimes this voice is loud enough or persuasive enough that I will follow through, to my later regret. This was truer in my younger days.

But as I've gotten older, I've learned not to blindly follow that voice. And I decide against it. But here's the point. The decision was made, and sometimes the behavior was implemented, before I had the chance to verbalize it. So, I was acting in opposition to that voice.

And it's not always the case where the voice was arguing the bad side, either. I have had times where my "voice" was telling me to do the right thing, yet I still did the wrong thing.

Going back to my commentator analogy. I have only one commentator. But there are multiple things going on within my brain at the same time. The commentator chooses which action or line of thought to follow, but that does not mean other lines of thought are not occurring at the same time. The key, though, is that the voice is only *commentating*, it is not *deciding*.

Further, the voice may suddenly change what line of thought it is following. Sometimes this is a "conscious" decision on my part. But that "decision" is not verbalized until after it is made.

Freud talked in terms of three levels of our conscious –

the Id, the ego and the superego. The "id" followed our basic instincts – the need for food, shelter, sex and to flee danger. The "superego" was our higher level of conscious. It would tell us the "right" thing to do. The ego was our self-awareness – essentially our "stream of conscious."

Others may state that it's like we have an angel on one shoulder and the devil on the other. Both give us input. And we must decide which direction to go. I am not convinced, though, that there are only two trains of thought going on, as I will often perceive three or more directions to go, and my "inner voice" may be directed in any of those directions and my behavior may end up going in another.

Here is the ultimate question. What part of this belongs to the "soul?" Is it that stream of conscious, that inner voice that conveniently speaks our language? Or is the soul the part of us that makes the actual decision?

We know emotions are mostly, if not entirely, biological in nature. We can manipulate them with chemicals and electrical stimulation. We know our conditioned behaviors are shaped by our environment, and thus also would seem to be biological in nature as they mimic conditioned responses of lower animals. We further know there is a part of our brain responsible for language. It is reasonable to assume that it may also be the origin of our "inner voice." Yet we also know people who have suffered brain damage to this area are still capable of intelligent thought, and even communication. Have they lost this "inner voice" or has it simply changed its nature?

But what about this higher-level decision maker? The one that will sometimes react contrary to our inner voice, or direct the inner voice to consider a different line of thinking? Where does it come from? Is it also strictly biological in nature, the product of our cerebral cortex, or is there something else that gives it direction and power?

We know we can influence how a person thinks by manipulating his or her environment, or by changing the chemicals within their body (i.e. drugs), or through conditioning. Is this also changing that person's soul?

What of our memories? They also appear to be chemically and biologically based. Do they become a part of the soul that survives? This is a question that really scares me. For without my memories, would it still be "me" that survives?

TEMPTATION

Going back to the issue of good vs. evil. I believe we all face temptation. And often that temptation may be to do something others would consider "bad." Sometimes this temptation is expressed by our "inner voice," while other times we simply are aware of it.

Perhaps this is what really distinguishes man from other animals on this planet. We know other animals have intelligences, some appear to be at least as smart as a three- or four-year old human (or older). When you think about it, that's pretty intelligent as they can certainly get into a lot of trouble! But here's the point. How often do you see, or even hear about an animal doing something that would appear to be a deliberate act of evil? (We had a cat growing up, Sparky, that would mercilessly tease my dog. Snoopy was terrified of her and she knew it. She would do things like when she heard someone calling for Snoopy, she would hide around the corner, only to jump out when Snoopy came running up. Or she would lay in the middle of the stairs, effectively blocking Snoopy from going up or down as the case may be. Snoopy would just start whining until we rescued her. More recently,

Holly and I have a cat, Lucky, that would terrorize another of our cats, Cleo. He never overtly attacked Cleo but would seem to "stalk" her. It was funny to watch. I am sure to Snoopy and Cleo, Sparky and Lucky were "evil." But to us, they were just funny.)

The point I am trying to make is that we humans are constantly faced with temptation and whether or not to act in a way others consider "evil." This goes back to my thoughts as to our purpose. Are we here to learn to fight temptation? To learn to distinguish "right" from "wrong"? Or is the struggle the purpose in itself?

I don't have the answers to any of these questions. But one thing is for sure. We will all learn them soon enough. I, for one, am not in that big a hurry to find out.

THE AFTERLIFE

NATURE OF THE AFTERLIFE

June 2017
We all want there to be an afterlife. The thought of simply ceasing to exist is very scary to us. And believe me, the closer I came to facing the end of my existence, the more I wanted to believe in an afterlife.

If we assume there is one, the question becomes, "What is the nature of the afterlife?" Is it a reward or punishment depending on what we do on our time on earth? In other words, is there a heaven and a hell?

ETERNAL LIFE

Whether or not there is an actual heaven or hell, one thing I simply cannot accept is that we are placed there for *eternity* and this is based on what we do on earth. To some, it does not have anything to do with how we lived our lives, but only that we accept Jesus as the Lord and Savior *and* accept that particular church (religion) as the one true religion.

I remember sitting in on a Southern Baptist service in western Kansas when I was visiting my relatives there. The minister was telling the story of how an elderly woman, *on her death bed*, "accepted Jesus and became a Baptist" *just before she died*. Isn't that wonderful, he said, her soul is now saved, amen. I'm sitting there thinking, "isn't it just as possible, her conversion just caused her death?"

There was no discussion as to how she lived her life. But you get the feeling that, according to the minister, she could have been a mass murderer as long as she accepted Christ before she died. On the other hand, she could have lived like Mother Teressa, but she would have been condemned to hell if she had not accepted Christ or become a Baptist. Thus, Gandhi is condemned to hell because he never became a Christian – or even the Pope may be so condemned because he is Catholic and not Baptist. Ridiculous!

First, I cannot accept we spend *the rest of eternity* in either place due to what we have done during our lives – no matter how good or bad that was. I cannot believe God is that unfair. It just does not make sense. Our time on earth, after all, is just a moment in the torrent of time.

Let's put some perspective to this. Instead of eternity, let's assume a much less severe punishment/reward. Let's say the amount of time is equal to the amount of time Earth has existed. Ok, say you live to be 100 – which the great majority of us do not do, and lets further assume science is right, and earth is 4.543 billion years old. This means your entire lifespan measures .000000022 of the time of earth's existence. This is less than one second compared to our 100-year life. That seems an extremely harsh punishment if you did something wrong. Especially if you are a Christian, or a believer in any religion where one of the main tenants is the concept of *forgiveness*. Are we saying God holds us to a much higher standard than he holds himself? Does not compute. (I will say that if hell does, in fact, exist, I suspect there is a special spot there reserved for the people who drive slow in the left lane.)

What does compute is the idea of using the *concept* of an afterlife as a mechanism to try control the corporal life. After all, who can argue against it? As one cannot prove (or disprove) there *is* an afterlife, one certainly cannot prove what you do in life affects it. So, it makes terrific sense to use the afterlife as a way of trying to control the masses, especially when these masses may be otherwise oppressed or living in poverty, etc. Thus, it seems much more reasonable the concepts of "heaven" and "hell" are more man-made constructs than divinely inspired.

My reasoning also takes me back to the concept our earth is the classroom for our souls and our life here is meant for the development of this "soul" of ours. It all fits, except for one thing. What are we expected to learn? And why? (Ok, that's two things). Of these two questions, the second is far more important than the first. For if we know the answer to the second, we can probably deduce the answer to the first.

What, indeed, are our souls "being trained" for? Is there yet another existence in which we participate that requires our having learned a key lesson(s) on earth? If we fail to learn the lesson, are we sent back to school? (Reincarnation). What presents do we get for graduating?

It seems to me one of the lessons has to involve at least understanding, if not controlling, our emotions. After all, experiencing emotional extremes is one thing we all share. Do our emotions, especially perhaps love and suffering, serve as the flames in the tempering of our souls?

EMOTIONAL SURVIVAL

Emotions, themselves, are an interesting story. Clearly there is a strong biological component to them. How much of what we feel emotionally comes from the mind as opposed to our biology? What part, if any, survives our death?

This leads me to a very scary thought. What if the reason we need to understand emotions during our life on earth is because we do not have any in our afterlife? Think about it. We know our emotions are heavily biological in nature – easily controlled and amplified by chemical (hormonal) means. Once our corporal bodies cease, would it not make sense our emotions also cease?

While some may welcome this thought, it also means we lose the concept of emotional attachment – i.e., love. Perhaps that is why there is so little communication between the afterlife and our current life. Our "souls" simply no longer have an emotional attachment to the world it left behind – including all the people (loved ones).

The thought of losing this emotional tie to my wife and kids (as well as my friends and family) is unbearable to me. It is almost as bad as the thought of completely ceasing to exist.

It would be even worse if our soul fails to retain our memories as well as our emotions. At this point, I argue that "I" would cease to exist. While on some level, I am happy at least part of me survives, it gives me little comfort. I've already forgotten enough things; I would hate to lose the rest!

But having no memory begs the question as to how would we learn? Isn't knowledge reliant on memory? Why learn a lesson we are going to forget once we pass the threshold? Thus, if we have no memory of our lives in the afterlife, it pretty much rules out the purpose of our life is to learn.

MORALITY

While I may not believe in heaven or hell, I have always tried to live my life as a "good" person. I strongly believe in the Golden Rule and try to treat others – all others – as I would like to be treated myself.

I hate hypocrites. This is perhaps the main reason I stay away from church as it is full of them. While many are there for pure reasons, so many others tend to go for appearances or worse, feel it is a "get out of jail free card" that makes up for all the bad things they do during the rest of the week. I don't need a minister to tell me how to be good. I know how. And I try to do it, not because of some mythical "heaven", but because I think it is simply the right thing to do.

This moral drive was strong, even back to my teen and college years. This, no doubt, helped contribute to my lack of popularity. I wasn't into doing things that I considered wrong – which includes drugs, disobedience, breaking rules, etc.

I am certainly not perfect. Far, far from it. I am very aware of my faults (see my Self Reflections).

I care deeply about politics, but not enough to do anything about them other than vote (which I do) and complain (which I also do). But I don't campaign or voice my opinion to anyone other than close friends or family or contribute to campaigns. Part of this is business related as I never discuss politics with clients (in fear they would quickly become ex-clients). Indeed, most of my clients probably think I am a devout Republican, because that's what they are, and I listen well to their complaints and proclamations.

Politically, I am mostly a centrist. More on the liberal side on social issues, but not to the extreme. More conservative on the financial side, but again, only slightly right of center, if at all.

Nowadays, it's especially hard to clearly define what a Republican is and what a Democrat is other than one is directly opposed to whatever the other one is promoting. (I say promoting, not believing, as too many times politicians will promote a viewpoint they do not believe in, simply because they feel it is politically – or financially – expedient). Indeed, Clinton, in many ways, would have been considered a good republican in that he shrunk government, got a lot of people off social welfare, and balanced the budget. Yet he was vilified by the Republicans. More recently, the republicans passed a massive tax cut that will add a trillion dollars or more to our national debt. This would have been unthinkable to the "traditional" Republican, who desire a smaller government and a much smaller debt. It seems it is more important to be loyal to the party – or donors -- than to the ideals they historically believed in.

On the other hand, I *try* to live up to a high moral and ethical standard. I don't always make it, but I do value its importance. As I mentioned, I adhere as much as I can to the Golden Rule. I try not to be influenced by society's prejudices and treat all people as equal. I always try to be kind and understanding. When friends and family (and often others) have problems, they know they can come to me for a sympathetic ear and that I will do my best to help them.

While I do not believe we face a judgement panel upon our death, where our life is evaluated and judged fit for heaven or bent for hell; I don't see any reason to take unnecessary chances! As a result, I have always tried to be good and hope that my good traits – in the long run – outweigh my faults. I am also hoping, perhaps, that while there may not be a heaven, it is possible that how we live our lives on Earth will influence what we do in the afterlife. Liken it to school, if we do well, we move on to the next grade. No telling what we get when we graduate.

MOMENT OF DEATH

July 2017

Here is another thought about the afterlife. I have always been amazed at how calm people seem to be when death appears eminent. Perhaps the most dramatic are those facing execution. I wonder why people are so complacent when they are given instructions that only make it easier for the executioners . . . e.g. standing still for a firing squad or kneeling with hands behind their heads when they know they are going to be executed.

Perhaps people are just so scared they are unable to do anything else but comply. Or perhaps it's because they know they are going to be killed, but they are afraid of suffering. So, by cooperating, they are assuring themselves of a quick death and the least amount of suffering. Or maybe they want their last impression made in life to be one of bravery.

I have always thought that, God forbid, if I was in a similar position, I would not want to make it easier on my killer. I would fight to the end, even though I know I am risking a worse death.

Maybe more people do fight. I am certainly not an expert on the subject. But it also occurs to me that perhaps in those moments, the calmness may be coming from God.

THE AFTERLIFE BEING

January 2018
In rereading the above, I realize I really haven't addressed what happens during the afterlife. Do we become ethereal beings? Do we even retain an individual consciousness? That is, are we even self-aware during the afterlife?

Traditionally when we talk of the afterlife, we have an image of a very human existence, complete with homes and family and an earth-like environment and existence. Certainly, that would seem to be most appealing to people in general. And it would be the easiest to understand. But is it at all realistic?

To have such an existence would imply some physicality to our existence. That is, we would need physical bodies and interact with a physical world. But if that's the case, where is it?

We are pretty sure it is not actually in the clouds, or we keep messing it up with our planes. Nor is it anywhere we can readily discern. It certainly is not on earth, or the moon. Nor it is likely to be on any planet or body in this solar system. So where?

It could be on another planet, I suppose. But then that leads to the possibility that earth is another planet's heaven or hell. Maybe we just trade souls. But that would also mean that the afterlife is NOT for eternity. Because no planet is likely to last an eternity . . . not if it is circling a sun. Stars all have life cycles and they will eventually explode and consume their planets.

Could it be in another dimension? Possibly, but again, it is difficult to imagine a physical world that lasts an eternity, given what we know of physics. So, either the afterlife does not last an eternity, or it is not in any way physical in nature. Either way, it most certainly is not the human-like existence we would like to think it is.

This brings up several other possibilities. We do not necessarily have to eliminate an actual physical existence. As pointed out, we could be reincarnated either on earth or somewhere else. But does this happen instantly? If not, what happens to our souls between incarnations?

Could it all be in our soul's minds, like the world in our dreams? As we have little or no concept of the passage of time in our dreams, this may make sense – especially if the initial afterlife is only a waystation for another existence down the line, whether it be reincarnation or another reality. In this case, we can have our homes, our lawns and our family as it is our memories and imagination at play.

That brings up the possibility these dreams become our heaven or hell. Could we endlessly remember our bad deeds or experience our good ones? But even if the afterlife is a dream-like reality, it still calls the question, what is doing the dreaming?

Just for fun, I will suggest a possibility of a physical reality where our souls may exist in our current universe. And that is dark matter. Astrophysicists now believe that dark matter, or matter that we cannot see, makes up as much as 95% of the mass in the universe. That is, matter that we really have no idea about its properties or nature, other than it takes up mass, outnumbers known matter by 20 to 1! That certainly could account for God and a lot of souls!

Perhaps we have no mass but do have a physical presence- like an energy form. Perhaps it is the force that Luke Skywalker masters. Whatever it is, it is most likely of the same physical, or non-physical nature that also makes up God. And it is quite possible, if not likely, that this existence is of a nature that is not perceivable by physical means (no mass, no energy).

There is another possibility, and it is one that I believed in when I was old enough to contemplate the nature of an afterlife – probably around ten or so. It occurred to me that maybe we are already a part of God. We are like individual cells to God's brain. Like a cell has its nucleus, we have our brains. And just like a cell would have very little concept of the body it is in; we have little concept of the being of which we are a part.

In this vision of the afterlife, we simply lose our physical shell and become reabsorbed into the collective that is God. As such, we may become more aware of the collective's thoughts and plans, while retaining some identity that defines our soul (or cell).

EVIDENCE

May 2017

In other chapters, I present a logical argument for an afterlife. But there is also evidence of a post-life existence we can consider.

I will present three bits of evidence. In each case, the evidence is *not* clear, but in fact, highly debatable. And one can easily argue one sees what they want to see in the evidence. Certainly, our motivation is high when considering the afterlife. I don't know anyone who really doesn't want there to be one, unless they are convinced it would not be favorable to them (i.e. they are going to hell).

RELIGIONS

While I don't consider the bible, or any other single written document that simply states there is an afterlife as evidence, I do think the preponderance of religious beliefs in the afterlife as the first bit of proof. Almost every major religion espouses a belief in the afterlife. After all, explaining why we are here and what happens after we die is one of the major reasons behind the *existence* of religions.

This is not meant to be a book on Theology. But I believe most religions have more in common with each other than differences. In fact, three of the major religions, Christianity, Judaism, and Islam, even share much of the same document – the Old Testament. Such is the nature of man we focus on our differences instead of what we have in common! I believe we are more likely to find the "truth" if we look more at what the religions have in common, than what they don't.

We are certainly motivated to *want* to have an afterlife. Not only do we want to continue to exist, but it provides more meaning to our mortal existence. It is especially important for those who have suffered greatly during their lives as they want to believe their suffering serves a purpose. Religious (and political) leaders also like to have not just the concept of an afterlife, but the belief our lives on earth will determine whether our eternal existence is pleasant (heaven) or very unpleasant (hell) as this helps motivate people to be "good" and "follow the rules" when their circumstance may suggest the alternative is better for their current life. Because almost all of us hate the thought of ourselves simply ceasing to exist, religions are formalizing what we *want* to believe.

So, the fact almost all religions state there is an afterlife may not, in itself, be very convincing. But it can also be said where there is a lot of smoke, there is usually a fire. Further, these religions all claim to have been divinely inspired – meaning somewhere down the line one of their religious leaders supposedly received *direct* communication with God and during this communication, the afterlife was confirmed. Thus, disputing these claims means doubting the very core of these religions, meaning everything else they teach is questionable at best. In other words, either all major religions are dead wrong (pun intended) or we must accept afterlife is a real possibility - only the details of that life are up for debate.

More importantly, if we are accepting of the existence of God, we must also at least be willing to consider God at the very least *influenced* the creation of the various religions. (I say "influence" because I find it hard to believe God created "one true religion" and all the others are false. I find it easier to believe God may have "touched" some people in a way they are more aware than others, but being human, these people interpret the touches in their own ways. The prophets all say they spoke to God. How can we tell which ones did and which ones didn't?)

SPIRITS

This brings me to the second bit of evidence to consider – spirits. No, not the kind you imbibe (although that can quickly lead to an afterlife experience, especially if you drive afterwards), but the kind that represent the dead. This includes ghosts (physical manifestations) as well as the spirits that seem to communicate directly with the living.

Do ghosts exist? A Harris Poll recently suggested 42% of Americans believe in ghosts. In other cultures, that number approaches 100%. The same study said that 61% of Americans believe someone else has experience with seeing a ghost, which seems contradictory. A 2009 study by Pew Research said 18% of Americans believe they have seen a ghost, while 29% believe they have communicated with a spirit of a deceased person. This number has been *increasing* over the years, even in the age of science and technology.

There are several shows on TV now documenting ghost sightings and offering "tangible" evidence of their existence (although much of this evidence is easy to fake). What is interesting, though, is the number of times ghosts are appearing in photos, when they were not seen by the naked eye. Indeed, I have had this experience myself, although not nearly as clearly as photos I've seen from others. Again, it is easy to fake – except when you are taking the picture yourself! Which I have done.

And there are literally thousands of places that are said to be "haunted", including the museum where my wife works. Some of these places come with stories and continued experiences that remain hard to explain by non-paranormal means.

Just as one unexplainable event does not prove the existence of ghosts, or of God, or of ESP, or of the afterlife; it is also true that debunking a single event does not *disprove* their existence, nor does it mean that *all* the evidence is faked. Sadly, we find this occurring all the time. It's like those people who seem to believe that an arctic blast in the winter somehow disproves global warming (hello, DC). We all tend to filter evidence to suit our own prejudices and beliefs.

One in five is an impressive number of people who claim they have seen a ghost (and that percentage is almost certainly much higher world-wide) and nearly one in three say they have communicated with a dead person. That is a lot of people to claim are making things up.

And no doubt many, if not most, of the "mediums" we find are charlatans. But there are also many who have come up with stories that are *extremely* hard to explain without resorting to the paranormal, including many instances where mediums have successfully helped in police investigations. But fear of ridicule keeps most of those who have experienced these things silent.

It is also true that if you are not wanting to make your fame and fortune through communicating with ghosts or spirits, you would be highly motivated to keeps such a talent secret. Can you imagine the number of people who would be begging you for help if they knew you could communicate with their deceased loved ones? While others would just think you're crazy. In either case, good luck having a normal career, relationship or life.

It may also be the case some of the "charlatans" are not complete fakes. Most "experts" agree psychic abilities are inconsistent. In other words, it is hard to produce on demand and to control it. Thus, those that may depend on psychic abilities to earn a living may be predisposed to "cheat" because they know they cannot count on their abilities to come through when needed.

I had two aunts who swore they heard my grandmother shout "I'm Free, I'm Free" at the moment of her death, when they were hundreds of miles away and did not know she died. (These stories were confirmed by their families as they reported what they heard before hearing about her death). My parents, however, failed to similarly inform me of their deaths. I had to discover their demise in a more conventional fashion.

I am not about to review all the evidence behind the existence of ghosts and spirits. There are literally thousands of books that have already done so. I doubt if any of them will change your mind. You either believe or you don't – at least until you've experienced one firsthand.

Skeptics are always going to dismiss the evidence. They will point out the known fakes and generalize they all must be fakes. They will disprove some physical evidence and thus claim all evidence must be false. But the truth is many of these instances of hauntings remain unexplained.

Perhaps as interesting as their existence is what their existence would be telling us about the afterlife. Why are there ghosts? Do we all become ghosts when we die? Does our "spirit" survive us intact, which allows us to communicate with the living as our past selves? Or do only certain people become ghosts – usually due to the circumstance of their death? Or only those already dressed in white? (Just kidding).

NATURE OF GHOSTS

Ghosts seem to come in two types: static and active. Static ghosts are ones that are either stationary or whose movements are very repetitive, while "active" ghosts appear to move around and interact with the environment in much the same way as the living. Thus, the static ghosts are essentially like recordings, playing back over and over again, while the active ones appear to be more "alive," and may even act with some intelligence. Some have postulated the static ghosts may be a recording of sorts of the "psychic energy" of the individual, usually at a very traumatic point – like their moment of death when this energy is broadcast. This "recording" then becomes attached to an inanimate object, whether it be a room or an artifact.

This phenomenon may be closely related to the psychic "auras" people claim to see that surround each and every one of us. While there appears to be a "base color" for each of us, these colors – and the shape and intensity of the aura – can change depending on the mood of the individual and the situation. I do not see auras myself, but I am impressed by the fact that when I've talked with various psychics, they agree on the color of my aura or on the color and shape of given individuals. This would seem to imply they are seeing something. The auras have also been associated with acupuncture points. Personally, I am neither a skeptic nor a believer, but I am open to the possibility.

"Active" ghosts are a different animal, so-to-speak. Their existence implies an intelligence still exists within the spiritual shell of the ghost. These are considered a more-or-less physical manifestation of the spirit of a dead person.

Undoubtedly, you probably know someone who has claimed to have heard from a dead person, whether it was a one-time phenomenon such as my aunt's hearing her mother at her death, or multiple times. The number of instances of similar experiences shared by people across the world and across times is just too staggering to simply ignore. Again, could it simply be a case of wish-fulfillment coupled with active imaginations? Possibly. But then, there are so many instances where the "spirit" has revealed information the individual communicating it would have no other way of knowing.

Our western society, though, tends to chastise people who talk about spirits, or psychic events, or other outlying phenomena (like UFO's). As a result, many people who *have* experienced them, refuse to admit it or talk about it for fear of ridicule or worse.

It is also possible society conditions us to reject psychic and/or spiritual input we might otherwise perceive. When my kids were very young (probably six and three), I conducted an ESP test with them using the Rhine deck of cards. While this was not done in a laboratory where conditions could be strictly monitored, I did my best to make sure they could not "cheat." The Rhine deck is composed of cards with various symbols, a circle, a square, wavy lines, plus sign, and a star. I shuffled the cards thoroughly, then placed a card behind a screen and asked them to guess what card it was. Their rate of accuracy was dramatically better than chance. But as they have gotten older, while I have not repeated the experiment, I have not seen any dramatic signs of psychic ability.

What if some mediums are right and they have communicated with the "spirit" of a deceased person? Not only would that confirm a life-after-death, at least for a period, but it also suggests we retain our identity and memory from our corporal existence. I must admit, this is very reassuring, as I could imagine an afterlife where our "soul" may succeed our living body, but our memories are not preserved. I argue, then, this existence really isn't *me* surviving any more than it is *me* lying six feet under, or possibly surviving as an organ in someone else's body.

NEAR DEATH EXPERIENCES

Another bit of evidence comes from the growing body of "near-death" experiences, which come after a person has been pronounced clinically dead. Again, there is a large body of literature on the subject and the reader is encouraged to investigate. But suffice it to say, the number of instances where the experiences are eerily similar is very hard to ignore. Indeed, we are now all familiar with the expression "go towards the light" which refers to the common near-death experience where one sees a tunnel with a bright light at the other end. In many of these cases, the individual often sees other people, usually dead relatives, at the other end of the tunnel either beckoning them on or telling them it's not yet their time.

Scientists have explained this phenomenon as the massive firing of neurons at the time of death. We have all had the experience of where, when we are dreaming, we seemingly experience an event that may last hours or even a day or longer, only to wake up and discover that only a few minutes have passed. This indicates our minds can compact a lot of perceived time into a very short amount of real time. Our minds are also very capable of constructing a reality around our perceptions. If the rods and cones in our eyes are all firing or the optic nerve is stimulated and our brain cannot understand the message, it may well create its own reality to explain what it is receiving. We are all aware of optical illusions (I studied them as a graduate student in perceptual psychology). Thus, the scientific explanation has merit. Except for the fact so many of these stories are very similar. If it were our brains interpreting signals it is receiving, one would suppose each brain would have its own interpretation. How then are the experiences so similar?

Again, I'm not necessarily trying to argue the validity of any of these notions. Each one of them has logical arguments against. But when one considers the totality of evidence, it becomes that much harder to deny the possibility of an afterlife. One thing though is sure, we will ALL know the answer soon enough. Let's just hope that we can appreciate the answer after we learn it!

FAITH AND LOGIC

I will add, though, one more logical argument for an afterlife. And that is the existence of God. If we are to believe in a supreme being that is somehow all-powerful and who has survived since the dawn of time, is it so hard to accept that we, too, have souls that may survive the fleeting moment in time we call a life?

Indeed, it goes back to the question of why we exist. If we believe in God, then it is logical to assume there is a meaning to our existence, (and vice-versa) even if that reason is beyond our understanding. If we further assume this reason is not simply for his amusement, than it is a logical extension to believing our corporal lives serve a higher purpose. The question becomes, is that purpose tied to humanity as a whole, or does it involve individuals.

To the degree we believe God interacts with our individual lives, we must believe there is a reason for Him doing so. A logical explanation would be he is helping us prepare for the future. That his interest is not in our mortal body, but in something that survives this existence – i.e., our "soul." And the existence of a soul strongly suggests the existence of an afterlife.

We have been taught about the existence of souls by various churches and religions. But it is somehow more comforting to me that there is also a logical argument for its existence rather than simply taking it "as a matter of faith," or simply the desire to survive death.

I cannot prove there is an afterlife, just as I cannot prove there is a God. But I do believe both things are true. And it is not just a matter of faith with me, but it also makes sense.

WHY?

WHY ARE WE HERE?

May 2017

Why *are* we here? What is the purpose of life? These are the questions mankind has been asking since the dawn of our existence. We all ask them at one time or another. These questions, though, tend to come into a lot sharper focus when you are facing the prospect of being permanently removed from the equation.

I have tried to answer these questions myself, using simple logic and my own observations. I certainly do not claim to have the answers but hope my thoughts may be provocative.

I start with the premise (conviction) God exists and he somehow is responsible for our existence. After all, if this is not true, if there was no guiding intelligence behind our coming into being, then the answer to the question is unanswerable. If there was no reason behind our creation, then why would there be a reason for our continuing existence? But I have come by my conviction of his existence, not because I was *told* he exists, but because I have *experienced* his presence and even *tested* his presence as I mentioned in previous chapters.

While I am convinced God exists, I am far from certain as to what is the nature of God. For now, we only must accept there was an intelligence and, thus, a purpose behind our creation and presumably our continued existence.

There are those who speculate we are just part of some very sophisticated "video" game. But then that is a purpose. We would be God's toys and our purpose is his entertainment. Let's hope that if that's true, he doesn't have a mean sister who destroys his toys just for the heck of it, or he doesn't get tired of us and toss us into the recycle bin or get tired of losing and hit the "reset" button.

The next step is equally important. Do I accept God, in some fashion, has been interacting in my personal life – like the miracle ring, etc. etc. As I previously discussed, if you examine each turning point event in my life, like the ring, you find the odds are overwhelming against these events being random. But when you look at the totality, in my opinion, the odds become a near certainty they are not random.

Ok, that leaves me with two main explanations *other* than chance. The first was that I or someone else, was somehow creating these events, perhaps psychically (ESP). The other was that they have a divine origin. Either of these explanations would be notable. And, to some extent, I happen to believe both may be true.

I can pretty much rule out that someone else, other than myself, was psychically behind these events simply because there is no one who has been around me all the times they occurred, and only my sisters, who I rarely see, have even been a part of my entire life through the entirety of these events. So that leaves me as a potential source.

I believe in ESP and psychic energy and lots of other things that are not now part of mainstream science but whose existence has overwhelming circumstantial evidence and, in the case of psychic phenomena, even some scientific evidence. Remember, I used to teach a university course on the topic. I even had the opportunity to work for a while with the American Society of Psychical Research, the birthplace of parapsychology, when we moved to Durham. And I also believe that I, personally, have very modest psychic abilities. An example of which is the degree to which Holly, and I are in sync. We regularly call each other *at exactly the same time.* I'm not talking about, "oh I was just thinking of calling you," which also happens frequently, but times where we will call and get a busy signal because the other is calling at the exact same instant. (And for you skeptics who think we might be listening to the same song on the radio and think of each other . . . these most often occur when Holly's at work where there is no radio and I never listen to the radio.). You only get a busy signal on cell phones if the two calls are simultaneous, otherwise it would go to voicemail. And I have lots and lots of other examples of minor stuff. (It has even saved me from a ticket or two when I get the sudden urge to slow down, only to discover a police car over the next hill. Unfortunately, it does not work 100% of the time as the number of tickets I *did* get will attest).

I also think that I might "project" psychic energy, although I certainly am not able to consciously control it. But it may be one of the reasons I am so successful at sales – either that, or I'm just really, really good. But I don't think so. I don't practice a lot of the sales techniques I've learned. In fact, I have tried to reject anything that to me would represent manipulation. This is part of the reason why I hate sales so much. I am afraid that subconsciously I may be influencing people. I understand that "influencing people" is pretty much the definition of sales. And I'm okay to the degree that I feel that I am influencing them to make the right decision *for them*, not for me. The trouble is, that line can get awfully blurry, especially when your bank account gets low.

Also, when I get angry, people get very scared. Now I realize it may be scary whenever someone loses their temper. And my appearance may be scary to a lot of people when I'm not angry. But people seem to really overreact to my outbursts – even when I merely raise my voice and fall way short of an all-out tantrum. And I am not a violent person. Just the opposite. I can remember maybe three times in my life when I struck someone physically in anger. Once was as a child, once was as a parent (I was very angry at my son and gave him a spanking when I saw him being mean to his cousins), and once in college – but it was accidental I made contact (not intentional).

But even if one were to suppose I had great psychic ability and the power to conceivably manipulate huge events (such a causing a 28" rainstorm), why would I do these things to hurt myself? Because half of these weird and unexplainable events have been to my benefit, but the other half were to my detriment. That is even harder to explain.

And while odds against these events being natural occurrences are staggering, assuming they are all circumstantial ignores the fact that each event had a significant and profound effect on my life – literally life changing. If everything was natural, wouldn't some of them be of neutral impact? Or even further helping the direction of my life, no matter which way it was going? But no, each event occurred at the either the height or depth of my cycle and was the principal cause of the cycle reversing direction.

Thus, if you accept that God is real, then you accept the *possibility* he could influence an individual's life in such a way as what has happened to me personally. Given that possibility and the facts presented above, then the only logical conclusion was that God, for whatever reason, has been behind these events.

Wow. This conclusion raises a whole bunch of other questions and possibilities.

The two questions that immediately come to mind are 1) why me? And 2) to what purpose?

WHY ME?

Let's tackle the first one. Why me?

Ok, let's examine some possibilities. First, God could be doing this *only* to me. Now I have an ego, but really? I'm not Trump, after all. Second, God singles out some individuals, but not others. Or Third, God takes a role in all our lives, we just may not be aware of it.

I think I can pretty much eliminate the first possibility. It would, essentially, presume the entire world was created for my benefit or that I alone was placed here for some special purpose. If that were the case, I can certainly imagine a much better world than what we have. One would also expect I would have made a much bigger impact on the world at large than I have.

Could I be one of a chosen few? I am Jewish, after all, the "chosen people." While I cannot rule out this possibility entirely, I can treat it with one of my favorite tools, perspective.

It does not seem reasonable that some people are singled out. After all, aren't *all* people, by definition, God's creation? Why would he then use some and not others?

But I do think his *influence* is going to be different in each person's life. This is because we all have our own purpose. Some may require more involvement with God than others, or more manipulation.

WHY? WHAT PURPOSE?

At this point, the first question, *why me*, dissolves into the second, to what purpose? Obviously, I was wrong in my youth and am not destined for "greatness." Nor do I seem to be headed in the direction of becoming a mass-murderer or other devil-incarnate.

I really can only come up with three main possibilities. The first is that I'm really in some kind of "purgatory", alternating between near bliss ("heaven") and the depths of depression ("hell"). The second is that I'm here to help someone else. And the third is that I'm here to learn something. Each of these has significant ramifications.

There is a funny show on TV right now, called "*The Good Place*" that basically lampoons our concepts of heaven, hell and purgatory. I bring this up because I think my currently being in purgatory is similarly laughable . . . or is it? It would mean heaven, hell and/or purgatory are literally here on earth, for one thing. (Or in our minds?) It would also mean I had to have had a previous existence for me to be so sentenced to purgatory. This, in turn, means there *is* life after death and reincarnation is a reality. Only our return to earth and our resulting life is predicated on what we did in a previous life. If we were bad, we are punished with our next existence. If good, we are rewarded.

This is similar to the Hindu belief system. Thus, while it may not be "purgatory" in the Catholic sense, it does mean our current life is based on our previous lives. And certainly, there is some colloquial evidence for this. Many people have undergone hypnosis and revealed details of previous lives they could not possibly have learnt in their current lives. Others have experienced "flash backs" and "Deja-vu" events that harkened to a previous life. Thus, the idea of reincarnation seems to have at least some merit.

The second possibility is my life here is really for the benefit of someone else. Perhaps I was brought into being only so I could help bring my kids into existence. And that it was not me bound for greatness, but my descendants. Or it could be that I have or will have a profound impact on someone else's life ("A Wonderful Life" comes to mind) that I may not even be aware of. (Maybe I saved a golf course that in turn helped save someone's sanity . . . ☐)

While this possibility may have merit, it also generates some interesting implications. Foremost is it implying God values some lives over others. If my sole purpose is to help another life, then doesn't that imply the other life is more important than my own? It also asks the question, "how does God even value lives?" What is the scale of importance in His mind?

It also raises the issue of predetermination vs. free will. If I was brought into the world because of what I was going to do, then it means that event was already known to God – or at least foreseen by him. He knew I would be needed to influence this "important" person, and thus he brought me into existence to follow this path.

While these implications do not eliminate the possibility the purpose of my life is to help others, it perhaps makes this possibility less attractive. I don't mean I find having a life's purpose as helping others is unattractive. Just the opposite. I would love to think that I have helped others as it would give my life more meaning. I have always tried to live by the Golden Rule (more on that later).

But these implications say nothing about an afterlife, which I naturally find disquieting, especially in my current situation. And it means my life has been predetermined, which leads to a lot of discontent. Further, if my life was predetermined, does that mean everyone's is? What about all the evil in the world? Is that predetermined as well? If so, why?

Indeed, one could argue if everything is predetermined, why would God create it in the first place? What would be the purpose in creating something that seems random but really isn't? There must be some free will involved or the purpose in living a predetermined life is for *us* to experience it. This, then means two things. One, we are somehow meant to "learn" from this experience, and two, there must be an existence beyond our human life cycle in order for us to be able to "apply" this knowledge we gain.

This brings me to the third possibility: I'm here to learn. Now this possibility is interesting. The natural question of "what am I supposed to learn" pales in comparison to the bigger question, why? It would certainly seem to imply what is being educated is my "soul" or "life-force" or whatever you want to call that thing that survives our death, and thus implies strongly such a thing really exists. Otherwise, it would make little sense to spend your life learning a lesson, only to die and have that knowledge go to dust.

It is also possible our lives may serve multiple purposes. My "life" is needed to help another's life – whether to be through genetics or an act of mine; while my "soul" is here to be educated for yet purpose in the afterlife. And, strange as it may seem, it could also mean that earth, as we know it, may really be a sort of purgatory for our soul. We were sent here to suffer and to learn.

While I can offer no "proof," I do believe I was put here to learn. That would best explain to me why my life has had so many dramatic twists and turns, without ever reaching a threshold. And certainly, I feel I *have* learned. Some may call it maturing, but I have become a lot less selfish, a lot more patient and understanding, more sympathetic to others, better able to cope when things go wrong, and have a deeper faith. I also like to think I have become wiser – in more places than just my rear end.

It may also be possible my soul is being "toughened" for some reason, by constantly cycling through ups and downs. (A life-long basic training?) But is not "toughening" another form of learning?

As humans, we all suffer. And we all must learn to cope with suffering and tragedy. It is also very hard to state one person suffers more than another. We can easily say one person has gone through worse *experiences*. But suffering is an *emotion*, and by its very nature *subjective*. And it is a lot more difficult to compare degrees of emotion from one to another. Again, I bring perspective into the equation. A baby "suffers" when he/she is not fed on time, or when his/her toy is lost. We may laugh at this and think this is hardly suffering, but to that baby or toddler who has experienced nothing worse, than that event *becomes* the worst thing they have ever experienced. To them, at that moment, they are suffering greatly.

Thus, it is wrong for us to minimize the degree someone may be suffering simply because the events they are "suffering from" do not seem to be major to us. They are to that person. And until that person develops perspective, or the event is no longer prominent in their thoughts, they will continue to suffer.

And perspective, I believe, is one of the biggest lessons I have learned. No matter how badly I feel, no matter how poorly I believe I am being treated, I do not have to look far to see others who have it so much worse. As they say, always count your blessings.

I also believe that emotional "suffering" is alleviated by

faith. If you believe your suffering has a purpose and/or that you will somehow be rewarded for it, either in this life or the next, then your emotional suffering may not be as intense as it would otherwise be. Perhaps this is part of the "toughening" process. Just like with Job, the stronger our faith, the less our ultimate suffering when we experience dramatic loss.

WHAT ARE THE LESSONS?

So, are we all here to learn? We all certainly experience the gamut of emotions. And perhaps that is one of the things we are here to learn – coping with our emotions. Or perhaps *experiencing* the emotions in the first place. Thus, it would seem we all have things we *can* and perhaps *should* be learning from our existence, but this is a long way from arguing that is why everyone is here.

Then again, it does not seem reasonable to create a world of humans just to benefit a few lucky "souls". Again, it would argue for God having a preference of one human over another, and that just does not seem to me to be very "God-like." It seems more logical, to me, that we *all* are here to learn, that is, we all have "souls" that are here to gain from the experience of living.

REPEATING CLASS

That brings up a couple other big questions. To what purpose is our souls being educated or "developed"? And are our souls – or at least some souls – repeating the education (reincarnation)? It would not be hard to imagine whose souls may have flunked the previous course . . . or on the way to flunking this one. You know who you are . . .

While I have never had an experience that convinces me I've had a previous life on earth, I will say both Holly and I felt an instant attraction to each other. We both were immediately comfortable with the other and felt it was as though we had known each other for a long time . . . and perhaps we had, in a previous life.

One could easily argue perhaps all our souls are recycled. That we are all subject to reincarnation – whether as humans is a further issue. But then again, if our souls are here to be "educated" and our souls are constantly being recycled through lives, we certainly must have pretty dumb souls. Because if history teaches us anything, it is that it constantly is repeating itself. We, as humans, are constantly making the same mistakes over and over. And if God's purpose is to educate our souls so that we can be put back on earth to better mankind with our more advanced souls, you would think he would give us a better memory of our past lessons.

This then, brings up another possibility. Our souls are being educated or developed on earth for a purpose *other* than humanity as we know it. In other words, our existence here on earth is just our school for the afterlife.

I should mention there is a fourth possibility. We are all here strictly for God's amusement . . . i.e. the video game theory. If this is true, it certainly has been a really long game . . . but then there is the possibility God created the world just moments ago and simply gave us our memories of the past . . . I could go on like this, but at some point, we must put our "faith" into something. My faith is that I am not here *solely* for God's enjoyment. (I say "solely" because I do think He has a sense of humor and I am too often the butt of it.) I have no doubt to God, humans are an endless source of amusement. Yet I find it hard to believe a being capable of creating the universe, including humanity and all its complexities, is subject to such a construct as boredom.

Leaving the fourth possibility aside for the moment, two of the other three possibilities require there to be an afterlife, while the third does not preclude its existence. Thus, the logical "scientist" in me believes an afterlife is "probable." Faith convinces me.

PURPOSE OF LIFE

May 2017

Let's go back to the purpose of our life. If our human existence is for our soul to "learn" as I postulated, then the question becomes, why?

If God knows everything, then the lessons would not be for his benefit. This, then would mean that our souls are not somehow a part of God, himself. Or at least, not in the traditional (human) physical way.

So, what are we supposed to learn, and why does God care?

I can think of a couple of possibilities.

The first is that we are being trained for some higher purpose. Perhaps our souls become soldiers in a war with the devil, should one exist. Or against other "gods".

Perhaps our souls in turn become teachers or facilitators, such as angels, that then help other souls develop, whether on earth or elsewhere. But if that's true, what is the "end" game? Is God just wanting us to become as good as we can become? Is he lonely and trying to develop near-equals? Are there other planes of existence of which we have no clue? And our souls "graduate" from one to another?

Perhaps what we think of as God is not a single entity in the same way we think. Perhaps, as I speculated above, God is more of a collective. In that construct, then perhaps God represents the highest level of existence. Our soul is thus being trained to become a part of that collective.

Being a part of a collective implies some individuality is retained. It is even possible we could be part of the collective and retain some free will. Perhaps we are each assigned a specific duty within the collective. And that goes back to the nature of our training.

It is logical to assume that if our souls are being "trained" or "educated" during our human lives, then there is a higher purpose for those souls after our human existence has ended. I have no idea what that is, but it would make sense that it is a much higher purpose as that would explain why so few of our "spirits" seem to remain on earth or try to communicate with the living. We would not be worried about our past, but our present and future.

Here is another thought about the "collective." Using the cell analogy, what if our physical lives are like a body's senses. While we are "living," we become part of the collective's perception of the physical universe. But we are not just sensing the physical reality, but also the emotional.

Another possibility is that our soul is being "tempered" rather than acquiring knowledge. It is being "toughened" for some unknown purpose. Might that purpose be, in some way, helping guide humanity in the future? Think about it. In many of our professions, we have to toughen ourselves in order to perform our job. Perhaps the most relevant are those professions dealing with death, such as doctors, soldiers and government leaders. In the case of doctors, they have to toughen themselves not only to tolerate gore, but also death. While they are constantly fighting against death, they could not perform well if every loss affects them in a way that prevents them from acting in the future. Indeed, they must toughen themselves so that they *can* act in an emergency without fearing loss.

Naturally soldiers have to be conditioned to accept not only death but killing. Killing another human goes against virtually every moral and religious principal. Yet, to do their job, they have to push past that to look at "the greater good." They are conditioned to understand if they do not do something otherwise abhorrent, something worse could or will happen to those they love.

Government leaders also have to make decisions that affect multitudes of human life. Put aside the tyrants who are only looking out for themselves. Government leaders often are put in situations where they must put some lives ahead of others. Potential harm can come to some in order to achieve a "greater good." This includes not only committing war, but such things as allocation of funds, medical care, etc. Again, I go back to Jimmy Carter. Perhaps his strong moral character prevented him from making decisions that would knowing harm some in order to help the many. The truth is in just about every political decision there are going to be winners and losers. You are constantly having to balance what is the "greater good." To do this, you either much be of a single mind, not caring about the consequences, or have toughened your character to accepting some pain to achieve greater gain.

Perhaps this is one of the purposes of our life. To toughen our souls so that they can make decisions post-life that push aside individual consequences or revulsion in order to help achieve a bigger goal.

At this point, I have no idea. I can only hope that my soul does survive my human existence, and, just as importantly, that soul retains the memories of my existence. But one thing I am pretty confident of, the afterlife will *not* resemble life on earth as we know it.

Consequences

As noted previously, I do not believe in a "heaven" or "hell" as they are commonly presented. But that brings up the question, "are there any *consequences* in the afterlife for our actions during our physical life?

I guess one could always say, "do you want to take the chance there aren't?" Yet, most of us do not take these potential consequences into consideration in our daily lives, expect for maybe one day a week.

Some may suggest even, that many of our churches are partly responsible for this. After all, they preach about atonement and how you can be forgiven, or how you can be "saved" if you just accept certain beliefs. Are there limits to this forgiveness? If not, why should we worry about doing the "right" things in life if we can just make up for it in the end.

Again, these beliefs just don't pass the Spock test. Why would God put so little value on doing the right things and so much value on a simple act, one that perhaps is being highly motivated by a sudden realization that one's life is ending soon. It would make more sense that God wants us to *try* to always do the right thing but knows that we are flawed and will not always meet that standard. In other words, it's in the effort not necessarily the results.

I don't think it is that simple. For one thing, it is not always clear what the "right" thing it is. We cannot possibly envision all the potential consequences of our actions. We can only judge on what we know at that time.

I *try* to do the right thing . . . most of the time. I do consider myself to have high morals and character. But I also know I have done many, many bad things in my life (like leaving my wife and children). I have a lot of faults, and these faults (such as my temper) have contributed to many actions I regret.

I do not think there is a heavenly Santa tracking our every behavior, assigning positive or negative points. Nor do I think you can "balance out" a bad act with a good one.

But that does not mean there are no post-life consequences to our actions. I believe our soul is here to learn. Thus, it seems reasonable that if our soul fails to learn the desired lesson(s), there is some consequence.

The lessons are not necessarily knowledge based but can be character. How do we react when faced with disaster? With pain? With poverty? With anguish? Do we rise above our situation and "carry on," or do we let it fester, eating away at our soul? Do we try to take the easy path, even if that path requires us to hurt others? Or do we value others as we do ourselves? Are we willing to make sacrifices for others? Do we care only for ourselves? Are we willing to harm others just to improve our own position?

Can we give ourselves to another fully with our love? Do we allow hatred into our hearts and soul?

But if there is no heaven or hell, you ask, then what would the consequences be?

Simply put, I suspect those consequences are well beyond our mortal understanding. But I do not think they are eternal, as in your short mortal existence determines your future for all eternity thereafter. What makes more sense is that if we do not learn our lessons or fail to develop our "soul" as we should, we face the same consequence we do in our earthly life. If you fail in school, you repeat the grade. Perhaps that is what happens. Perhaps our souls must progress through various "levels" and if we fail to achieve the level intended, we are sent back to repeat.

While this would seem to imply that we all are reincarnated, it does not necessarily mean that we come back in a form we would currently recognize.

IMMORTALITY

There is another consideration at work. Is it right to assume that any afterlife would necessarily be eternal? Are our souls necessarily immortal? Do they necessarily have only one existence after our mortal life? This does not necessarily mean reincarnation, but rather potentially evolving into another type of existence. Think of the caterpillar. It starts as a larva, becomes a butterfly then morphs into a caterpillar. Perhaps our death is the beginning of our "butterfly" stage. Who knows what the caterpillar stage will be like or what comes after? Perhaps eventually we are absorbed into the collective life force, but not before experiencing many different individual evolutions.

UNIVERSAL TRUTH

As I mentioned previously, I think it is inherently illogical to think we are alone in the universe. Indeed, it is far more reasonable to assume there are billions and billions of other planets with life, and a good percentage of these would include intelligent life.

One day, we will prove this beyond all doubt. It may even be possible that there are those who already know the truth (Area 51?). I happen to believe our planet has been visited in the past and that some of the UFOs that have been reported are extraterrestrial in origin. There certainly is a substantial amount of evidence. But it is human nature to reject those things that disagree with our world view.

Could our government know about extraterrestrials visiting earth? If you're open to the possibility, there certainly is a lot of evidence to support that contention. If it's true, I can understand why it would be the most closely guarded secret in history. I fully appreciate the impact that this knowledge would have on the general public should it become known that extraterrestrial UFOs are real.

Think about it. The implications are enormous. First, it would be an incredible blow to our collective ego. For one, it would mean we are *not* the most sophisticated or developed species. Wow.

Think of the military implications. We have a bad habit of being able to weaponize any advanced technology. (We also have a bad habit of using it for better porn . . .)

Imagine the political consequences. One may argue it might lead us to a global government as we need to unite in the face of a species with advanced and potentially dangerous technology. But then the people who have the knowledge about extraterrestrials may not *want* a global government. Wouldn't it be antipatriotic to try to dissolve our borders and our government? Might they also lose their jobs? Their power?

I was convinced when *Close Encounters of the Third Kind* came out it was part of a government plot to try and desensitize us to the possibility of aliens of the extraterrestrial kind being here. Further, that just because they are *alien* does not mean they are *evil* (as in the *Predator* and *Alien* movies). But alas, no announcement was forthcoming. (But I do think the world has become a lot more desensitized to the existence of other intelligent species.). More recently the government released actual footage of UFOs taken by Navy fighters. Yet the release of these videos hardly caused a ripple in the public consciousness – far less than a typical Trump tweet. Are we already desensitized?

The biggest consequence, though, may be what it would do to our world's religions. After all, they tend to be very homocentric – as in, the universe revolves around humans.

But does God have to be exclusively for humans? Wouldn't God also have created these other races, as he has the other planets and the universe as we know it?

So how does God's other creatures figure into our afterlife? It would be my speculation that the afterlife is *universal*. That we share it with souls from other races, creatures, planets, etc. And if that is true, then might our souls get reassigned? Some faiths believe we can be reincarnated as other species on earth – like a cat or a dog or even a butterfly. Then why couldn't our soul become ET? Just saying . . .

EPILOGUE

JUNE 2017

This Epilogue is presented in chronological order. It was written after the main part of the book. It is meant to chronicle my fight with cancer and its impact – as it happened. The dates reflect when each part was written.

June 4, 2017
As I write this, I am anxiously awaiting my appointment with Dr. Bilen on Tuesday (the 6th). This is the beginning of a very busy week, indeed, a busy summer. The day after my doctor visit and infusion treatment, I will be heading to Chicago to start a summer long consulting project for the Northbrook Park District. The following week, I will be heading to Dallas to potentially list a golf course. While there, I will get to visit my sister, Cheryl. I will later have to return to Chicago for a week to do the survey work for the study.

But back to the doctor's visit and why I am so anxious.

Two months ago, I received terrific news. The scans revealed the immunotherapy was working – even better than could be hoped! The tumors in my chest were *gone* and the tumor on my kidney had shrunk considerably.

Three weeks later, things began to change. The abdominal pain associated with my tumor which disappeared in March, was coming back. It began as just an annoyance. But it continued to grow in intensity. For the most part, it would only bother me at night, when I went to bed. As time went on, though, both the intensity increased as did the time I was affected. Eventually it got to the point where I once again had to turn to Percocet along with Ambien at night, in order to sleep.

Both Dr. Bilen and my sister were concerned but had good alternative explanations. Dr. Bilen was encouraged that the pain was intermittent. He believed it could be a sign my left kidney, the one with the tumor, was trying to start functioning again. I also found out from my sister, that abdominal pain is a side effect of Tecentriq, the immunotherapy drug. In short, it could be like the chemotherapy where there was a cumulative effect.

On the other hand, over the last few weeks I have also experienced extreme lower back pain. Initially I just thought this was a return of my back problems. But the pain is not the same – it is higher up on the spine. Adding to my anxiety is that urothelial carcinoma, which I have, can metastasize to the spine.

I am also feeling more fatigued, which has been growing worse and worse over the last two weeks. Again, this is a possible side effect of the immunotherapy. But with my busy schedule coming up, it is obviously a big concern.

One other thing. On Thursday, the first, I had my scans repeated. Normally I get them at Emory on the same day I see Dr. Bilen and have my therapy. But none of the Emory facilities could work me in on the sixth, so I had them done here in Columbus at the same facility I've used before.

Once again, I experienced a mild panic attack during the MRI scan. Now I have never had a panic attack in an MRI, even though I am claustrophobic. And this particular machine was both a wide and short bore, meaning it was about 2/3rds the length the traditional MRIs and also wider. Indeed, when my panic attack occurred, my head was sticking out of the machine.

I was able to finish the scan, the first of four. But I had to take a break. The technician did a great job calming me down. He even took me outside, so I could walk around. Fortunately, the other three scans were a lot quicker and I did not have a repeat performance.

The only other time I had a similar panic attack during a scan was during my initial PET scan at Emory. I attributed that attack to subconsciously knowing what the scan would find. Indeed, the scan revealed my cancer was not restricted to my kidney, but had metastasized to several spots in my chest, making it inoperable. It also meant I had the worst possible situation, a stage IV urothelial cancer. (The one study I found with a similar population to my situation had a ZERO percent 5-year survival record – and that was *after* surgery to remove the kidney, which I have not had.)

So, did my recent panic attack mean my subconscious was telling me the cancer was worsening? Or was I just so anxious about it that it caused the attack? I will learn for sure Tuesday. In the meantime, I'm in for a lot of anxiety filled moments.

So far, I have refrained from sharing my anxiety of this moment from both Facebook and from most of my family. I see no reason to get people alarmed over what may prove to be nothing.

June 6, 2017

I had a hard time sleeping last night. I was very nervous about what the scans would show. The pains I was feeling made me think the tumor was again intensifying. But intellectually I knew there were alternative explanations for them. I clung to hope.

The ride up was filled with somewhat strained conversation between Holly and me. While we tried to stay away from the elephant, we knew it dominated both our thoughts. Finally, I asked Holly what she thought would happen. She said confidently she felt it was going to be a positive result. I assumed she meant the tumor had shrunk and not that she would soon be free of me. I told her honestly, I didn't know. My body was telling me one thing and my mind another.

After the obligatory blood sucking and a hurried lunch, we found ourselves in Dr Bilen's exam room, awaiting his arrival. I'm not sure I've ever been that nervous, although I would like to think I remained calm on the outside. (I would not have trusted me with a hot cup of coffee at that time, though).

It seemed like we waited for hours. But it was probably more like five minutes. Finally, he arrived. He looked at me, then Holly. He was solemn. But then he broke into a wide grin. "I haven't heard from our radiologist yet about the MRI's" he began. I had overnighted the disc with the scans right after I had them taken so he could have them looked at by the Emory Radiologists. But the place where I had the scans done, Columbus Diagnostics, had sent Dr. Bilen a report from *their* radiologist. Dr. Bilen continued, "But I have read the report from the radiologist in Columbus." Dramatic pause. "The CT scans again showed no evidence of the tumors in the chest." Huge sigh of relief. But that left the big one – the one on my kidney that started this whole mess. Another dramatic pause. "Based on the report I read about the MRI, ***they could find no evidence of the tumor on the kidney***." Just like that, the cancer appeared to be gone! Even Dr. Bilen could not believe the results, although cautioning he wanted to wait to hear from the Emory radiologists before he got overly excited. But too late for Holly and me. We were already shouting and celebrating! This would be miraculous! Even if the Emory report came back with signs of a tumor, it was clear it must have continued to shrink.

Dr. Bilen went on to explain that a new study, published just two weeks ago, had established a strong link between the treatment I was on and increased pain. Thus, it was very likely the pain I was feeling was due to the treatment and not the disease. Not a problem. I am more than happy to make that tradeoff. I can handle the pain. I was not quite ready to handle not being here anymore.

While this is incredible news, both Holly and I realize we are not out of the woods. First, and most important, the cancer can return at any time, and has a nasty habit of doing just that. But second, I am going to have to continue getting the immunotherapy treatments – probably for at least a year. This means I am going to continue to have to put up with the pain and other side effects of that therapy. But all in all, it was incredible news!

This year, D-Day for me, meant "**D**one with cancer!".

June 8th, 2017
The day after the meeting with Dr. Bilen, I was on a plane to Chicago for my first consulting job since losing the management contract. In fact, since that was managing and not

consulting, it was my first actual consulting job in almost exactly a year. I would also be reuniting with my good friend Jeff Braeur and Paul, who would be helping me on the assignment. Yes, *that* Paul. I can't help myself. I just can't hold a grudge. While I cannot forget what he did, I can understand he *likely* did it out of loyalty to our client, rather than to me. And I can understand, Howard was investing millions of dollars. Would you want to put everything in the hands of someone who was not likely to be around in a couple of months?

The site visit went great. We also managed to have a good time while we were there. For Jeff, it was a return home as he grew up in Chicago. In fact, he had even done some work at the facility we were helping and his first real job in the industry was at one of their closest competitors. Jeff made sure we had the full "Chicago experience" with hot dogs, Italian beef sandwiches, deep dish pizza and a Cubs game – my first at Wrigley. It was wonderful.

Physically, I was very beat, though. I still get fatigued very easily and the pain in my back and abdomen continued to bother me a lot. And just to top it off, my neck and knee also let me know they were there in a most obnoxious way. But it was nothing I could not put up with, given the situation. And I never felt the need to talk about my situation with our clients.

Dr. Bilen emailed me today the confirmation. The Emory radiologists confirmed the previous findings. There was no evidence of *any* tumor remaining in my body!

July – August 2017

July 10, 2017
The pain is still there. Every night. It's very strange because it does not bother me during the day. But after dinner, it will start and then slowly build. It peaks when I go to bed . . . most nights forcing me to take a pain pill, which I hate doing.

It feels like the same pain I had when I had the tumor. But the tumor is gone! Yet the pain remains as though a reminder of what might have been.

I tell my wife it is a blessing. It is a more than fair trade – my life for some pain. I'll take that trade . . . at least today. Who knows how I'll feel after another year of it?

Apparently, the pain is a side effect of the Tecentriq. Dr. Bilen mentioned a study that had just come out a couple of weeks before my last treatment noting that pain was a common side-effect of the drug. However, in the literature it was noted as a general pain, while mine is very specific – apparently targeting areas where I was already experiencing pain – like my abdomen from cancer, and my back, etc.

The pain I can deal with, though. But what has been much harder to deal with is that my insomnia has returned. The same frustrating insomnia I had exactly a year ago, when we didn't know what was wrong with me. The insomnia that refuses to bow to any treatment. The insomnia that makes me feel like I have "restless body syndrome." The one that is currently driving me crazy!

Fortunately, it is not nearly as severe as last year. But it is bad enough.

For the last several weeks, I have been going to bed at my regular time, which is about 9 pm to 9:30 pm. But I won't fall asleep until 3 or 4 am – only to wake up at 6:30.

One night, I didn't get any sleep at all.

I had been treating it with Ambien with some success. But my doctor and the literature have both warned me about getting addicted to Ambien and that it can interact with opioids (the Percocet I take at night for the pain). So, I am leery of taking it every night. As a result, I have been alternating taking Percocet and Tramadol; and between Ambien and Melatonin. Unfortunately, though, the Melatonin seems to have no effect on me. And so, I type until I get so fatigued, I can't type anymore. Or I play games on the phone until I can't see anymore. Then I just lay there.

What is not helping is the fact I've been of the belief the insomnia last year was my body's way of telling me something was wrong . . . which it was. But now I'm supposedly cancer-free, yet the insomnia has returned. What is the message that it is telling me this time?

The logical argument is the insomnia is a reaction to stress. Last year, the stress was caused because I was suffering from an unknown ailment, plus we were having all those financial issues. This year, the stress may be caused by having so many jobs going on at once. Which, to me, is a good stress and one that I normally thrive upon. That is why I have a hard time believing it to be the case. I've been under a lot more stress than I am today and did not have insomnia to this degree. It was always my "normal" insomnia caused by my brain not wanting to stop thinking . . . which the Ambien was always successful at treating.

And, to be honest, that's the way this insomnia bought started. The brain not wanting to shut off as I kept thinking about work issues. Only the Ambien did not work on it. Further, it then evolved into this restless body thing, which is incredibly frustrating as it makes it almost impossible to lie still – normally required in order to sleep!

Ironically it may also be my fear of the "bad" insomnia is causing it to manifest. This fear creates an anxiety about having anxiety. A vicious circle.

The good news is my daughter Elizabeth is in town visiting this week. It is always wonderful having her (and or her brother). This time, though, I am really putting her to work! Not so much physical labor like I needed her previous visits but assisting me with the research on my golf projects. It is wonderful to have her help!

July 22nd, 2017

Elizabeth left today. It was so wonderful having her. It always is. This time, I hired her to help me with my Northbrook project. I know I put in a lot more work into these projects than I need to, but I can't help it. I feel I owe them my best effort. Besides, I enjoy it. It's like solving a murder mystery as I dig deep to find the clues to solving the crime. Although here there is no crime, just trying to figure out how to best improve performance.

The work requires a lot of research, most of which can be done using the web. I put Lizzy to work doing much of the more mundane research not requiring any special knowledge to do, just good sense and research skills – which she has in abundance.

Yesterday, Lizzy accompanied me to Atlanta for my immuno treatment. This is the second time she has gone with me to Winship. The first was when she and Matt had come at Christmas and both came, which not only was a great morale boost for me, but it also gave them the opportunity to better understand what I was going through.

The circumstances for this visit, though, were radically different from the last time Lizzy came. Back then, we were all under the impression it was likely my last Christmas. And

I both looked and felt like it. Although I didn't know it at the time, my prospects were even dimmer than I thought as my tumors were growing again.

But this time, I am tumor-free. The treatments are to make sure it stays that way.

I remember very clearly the first time I saw Dr. Bilen. He never told me just how long the odds were that I faced. But he did tell me that "we will never get never get rid of the cancer." Our hope was to slow it down and prolong my life "a year or two." Yet here I am, cancer free (at least as far as we can tell).

Sadly, we did not get to see Dr. Bilen this visit. But we did see one of his excellent Nurse Practitioners. I asked her what the odds were of the cancer returning. She admitted no one knew. The treatment I am on is so new there haven't been any long-term studies. But once again, the staff there proved just how wonderful they were. She excused herself for a couple of minutes. When she returned, she told me she just did a quick literature review of the latest studies. There was a recent study (released in the last few weeks) that followed the treatment of 125 patients with my exact cancer and immunotherapy. Only 7% of the patients had complete remission like me. But for the 7%, the cancer has not returned. However, the study was published after only 46 weeks – not even a year. And that's the longest of any study so far. So, we don't know. We can only hope.

On another note, I ended the Lexapro experiment and went back to Wellbutrin. I had been on Wellbutrin for the past ten years, but stopped taking it last summer, fearing it was contributing to whatever was going on with me. And since the insomnia stopped, I attributed some of it to the Wellbutrin. Unfortunately, this created a lot of other problems as my ADHD became worse and my temper and patience a lot shorter. This, no doubt, contributed to the issues I had at Southern Hills. I needed something. Now I'm back on the Wellbutrin, and things are returning to the old "normal."

August 11th, 2017
Yesterday was my 63rd birthday. Having had sixty-two previously, it would not normally be a cause for great celebration. But what made this day particularly special for me was that I was here to celebrate it. Because not too long ago, the odds were against it. So, yes, it was special.

Unfortunately, I am so overwhelmed with work right now, I really did not have an opportunity to do much celebrating, other than going out to dinner with my wonderful wife. But the day was an important milestone for me, nonetheless.

As I write this, I am sitting in the treatment chair in the infusion lab at Emory's Winship Cancer Center awaiting treatment – which I get now once every three weeks. I am used to the routine. I will say that I am particularly grateful for the invention of the "portal" that is now implanted in my chest as it spares my arms from becoming pincushions. Now the pincushion is a square inch on my chest.

I am here alone as Holly and I decided she did not have to come to the treatments anymore. Why should she have to take another day off for something so routine, with no side effects requiring her assistance.

The treatment itself is only thirty minutes long and involves being hooked up to an IV bag attached to said portal through a series of tubes and valves. Very impressive looking I must say. However, the entire ordeal takes all day. My bloodwork was scheduled for 8:30 in the morning, meaning I had to leave home at 6 am in order to fight Atlanta rush hour traffic to get here. Then came the doctor's appointment, where they review the lab results (I am amazed at how fast they are able to get them – in about an hour!) and give me their blessing and whatever good voodoo they have. Next, I see my psychiatrist, Dr. Baer, who is a wonderful lady. She is trying to help me with my insomnia that has been plaguing me the past two months. So far, without great success.

She is wanting to take me off Ambien, which is the only thing that has helped me get some sleep. She is concerned about the drug reaction between Ambien and opioids. Even though I only take a pain pill at night, she is concerned it may be an issue. So, I tell her that I try to take the Percocet about once every three days now – taking the tramadol instead. I then learn that Tramadol is also an opioid, which I did not know. So, my strategy was not very good! Now I must find something else to help with the pain, so I can sleep.

The doctors and nurses here always ask about my pain level and what issues I am having with the medicine. But I feel conflicted in telling them about all my pains and sufferings. Because none of them compare to what I have already suffered through . . . and apparently beaten. To complain about a little pain (ok moderate pain at times) seems somehow ungrateful. I do tell them what I am feeling, though, because I know it is important. But I also make sure to tell them that I am not complaining! I definitely got the better side of that bargain.

[Update: The alternative pain medicine my regular doctor prescribed was a high dose of ibuprofen. However, when Dr. Bilen found out, he told me to stop taking it immediately. Turns out ibuprofen is hard on the kidneys. And since I now have only one, that's a problem.]

September – November 10, 2017

September 22, 2017

Today was the first set of scans since getting the "all clear" back in June. Naturally, I was very nervous going in. I was still having abdominal pain, although not nearly as severe as before. In fact, I probably only had to take a pain pill maybe a couple of times a week (I occasionally also need one for my other chronic issues like my neck and back.)

These scans were done back at Emory, at the downtown hospital where I normally have the scans. This makes for a long day as we must leave around 5:30 am to get to the hospital by 8 – given the Atlanta rush hour. Holly goes with me on the scan visits. She is there for support and to hear the results firsthand, and in case she has to kill the doctor if he gives us bad news.

In this case, there was no "Dr." Dr. Bilen is out of town, so the report was given to us by his very capable nurse practitioner, Greta. We were fully expecting to hear there had been no change from the last scan, as that one had already given us the all clear.

She began by telling us "Good news, the tumors are continuing to shrink . . ." Holly and I looked at each other. What did she mean, "continuing to shrink?" The last scan said they were GONE. She continued, "and the lymph node near the kidney has also continued to shrink. The tumor on the kidney is now just a cm in diameter . . ."

I had to ask, "but the last scan said it was gone! Does this mean it has come back?"

She reassured us the tumor was shrinking as evidenced

by the other measurements – like the lymph node. And that it was likely the previous scan simply missed it. Perhaps the other MRI was not as sensitive.

This is twice now, with the same tumor, a scan (or the radiologist reading it) failed to detect it. Of course, the first one was most critical. But I can't help but wonder how often this occurs? We put so much faith in these expensive machines we tend to believe they are infallible – the last word. And, as my own personal experience has shown, Doctors are just as susceptible as us patients in misplacing our faith in them.

But now I must readjust. I had told everyone I was miraculously cancer-free. I am not. Although the miracle is only slightly less impressive as I am *almost* cancer free. The only remaining tumor is the original one on my kidney, and it's a lot smaller. But still, I feel guilty about telling people the good news, only to have to come back with a more cautionary tale. Yet I am still very thankful we are making great progress!

However, Greta wasn't done . . . "We also found a spot on your prostrate. It could be nothing, but on your next visit, we will do a PSA test."

Talk about a double whammy, not only was I not rid of my urothelial cancer, but now I might have a second cancer? I knew prostate cancer was very treatable, especially if it's caught early enough – but my father-in-law (another John) had *just* died from prostate cancer, so I also knew what could happen.

My father-in-law's passing was hard. He was loved by everyone who knew him. He had a wonderful sense of humor. He had been in the Air Force (like my father, although much later – for the Korean War), and then continued his life in public service by being a fireman for Beverly Farms, a suburb on Boston's northern shore. He would retire as Captain. And he loved golf. I remember our rounds together very fondly. My kids adored him. And I know the fact he died from cancer and that I also have cancer weighed heavily on their shoulders.

October 17, 2017

This is my first infusion visit since the last scan. It is also the first time I get to talk to Dr. Bilen in person (although he called me the Monday after the scan to again put my mind at rest). Dr. Bilen reassured me we are making progress and that it was not uncommon for scans to miss tumors this small (which is good that it was now so small as to be hard to detect). But it also may be indicative of the difference in equipment.

Dr. Bilen seemed a bit more concerned about the spot on my prostrate, calling it a lesion. He is not worried, knowing if it was cancer it should be readily treatable. Nonetheless he will be presenting it to the tumor board next week, which includes a urologist. It is possible they may want to do a biopsy.

At the time Dr. Bilen talked to me, the PSA result was not back. I got that result a few hours later, when I was doing the infusion. My PSA is normal. Whew. But then, what is causing the lesion and why is it only now showing up? And could it have been responsible for my pain in that region two years ago?

The nursing staff in the infusion center were, as always, top notch. They are very good in both what they do and in comforting the patients.

November 10, 2017

Here I am once again at the infusion center. The process has become routine . . . the drive to Atlanta, fighting rush hour traffic, lunch at Romeo's (where I usually have a delicious Philly steak sandwich for lunch), then lab, then killing about an hour - often by reading in the nice patient/family room they have, then the visit with Dr. Bilen, and finally down to the fusion lab. After the infusion, I head back to Romeo's where I pick up a pizza (authentic New York style) for Holly and me to have for dinner, then battle rush hour and head home. Really, the only concern I had this time was that spot on the prostate. Last time, Dr. Bilen said he would present it to the tumor board, which includes a urologist. Since he did not call me, I knew the news was good. But still I wanted to hear it.

Dr. Bilen told me they went back and reviewed my previous MRI's and discovered the lesion had been present. It did not appear to be increasing in size. And since the PSA test was normal, they were not that concerned about it. Since I was getting scans every three months and he was adding PSA's to my blood tests, which were every three weeks, we would know quickly if the lesion starts to grow, or my PSA increases. At that time, a biopsy would be needed.

I asked him if he thought it was cancer, and he didn't really say "yes" or "no", instead saying it was nothing to be too worried about now and that if it does change, it was very treatable. That will have to do for now.

Between the last visit and this one, Holly and I took our long-awaited trip to the west coast. This was a trip I had started planning when I first learned I had cancer. It was something I really wanted to do and knowing I might not get another chance, I wanted to do it as soon as possible.

Originally, we had planned on doing it this past summer. But given my health had improved greatly and both Holly and I were extremely busy, we decided to postpone the trip until after Holly's big fund raiser, "Death by Chocolate," which was on Friday the 13th of October this year. (It went extremely well. I helped by becoming "The Great Selbini", dressing as a gypsy and doing Tarot card readings. I had played around with Tarot cards in college but had not done anything with them since. So, I spent several weeks studying and relearning the deck. I could have used another two weeks! But I did the best I could, and it seemed to be enough. I really freaked out several of the people I gave readings to, including getting one in tears (of joy). So, I thought it went well . . .)

We departed the day after my last infusion on Oct. 17th. We first flew to Seattle, where we spent two nights with Holly's friends, Amy and Buzz, who lived on Bainbridge Island. From there, we drove down the coast to Portland, where Juliette lives with her husband, Michael. Their daughter, Sarah, also lives in Portland. Matt flew in for the weekend as he had wanted to visit them as well. (In fact, Holly and I picked him up at the airport on our way to Juliette's.) We also dropped him off at the airport at the conclusion of our visit.

From there, we drove down to Milford for a night, before heading down the coast to Healdsburg where we stayed at a wonderful bed and breakfast. (We had been very nervous about that stay because Healdsburg was right between two of the major wildfires that plagued California this fall. Fortunately, it was fine where we were). We visited a couple of wineries before retiring quite happy.

Next, we drove down the coast to San Francisco where we spent the day before heading to my best friend's house in San Jose. We spent two nights with Jeff and Akiko, before heading again down the coast to Los Angeles, and staying four days with my son, Matt.

The twelve-day trip was the longest vacation I had taken

since my trip to England in 1975. (I think the next longest was a week, which I did many times.) It was a fantastic trip, full of fun, family, and fantastic views. As I love photography, I took a lot of pictures – and I mean *a lot*. Probably over 2,000. Thank goodness for digital cameras! Some of them were really good . . . law of averages.

A few words about my best friend, Jeff. He and I grew up together. He lived a few houses down from me in Mission, a Kansas-side suburb of Kansas City. Jeff and I were almost always together – whether at his house, my house, school or playing in the neighborhood. We were so close it was as though we were brothers.

Jeff moved away when I was thirteen. I was absolutely crushed. His departure coincided with the worst two years of my life – 7th and 8th grade, where I literally came home nearly every day crying. He had always been my anchor and then he was gone . . .

We kept in touch, writing the occasional letter and a rare phone call. This was in the 1960's – the dark ages before there was the internet, email and Facebook. If you wanted to talk to someone in another state (he moved to Indianapolis), you either wrote a letter, or made a long-distance phone call. And back in those dark days – you paid for long-distance . . . by the minute. So, our calls were infrequent and short. But, to be truthful, I have never been good about keeping in contact with people. I don't write (even email) enough, rarely call, and even though I am on Facebook, I rarely check it and even more rarely post on it.

It was about five years before I got to see Jeff again after he moved. It was the summer before my Freshman year at college. I talked my parents into letting me take a bus to go visit him. When I got there, it was as though he had left the day before. There was no awkwardness. We were instantly as close as we ever were. I drove there the next summer and the same thing happened.

It was a few more years before we saw each other again. It was 1976. I had gone to England to visit my mother's family. It was only my second visit to my mother's homeland. (The first was when I was thirteen and was with my mom and my sisters. This trip was solo. I did not know it at the time, but it was the last time I was able to go . . . something I am deeply sorry about). All her family is still there. Anyway, the night I got back from England I called my parents to tell them I was back home (I was living in Lawrence at the time) when my mother asked if I had heard from Jeff. I said, "of course not, I just got home." She told me I needed to call him right away. So, I did. It turns out that he was getting married in three days! He was now living in Los Angeles with his girlfriend, Akiko. Akiko, who is Japanese, had her parents visiting them so they decided this was the best time to get married. I was on a plane the next day to Los Angeles. Boy, did I feel like a jetsetter! And I was best man. (Although, I was not able to do a key best man duty . . . organize a bachelor's party. I not only arrived the day before the wedding, but I did not know anyone there besides Jeff and I certainly did not know the town. If I remember right, there really wasn't one because of visiting families and the rushed wedding.)

It was eight years before we saw each other again. This time, Jeff returned the favor and was at my side during my marriage to Ann, serving as my best man. Again, it was as though he had never left.

Over the next thirty-three years, we probably saw each other five or six times. Our correspondence consists of xmas cards (and his infamous Christmas, or rather "holiday" letters, as he's Jewish) and a couple of phone calls a year. We call each other on our birthdays and then usually the winner of the Chiefs-Raiders game would call the loser to rub it in. (I got to make more calls!) Sadly, when Jeff moved to Los Angeles, he went over to the dark side and became a Raider's fan, who were playing there at that time. The Raiders are the archenemy of the Chiefs –like KU-MU, or UNC-Duke. From LA, Jeff and Akiko would spend several years in Hawaii, before moving to San Jose, while the Raiders had moved back to Oakland. His unfortunate fandom only intensified.

We have gotten to see each other more frequently over the past ten years. I did a couple of projects in the San Francisco area and got to see them. I saw him briefly when they were traveling and had a layover in Dallas when we were living in the Dallas area. We met once in Las Vegas. And last year, they invited us to stay with us a few days when they had a time-share vacation in the mountains of South Carolina. And again, every time we get together it's like the old days. Anyway, it was a wonderful visit. Indeed, the whole trip was fantastic.

We finished the trip by spending several days with my son in Los Angeles. We stayed with him in his small one-bedroom un-air-conditioned apartment. But it was in Hollywood, just a couple of blocks from Hollywood Boulevard. Matt turned out to be an excellent tour guide.

November 10 – December 2017

November 17, 2017

I am now into my sixth month since being told (wrongly) the tumors were gone. A lot has happened in that time. For one thing, I was kept extremely busy all summer with work . . . It was probably the busiest summer I've had. Thank goodness I was doing so much better physically, or I would never have been able to handle it. Even so, I was not able to put in the hours I normally do (although I did put in eight to ten each day).

Currently, I have only one project I'm working on, and it should be finished by early next week. I have deliberately not solicited any work as I think I need a couple of months to "recharge" my batteries. Unfortunately, we are nowhere near being in a position where I can "retire," not that I would if I could. Fact is, I really enjoy what I do and would miss it. But I also don't want to overstress myself in the future. I no longer have visions of building a large company, etc. I am quite satisfied remaining an independent consultant. But I will need to get busy after the first of the year. I can't afford to go too long without significant income. But this slow-down period will give me the time to work on the book, get my businesses (golf consulting and the brokerage) better organized, and maybe even (gasp!) clean my office.

Physically, I'm doing so much better than in June, and certainly before then. But while the pain has greatly diminished, it has not gone away completely by any means. It still bothers me, mostly at night. I must keep a pillow on my side to protect it . . . mostly against Ferris, one of our cats, who likes to demand attention by ramming his head into your body. However, my other ailments, particularly my back, have been more debilitating than the tumor. I suspect the Tecentriq may be accentuating my back and neck pain. It may also be responsible for the dry, itchy skin on my back. But hell, that's one great tradeoff I would take any time! Most importantly, I'm able to get around and do most of the things I normally would do.

The worst thing, though, are the anxiety "flashbacks". These occur mostly at night and are associated with the tumor pain in my left kidney. I will suddenly have sort of an emotional flashback to when that pain meant I was not likely to be around very much longer. Because they happen at night when I'm in the bed, it keeps me awake. Most of the time I can distract myself by playing a game or something. Sometimes I will take a sleeping pill. But again, I can't complain (much) as these are *flashbacks* as opposed to the true anxiety I was feeling a year ago. Still, I sometimes can't help but be concerned that maybe the cancer is coming back. I realize I will probably have to live with this fear for the rest of my life. So hopefully I will be bothered by it for a long, long time!

One thing my recovery has cost me is a financial windfall from a malpractice suit. Apparently my getting well ruined my chance at getting a good settlement . . . at least my attorney appears to think so as I have not heard from him in months. Oh well. I'll take the trade-off.

Thanksgiving 2017
Holly and I traveled to Dallas to spend Thanksgiving with Cheryl and her husband Richard. They always do a big Thanksgiving dinner. Her daughter, Rebecca and her husband, Jon, and their son (and my sister's only grandchild),

Colton also came for the dinner as did their close friends, who happened to have three children of their own. It was certainly a full house. And it was a wonderful escape.

We stayed until Saturday morning, then flew back home that afternoon. It was a great trip. Both Holly and I enjoyed it immensely, although we are carrying too much of it back with us – around our waist. We ate well! Not only is Richard an outstanding cook (he did a Smoked Turkey), but Cheryl forgot Richard bought a turkey and so bought another one, which she baked. And, surprisingly, she did a great job too! (Richard is most definitely the cook in that family).

Sadly, both Holly and I were under the weather for the trip, suffering from head colds. But I can't complain. I don't think I ever will complain again about sniffles or colds. When you've had the Big C, everything else becomes a mere inconvenience. Ok, I realize that my mere mentioning my various pains comes across as complaining, and then I say I'm not complaining. I really don't discuss these issues with those around me. But somehow it seems appropriate in this book as I am trying to portray a realistic picture as to what someone goes through in their fight with cancer. Do I try to put up a brave front and give you an unrealistic picture, or am I to be more honest, but try to convey that I am very, very grateful to still be able to feel pain? I opted for the latter. I hope you understand.

But speaking of the Big C, my tumor has been bothering me a lot more lately. I say it's my tumor, but I don't really know. I just know it's my kidney area.

The pain has slowly intensified over the past few weeks. It still comes and goes in intensity – sometimes barely noticeable (unless something pokes it, like one of our cats begging for attention – yes, I mean you Ferris), but other times debilitating . . . although nowhere near the degree it was before.

But I can't lie, it does concern me. Anytime I feel the pain, I am reminded about the cancer. And when the pain increases, there is always the concern the cancer is once again growing . . . and then the fear starts welling up again. I even have had a mini-panic attack at night. Fortunately, a little Ambien, combined with Spider Solitaire, is able to distract me until I can fall asleep.

Rationally, I know that it's not likely the cancer is growing again. After all, I went through this before . . . last June . . . right before being told the cancer had disappeared (they were wrong, but it still had diminished tremendously), so I know the pain can be intense without necessarily meaning the cancer is responsibly . . . at least directly. But every twinge carries both a physical and an emotional pain. At least I won't have to wait long until I know for sure. My next scans are schedule about four weeks away . . . on December 22nd. Hopefully, they will provide a great Christmas gift to me and my family.

December 4th, 2017

The pain has gotten worse the past few days. I've come to expect it now. I had another immunotherapy treatment on Friday. And I have begun to realize the pain may be associated with the treatments. It seems to spike shortly after the treatments (a day or two), then gradually recede. That seems to be what is happening this time. I was hurting the most on Saturday. It eased off some yesterday and a little more today.

That does not stop me from worrying. What if the cancer has started growing again? Other than the tumor growing, what else could be causing the pain?

We also had to move the scans back to January 12th because they could not get me in for the scans on the 22nd. So, I am going to have to wait another three weeks to learn for sure what is happening with my tumor.

The pain is once again at the point where anything jostling my stomach causes a sharp pain. Like last year, riding in a golf cart can be a very painful experience now. (Prior to the cancer, it used to be painful only because of my score and needing to make frequent stops). But when the pain is bad, riding in a car can be a bad experience as well. Even with good shock absorbers, I feel every single bump and swerve. Thank goodness I don't drive a truck!

However, if this follows the pattern of the past few months, the pain will gradually ease off over the next few days – to the point where it is not very noticeable during the day (unless I really aggravate it). But I still will likely experience the "sundowner" syndrome, where the pain starts intensifying in the late afternoon and early evening – reaching peak levels when I finally go to bed.

One thing that struck me this time when I was plugged into the infusion tubes, was just how surreal this whole experience has been. Never had I ever imagined myself being dependent on chemicals being pumped into me via these plastic tubes. Nor had I ever imagined myself with cancer. But here we are!

I think the absurdity of it all strikes me more now that I'm doing better. When you're in great pain, your concern is just to moderate the pain. You don't really think about the consequences or seeing the big picture. Now it just all seems so surreal.

Christmas, 2017
Fourteen months ago, there was serious doubt as to whether I would even see one more Christmas, let alone two. The fact I am still here writing these words is my own personal miracle and the best Christmas present. And don't think for a mo-

ment I do not appreciate that fact. I most certainly do . . . and will continue to do so, no matter how long I have remaining.

Both kids came for Christmas, with Lizzy staying a week and Matt a couple of days. They both left on Christmas day to go to their mom's. But it was wonderful, as always, having them here.

It is also wonderful not having to worry about the immediate future. I don't know that I am cancer-free. I won't know until my next set of scans on January 12th. But I do know I am feeling better. And I am certainly a lot more optimistic. The pain is still there, reminding me of what I've been through. But the pain does not necessarily mean the tumor is still there. It wrecked a lot of havoc when it was growing rapidly within . . . including essentially destroying my left kidney. It may take time for that part of my body to heal.

December 30, 2017

Holly's been sick for a couple of weeks. It seems like a bad head cold/virus. It got so bad; she *voluntarily* went to the Doctor last Wednesday – which is about the only time I've known her to do that. Normally I must beg her to go. But she's been generous. She gave it to me.

I think my ramped-up immune system has spared me the worst of it, though. As I do not seem to be in as bad a shape as she was at its worst. Fortunately, the medicine the Doctor gave her is working and she is doing much better.

My cold, too, is doing better. But that is not why I am writing today. The reason I'm writing is that I'm in great pain, this time from the tumor area. This is completely unexpected as it is happening during the day and not the night. Plus, it is the most severe it's been since at least May. Bad enough that I've had to take a Percocet. I am writing this as I'm waiting for it to kick in, which I hope it does soon!

The worst thing about these pain attacks is not the pain itself, which is manageable. It is that it conjures up memories of why I got the pain in the first place. And, naturally, this raises the fears of "what if the cancer is back? And the tumor is growing again?"

I do my best to rationalize the pain, both for my sake and Holly's, as she gets very upset when I'm hurting there. (When the pain is in my back, that's perfectly ok with her, at least that's what she says.) We are both all too aware of what it would mean if the tumor is growing again. We've already been through Options A and B. The good options are gone. But there is always a plan C and D. Dr. Bilen always has options.

We will know soon enough. The next scans are thirteen days away.

January - February 2018

January 15, 2018
Last Friday were my latest scans. The day got off to an auspicious start. Holly and I were up at 4 am in order to get to downtown Atlanta by 7 am. When I get the scans, they usually set up the scans at the downtown Emory hospital, then I go back to the campus Winship center for my doctor's visit and infusion. What is amazing is that, even though I will have had the scans only an hour or so before my doctor's appointment, they will already have the results by the time I get there.

I have also learned from experience to have the lab before the scans. This is because the scans require contrast. If I have the labs before the scans, they can access my port for the contrast. Otherwise, I am stuck (literally) with an IV, and you know how I love to have a needle in my arm.

Holly and I arrived *before* 7 am, which is when the lab opens. So, we were first in line. That's when the fun started.

When I gave the receptionist my information, she told me while she could find the appointment, the doctor never sent the lab request, so they could not draw my blood! Further, they could not call to get them to send the request as the doctor's office was not open that early. Sadly, it took them thirty minutes to discover all this. I was able, however, to talk them into going ahead and putting in the port access, so at least I would avoid the needle. But because of all the paperwork delays, I was now twenty minutes late for my MRI appointment.

We headed downstairs to outpatient radiology on the 8th

floor. Fortunately, I was able to get right in for the CT scan, which only takes a few minutes. When finished, they had me go back to the waiting room to join Holly while we waited for the MRI.

After about fifteen minutes, the receptionist called me over. There was a problem. The MRI machine was broken! This could take fifteen minutes to fix, or it could be an all-day thing. Given my tight schedule, I really did not want to wait long – and I certainly did not want to have to come back. I was understandably concerned with what the scans might show.

However, I remembered that the hospital had a 2nd radiology lab downstairs, which was used for both inpatient and outpatient. I told the receptionist my situation and pleaded with her to see if she could get me in downstairs.

Amazingly, after about another fifteen minutes, she called me back up and told me they were able to get me in downstairs! She escorted us to the staff elevator, which would take us straight there and avoid us having to change elevators.

My good luck continued as they got me in right away downstairs. However, by the time I was done, we were pushing against my doctor's appointment time, and I still had to have my lab work.

Instead of returning upstairs to try to get my labs done and risk another long delay, I figured my best chance was to go to the campus Winship center, where at least they knew me and Dr. Bilen.

We got there with a little time to spare before my doctor's appointment. But again, we ran up against another roadblock. Apparently, the system did not like me having an appointment scheduled at one place and then have it done at another. Incredibly, it took forty-five minutes for them to straighten out this snafu – and get the doctor's orders. Now we are about forty-five minutes late for the Doctor.

Now waiting forty-five minutes is nothing unusual with Doctor visits. But it seems like an eternity when you are extremely concerned about the news that the Doctor will be giving you.

After another twenty-minute wait, we were sent back to one of Dr. Bilen's exam rooms. Unfortunately, Dr. Bilen was not available. But one of his assistance, Else, was and she saw us immediately. Both of his assistants (I think they are nurse practitioners, although they may be residents) are quite capable and very nice.

She then gave us the good news. The scans showed that, again, there was no evidence of tumors in my chest. Further, the tumor on my kidney was continuing to shrink. It was still there, but it was smaller. We were still winning!

We were now about an hour late for the infusion treatment. But we were both hungry, so instead of going right there, we made a detour to the cafeteria for lunch. There, we were happy to find lunch items that fit into our newly started Adkins diet. I felt that the infusion lab would take me even if I was late, which, fortunately, they did.

The scan results were not the only good news I got that week. The day before the scans, I received a call from the City of Detroit. This was with regards to the proposal I had submitted exactly one minute before the deadline. They were calling to ask if we could come in for an interview on Tuesday. She let on, though, that we were the *only* company being interviewed. This meant that as long as we did not screw it up during the interview, the job was ours! It would easily be the biggest job of my career.

So here I am writing this in the Atlanta airport, waiting for my flight to Detroit, where it is a balmy twenty degrees and snowing! Not exactly the most desirable place to be in the middle of January for someone living in Georgia. But I do not mind one bit, as the opportunity is well worth any minor discomfort.

January 22, 2018

I'm having trouble sleeping again. Nothing new. And so far, the Ambien is solving the problem. But it's still very annoying. But you get to the point where you are almost dreading going to bed because you're afraid of the insomnia – even though you are dead tired (forgive the expression.)

What's especially annoying is that my nose is getting clogged up at night. Now that might seem like a minor thing, and it is. And it used to be for me as well. But it isn't anymore – at least when it happens in the middle of the night. This is because I still remember the panics that a stuffed-up nose would cause me at the height of my illness – where the inability to breathe would cause thoughts of death . . . and these thoughts were not pleasant, to say the least. And while the panics I am having now are not nearly as bad, they still are mindful of the ones I used to have, and I get scared that they are coming back. I believe these panic attacks are a minor version of PTSD.

The bottom line is that even though physically, I am so much better – and hopefully on my way to total remission, I still have a way to go to recover mentally.

On the positive side, it does appear more likely that the Detroit management contract will come to fruition as we're the vendor of choice and we've cleared most of the hurdles. We are also the vendor of choice for the management contract for Northwood Golf Course in Rhinelander, WI. Yep, both contracts will be partnerships with Paul. His company will be the company of record for Detroit, given the need for all the vendor relationships, etc.; while I will be the vendor of record for Rhinelander. But both contracts have to be approved the respective City Councils, so nothing is definite. And if there is one thing my life has taught me – never count my eggs before they have hatched, counted and cleared by the doctor.

February 2nd, 2018
Graduation Day! Of sorts anyway. No, I'm not talking about the Groundhog who saw his shadow, despite a forecast of snow, but my own Graduation at Emory. Dr. Bilen's assistant, Greta, told me today that they don't want to see me again . . . for six weeks. I still must have treatments every three weeks, but I get to skip seeing the doctor on every other visit. Yes, it's a small milestone. But a milestone just the same! I'll take every single one that I can. Of course, it could simply mean they are tired of seeing me so often . . .

Next week, I'm traveling to Minneapolis and then to Detroit . . . both for business. We are being interviewed for a major project for Ramsey County (St. Paul) that would easily be the biggest project I have done under Sirius. If successful, it will be the three amigos again . . . Jeff, Paul and I. Jeff is joining me for the interview.

Then it's on to Detroit. We have been awarded the management contract for the City's three municipal golf courses. It's a two-year deal, but still it's a huge deal. And once again, I am partnering with Paul. The chose us because of the proposal that I submitted. However, we will execute the contract under Signal – Paul's company – because of his vendor contacts, etc. But that's fine with me. We will be equal partners on the deal. I did make sure Paul and I had a written contract, however. It includes a $20,000 penalty should either of us unilaterally cancel the contract. I may be a fool, but I am not a complete idiot.

It is so ironic. Exactly a year ago, I was losing the one management contract I had, and the future was extremely bleak. Now, while I'm not cancer-free, I am close. Physically, the cancer is not affecting me hardly at all. And now I have a new management contract that will pay significantly more and is more prestigious with three courses instead of one. And because it is a major city, it can easily lead to a lot more contracts. I am also one of two finalists for another management contract for the City of Rhineland, Wisconsin, and we are a finalist for this huge Ramsey County consulting project. What a difference a year makes.

As I am writing this, none of those jobs are guaranteed. Not even Detroit. While we have a signed contract, it must be approved by the City Council, and it hasn't been yet. In fact, I cannot even talk to anyone about it until it has been scheduled with the City Council. But it is highly unlikely the City Council would go against the recommendations of its staff.

The other two jobs are much less certain. But if I could get just one, it would be a great year . . . and this is only February. I would say, "wish me luck," but by the time you've read this, the decision has long been made – and the projects likely concluded. But I will take the good luck all the same.

Another bit of historical reflection. I just realized that I did not play a single round of golf in 2017. Why is that significant? Well, I am in the golf business after all. And it's probably the first year since I was about six that I did not play a single round of golf. (Since getting into the golf business, I really don't get to play that much . . . usually 10 rounds or less a year. This is less than half what I played before.)

Not all the blame goes to the cancer. My bad back was also a major factor. But I am hoping that I can play some this year.

MARCH 2018

March 12, 2018

I am writing this on the airplane, on my way to Detroit. This contract has proven to be challenging as the current vendor is pulling out all the dirty tricks, trying to prevent the City from going with us. They were making up all sorts of nasty stuff. Fortunately, everyone in City administration, from the Mayor on down, does not want them back and wants us. Now we go before the City Council tomorrow to get their approval. We finally made it through the subcommittee last week (unanimously).

I also am awaiting the final contract for the consulting project for Ramsey County, Minnesota. Not only were we selected over all the top consulting firms in the country, but I learned we were also the most expensive. Although after being selected, they have asked me to reduce my fee a bit, which I was happy to do as they were willing to forego a printed report.

Ok, that's the good news. The bad news is that on my flight back from Detroit last Friday, my kidney pain returned – with a vengeance. It really bothered me for the rest of the day, before easing off Saturday. But there is still pain there – for the first time since the first of the year.

Naturally, this pain is causing me great consternation . . . Is the tumor growing again? It certainly would fit in with God's wicked sense of humor . . . letting me win these two big contracts, then having the cancer return. Grrr.

But I also realize there could be alternative explanations. Indeed, the pain may even be a sign of healing. I'll learn more this Friday when I return to see Dr. Bilen. My blood test results have been trending better. If it takes a step back, that would be bad. I'm not due for another set of scans for twelve weeks, though. Let's hope that the pain is long gone by then.

March 19, 2018

Here I am again at the Atlanta airport, once again awaiting my flight to Detroit, where, once again, we will be presenting to City Council to get our management contract approved. Thanks to more dirty tricks and politics (they go together), the City Council failed to approve our contract on a split four to four vote last week. But the 9th member, who was absent, would have been a Yes vote. So, they have asked for a re-vote, which is a one-time thing. If we don't get it tomorrow, it is over.

I could easily write a book about our experiences with the City with regards to this contact. It certainly has been politics at its worse. Perhaps I will be able to write more about this later. I am certainly hoping that I will be around for a sequel!

That is far from certain, however, as the abdominal pain has continued. I have had to take my pain medicine more frequently. Further, the pain is once again always present, it just varies in intensity.

I went to see Dr. Bilen on Friday. While my blood work has continued to improve, he was concerned enough about my pain to move up my planned scans a month. I am now waiting to hear back from Emory as when we tried to schedule Friday, there were no openings on April 6th.

There is also the possibility that the pains have been exacerbated due to the stress from the contract negotiations. Stress seems to have a much worse effect on me than ever before.

March 27, 2018

I am writing this on a plane as I'm once again winging my way to Detroit. This trip is different from the previous ones, though, as this time I am returning as one of the principles of the management entity for the Detroit Municipal golf courses!

The dirty politics that went on behind the scene was unbelievable. I've never seen a City Council so acrimonious to the City Administration. Normally, if City Administration *unanimously* approves a contract, then it is rubber stamped by City Council. But in this case, it had to go through a subcommittee first. That took three weeks of heavy politicking as the company we were replacing was fighting hard . . . and dirty. They could not find any skeletons in our closet, so they resorted to simply lying . . . But taking a cue from our current President, they felt that if they lied loud enough, it would be perceived as truth. And it worked . . . at least for a while.

Again, the story would make a whole book. Let's just jump ahead. The four "no" votes from the previous week gave what sounded mostly likely campaign speeches as to why their vote was "no." Then the vote was called, and we were approved 5-4.

This all happened on Tuesday, the 20th. Now the real fun began! We were to take over operations on the 22nd. We had less than forty-eight hours to prepare.

One of the arguments the opposition had been making was that they were the only company that could possibly open the courses on time as they were currently in place. And certainly, a small company from North Carolina (and Georgia) could not possible do it, so the courses would be closed for a prolonged period.

I was darned if I was going to let that happen!

While Paul and I could not sign any contracts until our contract was approved, we could still work behind the scenes to try and get as much in place as possible, so we could move quickly when we did get the approval.

Two of the most important items was making sure we could get carts in and have staff to operate the courses. As the current vendor was leasing the facility, virtually all the equipment was theirs, so we assumed we would have virtually nothing to work with . . . and boy, were we right!

We were also handicapped by the fact the City did not want us visiting the facilities until at least the contract had been approved, and then, only when they were doing *their* survey. This seemed absurd to me. They were asking us, essentially, to take over managing three facilities without knowing what was there! Or what condition they were in! Or what we would need!

We were helped because they had only opened one of the three courses, so there was only pressure to keep that one open. And the weather was not exactly the best. The temperature was in the low 40s.

We found a great cart vendor and arranged to get a cart delivery of some carts that Friday morning (our first day of operations).

We were also fortunate in that a couple of the current management company's managers had reached out to us to see if they could continue with us. (We were not allowed to make the first contact). They, in turn, were able to get other staff interested. So, I had a meeting with a lot of the former employees on Wednesday. They were all eager to get started.

Another thing we had in our favor . . . the former management company was pretty much universally hated. Thus, we had lots of people within the community that were willing to help. One of them was First Tee of Detroit, who had recommended a person to us as a possible overall operations manager.

Karen was a perfect match. She was extremely qualified, having run all the facilities for American Golf, who managed them prior to the vendor we were replacing. She was well liked, especially by the City. She had even received recognition from City Council back when she operated the courses. Further, she was the first black member of the LPGA in Michigan.

Paul, unfortunately, had to leave Tuesday night. Thus, it was Karen and I that had to do all the running around. Paul worked in the background, like with the carts and trying to get us a POS system in time. But we knew it would not be ready Friday.

So, we went shopping. Buying everything we needed to get open, including chairs, a cash register, a computer, office supplies, cleaning supplies, food and beverage inventory (drinks and snacks), etc. I even arranged for delivery of some merchandise. And with the help of First Tee, we had a good work crew in place to help us clean the place up and get ready quickly.

But the current vendor was not through with their dirty tricks. When we arrived early Friday morning, not only did we find the clubhouse a mess (expected), and the equipment gone (expected), we also found:

- The phone lines were CUT
- The granite tee markers were gone
- The flags were missing
- The irrigation pump was gone
- The irrigation control boxes were locked, with no keys left.

In all my years of consulting in the golf business, I never heard of a management company having so little regard for their customers and so much hatred to being kicked out that they would do anything to sabotage the operation for the next operator.

We were *not* to be deterred. And this is where the community kicked in. We had lots of volunteers, including people from the First Tee, in there helping us get the place clean. The cart vendor, who also sold maintenance equipment, called area superintendents. We got two country clubs to lend us flags and cup cutters (they were not open yet for the season).

As to phones, I got the brilliant idea of having the phones forwarded to one of my cell phones (I have two, one for business, one for personal.). I then recorded a message telling people we were open, but our phone and internet was down, but would be up later in the week.

We opened on time! We did not get a lot of play that day (twenty-two rounds), but it was the principal of it. And on Saturday, with the temperature even colder, we did fifty-two rounds and another forty-three on Sunday. Not bad for not having working phones or website!

What really made it worthwhile was that later Friday morning we had a meeting with the City and the previous vendor to discuss the transition. This meeting, naturally, should have been held *before* the transition, but they insisted on doing it Friday.

So, the owner of the previous management company was at this meeting. He had a smug look on his face as he fully expected he had the City over a barrel. He was wanting the City to buy back from him everything he stole and at his prices. But during the discussion, I just happened to let it "slip" we were open. The look on his face was well worth all the trouble we had gone through. Poof went his leverage.

Later, I had lunch with one of the CEOs for the City. And his grin when I told him that we were open, was almost as rewarding.

Unfortunately, I had to leave town right after that meeting. So now I'm on my way back. Paul arrived yesterday and has certainly been busy these past two days. He also brought his right-hand man with him to help with the training and getting things set up.

Meanwhile, this past weekend was my wife's big event at the museum, Riverblast. Which was why I had to return Friday as I had promised to help. Further, my son, Matt, was coming into town Sunday. He had a wedding in Atlanta Saturday and extended his trip, so he could spend a couple of days with us.

Matt was also kind enough to help us around the house, which was greatly appreciated (especially cleaning the six cat litter boxes!).

Another bit of good news. The cancer pain has diminished substantially! I can still feel it, but it is no longer causing me a lot of pain. This gives me more confidence heading into the scans, which will be next Friday (the 6th).

New Year's Eve, 2018

It's been a long, long time since my last entry. This has been due to a couple of factors. One, I've been really, really busy. Two, a lot of what I would say would have been repetitive as to the cancer. And three, well, I was afraid of what I would write.

Let's just say it has been an interesting year. Like in the Chinese curse "may you live in interesting times." Although not all of it has been bad.

Physically, not much has changed. In August, we decided to take a two-month break in the treatments. But when the pain came back with a vengeance, Dr. Bilen decided to return us to our previous schedule (treatment every three weeks, Doctor visit every six.) The tumor has stubbornly remained, although it has not shown any signs of growth. Given that we have not done a biopsy, it is possible what is showing up on the MRI's is really scar tissue. But Dr. Bilen does not want to take that chance. We are in uncharted territory. In a month, it will have been two years since I first started on Tecentriq. There simply are not any studies showing what the long-term effects of it may be -- or the likelihood of the tumors returning. In this regard, I am a pioneer! Like my childhood, Captain Kirk, I am going where no man has gone before . . . Ok, now I may be guilty of overacting just a little (sound familiar, Mr. Shatner?)

The pain in my side is still there. It comes and goes. The locus of the pain moves around a bit, but the general area is the same. We still have no idea what is causing it, other than it may be a side effect of the Tecentriq. However, there is also speculation that the pain may not have anything to do with the cancer, but is because of my bad back, which may be pinching a nerve.

I still occasionally have fear "flashbacks" at night, but the frequency has greatly diminished. And, other than the trip to Atlanta every three weeks, my life is back to normal . . . which is to say, mostly chaotic.

My dreams about getting a windfall from a potential malpractice suit naturally fizzled right as I was getting going with Detroit. Indeed, *two weeks* before the two-year deadline for filing a malpractice suit, my attorney calls and tells me they are withdrawing from the case. Wonderful. Apparently, they consulted another radiologist and oncologist. While they confirmed the CT scan done in June 2016 indeed showed a tumor, indicating *malpractice occurred*, the oncologist said because it also showed the lymph node was affected, I was likely already Stage IV and thus, earlier treatment may not have had an impact. Bottom line, the attorneys would not be able to get a big enough settlement to make it worth *their* while (and expense) to pursue. And with only two weeks left, there was no time to get another attorney involved.

Meanwhile, I could write an entire book on Detroit. This was a fiasco from the get-go. I guess it is a classic case of being careful what you ask for.

I have already described the drama associated with getting the contract approved. Little did I realize it was only the opening act. Shortly after opening I was to learn that almost everything the City had led us to believe was going to happen was not.

First, none of the people who were responsible for hiring us were going to be involved in working with us. The entire Parks and Recreation department was reorganized and put under a different City department. Further, we were told by the new manager *that we were to have NO contact with those that hired us*. Talk about inter-department rivalry! But that was only the beginning.

Our new boss assigned a liaison whose job was to act as an interface between us and the City. After all, it had been over twenty years since the City had been responsible for operating the golf courses (they had been leased out). The person assigned this job was a former Superintendent who had worked on one of the city's courses (which the City no longer owned, due to shady dealings), twenty years ago when the City still operated them. She had not been a superintendent since.

Initially, we got along well. We both had a common goal, after all, of making the courses better. But there was something she said during our first meeting that bothered me. She kept talking (and boy, can she talk! She could be a professional talker) about how important this was to *her* and what it would mean for *her* career.

It quickly became obvious she had a completely different interpretation of her job. She took it to mean she was our *boss*. And she wanted to be involved in *every* decision. And I mean every single one. She even wanted to approve office supply orders!

Paul, though, was paranoid about complaining. After all, the equipment, including both the maintenance equipment and the carts, were in his company's name. Thus, he was responsible for over $1,000,000 worth of equipment. If the City cancelled our contract, he would be in *serious* trouble.

But during one of our meetings with our liaison and her boss, and her boss's boss (the Department manager), I got the big boss to state unequivocally we did not have to submit every order for her approval prior to purchase. I even got him to state it twice, while she was there. But no sooner than when the meeting was over then she calls us over and tells us no matter what the boss says, she still wants to see all the orders first!

The whole premise was preposterous. The reason one hires a management company is because you want the professional expertise to manage the course most efficiently. If they were going to micromanage everything, why were we there in the first place?

It got worse.

The main reason I was told we were hired was because of the marketing plan I had put in our RFP response. Indeed, right before our interview, I had an inspiration for a new branding campaign and a new logo. The previous operator was all about promoting himself. He named the company after himself and had his name on everything. I wanted to take the opposite approach. Not only did I not want it to be about Paul or myself, I did not want it to be about our company's. Instead, I came up with "Golf Detroit." That would be the management company's public façade. I then came up with what I thought was a very clever logo. I had a cartoon car with golf clubs in the back. The car had a grin out of its grill. I took the concept to an artist who worked part-time at Holly's museum and he was able to come up with a great drawing. We presented it at the interview. They loved it!

But that was the old team. The new team was a different story. They were not in love with the idea, but gave in. But our new liaison seriously objected to the color scheme in our logo. (Red car with blue lettering). She wanted a green car. Apparently, she (and her immediate supervisor) both went to Michigan State – whose color is, you guessed it, green. And the colors I had chosen were too close to their arch-rival, Michigan. Geez. Paul wanted me to change the color to green. Instead, I altered the logo to include all three colors. But that was the least of the problems.

Next, the new management told us we could not change the pricing. This had been a significant part of our marketing plan! But the new boss said we had to use the existing pricing structure – everything was to be the same as the previous year!

It got worse once we opened. I wanted to issue a press release right after our first day of operation. After all, it had been major news (front page, lead story, etc.) that the mayor had threatened to close the courses. And the previous operator had claimed we could not possibly open on time. Yet we did. This should be shouted from the rooftops! What a great PR opportunity. Only the City did not agree.

Next, one of the things the previous operator was willing to sell us was the websites and domains for the golf courses. He only wanted $2,000, which, in my opinion, was well worth it. The City did not agree. So now everyone who went to the old websites were being redirected to the previous operator's main website. I had already secured new domains; in case this would happen. And we were able to get a new website up quickly. But because the City would not let us do any promotion, how were people going to find the new website? Or even know we were open?

Further, we were told that we were NOT to do any marketing without getting it approved by the City. (Again, weren't we hired for *our* expertise?). This was a big problem. Because cities were not known for quick responses, or their marketing expertise . . . and this was especially true with Detroit. Indeed, it would take six weeks before I was even able to *meet* with the marketing manager, not to mention being able to do any advertising. They did not want us to do much advertising. They were afraid the courses were not ready. And they were right, to a degree. The courses were not in great shape. But then again, the previous operator had left them in horrible condition.

In my agreement with Paul, I was responsible for marketing and golf operations. He was handling course maintenance and accounting. Only now I was not able to do any marketing. Fortunately, things were going well, for the most part, with operations. I was onsite for most of the next two months.

As noted, we had Rackham, the main course, opened on the first day of our contract. We discovered the previous operator had done more dirty tricks at the other courses – including physically cutting phone lines and sabotaging the plumbing), but we still got them open on schedule.

Things were not going as well on Paul's side of things. First, our "liaison" had talked Paul into using her preferred vendor for the maintenance equipment. Big mistake. Unlike the vendor we had chosen for the carts, who moved mountains to get us the carts we needed. The maintenance vendor did little extra to help. We were able to get a few pieces of equipment, but we now had three courses to operate and we needed a lot! It would take nearly three months until we got everything we needed.

Initially it was not that big a deal. After all, grass does not grow much in March and April in Detroit. But that is not the case in May. While we were able to scrounge around for greens mowers and were able to get the fairways cut. We did not have the mowers to also cut the tees and roughs. Things quickly got very bad. And the enthusiasm we had built from our customers who had been ecstatic with our take-over and vastly improved customer service was now souring with the poor course conditions.

Meanwhile, there was another golf property up for lease in Detroit. It was the driving range on Belle Isle. This had once been owned by the City and had included a lighted Par

3. The main golf course closed years ago. But the facility still had a six-hole "chip and putt" course. When Detroit had gone through its bankruptcy, it leased the entire Island to the State, including the driving range. The State made the Island into a State Park and charged admission. Which does not help the driving range.

The State had subleased the driving range to various operators. It was now up for a new lease. When I learned about it, I approached Paul. I thought it would make a great addition. I felt we could do some marketing and turn it around (the previous operator had done little). Paul agreed. We then asked the City for their opinion (this was the original team that hired us). They, too, thought it was a great idea. In fact, one of them was on the committee that would be making the decision!

So, we submitted a proposal. This was in mid-February, after the City had hired us, but before all the public meetings were held to get the Council's approval. The contract with Belle Isle was to start April 1st. The State told everyone in a prebid meeting that they would decide by the second week in March. It didn't happen.

We finally were given word we had the contract on April 5th, five days after the range was to open. And, because it had been leased, we needed to get all the equipment. Fortunately, the State was willing to give us several weeks to get ready as the facility was in poor condition.

The proposal was for Signal and Sirius to form a joint venture, much like we proposed for the City. But again, Paul insisted we put the contract in Signal's name. Because we needed to move at light speed, and because we needed to invest money that I did not have, I agreed. However, this time, unlike with Detroit, I did not insist on us having a written contract between us.

One of the big issues at Belle Isle was the irrigation system. It turned out not to work. Again, this was Paul's area of expertise and responsibility. But by the time he reacted, the greens on the short course were all dead . . . completely dead. As in, we just lost one of the major parts of our operation.

Meanwhile, Paul and I were not getting paid by Detroit. Moreover, our contract with the City did not include any reimbursements for travel. When we were still working with the "old" team, it had been strongly suggested that we get an apartment in the City. Detroit is extremely sensitive about doing business with Detroit located vendors. I don't mean Detroit metro; I mean Detroit City. Indeed, we were told we had to give extreme priority to using Detroit vendors whenever possible, even if they were a lot more expensive. Since Detroit was paying the bills and we worked for them, we had no choice.

However, by renting an apartment, we would now become "Detroit" vendors. This would give us a serious advantage when the "real" management contract came up in two years. (We were working on an "interim" two-year contract. After that, the City intended to do a long-term contract with a vendor who would also contribute significantly to the needed capital improvements.) As we would be the only company located in Detroit, or at least having an office in Detroit, we would be given a priority. And not a small one. Typically, this carries a whopping 40% of their weighting. One of the old management team members had an in with one of the downtown apartment complexes, and we each rented a one-bedroom apartment there. (He also lived there). The apartment was decent. It was notable as one wall was solid window. I had a ninth-floor apartment that faced Ford field. Nice view.

Our leases started April 1st. I drove up this trip, having purchased the bare necessities to get me by, including an inflatable mattress. That first day, I got really lucky. I went down to the lounge and saw a flyer on the table from someone in the building wanting to sell all their furniture. It proved to be an estate deal. But I was able to get a real bed, couch, tables, lamps, etc. for about $600. And it was nice stuff too. Indeed. the mattress and box springs were practically brand new.

Meanwhile, the City put out a bid for a construction manager to manage the $2 million in capital improvements they had promised to make over the next two years in the courses. Naturally, Paul went after that contract. And he certainly would be a natural. Paul promised me if he got the contract. he would then be able to pick up some, if not all of my travel expenses. That would be really helpful to me as my travel costs were extensive, well in excess of what I should have been earning to this point.

Meanwhile, we still had not been paid a cent by the City. It was now June. Not only had we not gotten any of our management contract, the City had not reimbursed for any of our operating expenses. In our contract, we were to lay out for all operating expenses (equipment, payroll, advertising, etc.). The City would then reimburse us. We had been assured that they would do this expeditiously. Right.

This affected Paul much more than me, as his company was fronting all the operating money (remember, he insisted on having the contract in his company's name). Still, I had paid for about $10,000 worth of supplies (when we were getting opening supplies) and had another $10 grand I had laid out in travel expenses. I was not really in position to lay out that kind of money!

Meanwhile, it was now early June and we needed to start

on the Ramsey County contract. We had set up in April that our first site visit would be June 5th. On June 4th, I get a phone call from Jeff. *He* informed me Paul was not going to be able to make it. Jeff felt it would be ok, because he certainly knew enough about agronomy, and he could do the soil samples and handle the inspections and interviews with the course superintendents. Paul would visit the courses later and look at the samples and review the information and pictures Jeff provided.

Given that we were to start the next day, I had little choice. But I was miffed, especially since I had already paid Paul part of his fee up front. But I was especially upset that Paul did not call me, but instead worked through Jeff.

Meanwhile, Paul could not make up his mind how to handle the maintenance at Belle Isle. The previous vendor had contracted it out. Which would have made it simple. Our manager had a superintendent he wanted to hire. But Paul hesitated. The hesitation cost us the opportunity. So we hired an inexperienced worker to mow and had our manager, who was not a superintendent, oversee him. Big mistake. The worker put regular gas in a diesel engine, ruining our tractor. Plus *all* the greens mysteriously died. (It is possible it was sabotage, but we have no proof). So now one of our main sources of revenue was lost for the year. (Again, maintenance was Paul's area of responsibility).

I was in Minneapolis through Friday afternoon, then flew back to Detroit as we had a big "block party"/grand opening celebration at one of the courses. This was one thing the City did get behind and promoted, and I wanted to make sure I was there. (Paul did not make it). This was the 2nd of two we had.

Unfortunately, at the celebration, I had a row with the liaison over pricing. Her boss had approved of my plan to return to the summer pricing that was supposed to be in place. However, she disagreed. And it got ugly, with her calling me names, etc. She was dissing everything about me, making it very personal, and insulting me both personally and professionally. I have my limits.

Two days later, I get an *email* from Paul saying he was terminating our contract. I was out. Again. I was devastated . . . again.

In my mind, the liaison was behind this. I felt Paul was so paranoid about losing the contract the easiest thing to do was to get rid of me.

Paul said he was only terminating the Detroit contract. He still wanted me as a partner in Belle Isle. The reason, though, was not because he valued my expertise, it was because he was losing money on the project and wanted me to start contributing financially.

At this point, I was extremely conflicted. On the one hand, I could certainly understand Paul's position. He could ill afford to have the contract cancelled. And if he truly believed that was in danger, I could understand, sort of, his decision. I did not agree with it, but I understood it. Plus, by this time I was very vested in the golf courses. I wanted them to succeed. And I felt Paul, even without me, was better than if the City took it over completely.

My first inclination was to write a "tell-all" letter. I was furious with the City and how they were handling us, especially the micromanaging. I was especially upset with the "liaison." At that moment, I was wanting to send this letter, not only to the big boss, but also to the City Council and to the press. And because it contained a lot of embarrassing things for the City, it would cause a lot of problems. Indeed, I realized it could get Paul fired. Is that what I wanted? I talked to the person I had befriended that had been part of the "old team." He convinced me not to send the letter. The compromise I made was that I wrote a toned-down letter, concentrating on the issues with the liaison, and sent it to both him and Paul. My thinking was that if a future issue developed, which was likely, they would have this as more evidence.

My contract with Paul called for a $20,000 buy-out, which would make me whole. By this time, he had also gotten the first reimbursement from the City, so he was able to reimburse me for the supplies I had laid out. He also agreed to purchase the furniture I had bought for my apartment, and to pay any cancellation fees. He told me he would pay the $20k by July 15th.

I was scheduled to make another trip to Detroit the following week. As had been my habit, I drove. I liked driving as it gave me a lot of flexibility in scheduling. I could stay as long as I needed. This was a lot easier since I had an apartment there. It was also cheaper.

Since I was still involved in Belle Isle, I made another trip to Detroit a couple of weeks later. This was a short trip, though, because I only had one facility to visit.

July 15 came and went, and no check. Further, Paul was not doing anything he had agreed to do on our other project, Ramsey County. And, he was asking me to contribute money for Belle Isle, which I had never agreed to do.

While I had always wanted to give Paul the benefit of the doubt, this was becoming impossible. He played a major role in my firing at Tempest. And he took over the management contract.

He had agreed to pay me a finder's fee for the Tempest contract. He never did. When we won the Belle Isle contract, he agreed my share of the financial contribution would be the finder's fee he never paid.

He backed out of Ramsey County, even after I had paid him an advance. And he never talked directly to me about it. He would later refund the advance – by paying it to Jeff, not me. So, what am I to think about him terminating this contract? Now he gets both his share and mine. Suddenly, for him, this contract becomes lucrative. And he still has the inside tract to the "big" contract.

I had to threaten legal action to get Paul to pay me anything. He paid me a little in August. And more in October. But as of this writing, he still owes me over $10,000. I guess I was the PT Barnum's sucker born August 10, 1954.

I took his non-compliance with the terms of our Detroit contract to assume it cancels our non-written agreement with Belle Isle. I had previously told him, back in early July, that once he paid me what he owed, I would be willing to contribute some to Belle Isle, as well as continue managing. Not anymore. He's on his own.

But, in a way, it worked out ok for me. Not financially. But it freed up a lot of time! And the project for Ramsey County demanded my time. In fact, I worked about sixty hours or more each week from mid-July through early December on this project. I finished the draft report on December 4th. The report was 550 odd pages long – single spaced. Enough for *two* doctoral dissertations!

I just recently received the corrections from the County. The final final is due January 15th. I honestly think it was my best work. It certainly has taken the most effort. My biggest regret though, is that I let Jeff talk me into not having another agronomist visit the facility. By the time it was clear Paul was not going to fulfill his obligation (August), it was too late to bring someone else in. Jeff had an agronomist, who was well qualified, review his notes, pictures, etc. But he was not be able to visit the courses in time (or within my budget). And while I had told the County what was going on, they did not object until *after* our presentation, when it was much too late to do anything about it.

I had two proposals for consulting jobs in October but did not get either. (I had not even *looked* at other opportunities until then). Now that I am catching up on the brokerage side, I will start looking for more consulting opportunities.

However, my whole attitude is different than Pre-C. I don't want to work myself to death. That's going to come anyway without my hurrying it up any. I can't afford to retire. But I can scale back and do some of the things I have been wanting to do – like finishing this book.

SOCIAL SECURITY

A quick note on Social Security. When I lost my job at Southern Hills, I applied for SS disability insurance, but was quickly denied. The main issue was that I had not paid into SS the last couple of years due to showing losses on my tax returns from my businesses.

Fearing I may not be able to work again, I decided to take early retirement benefits, which I was entitled to. Although my benefits were not substantial given all my self-employment years when I paid little into the system.

However, I found out there was a big string attached to early retirement. It did not mean anything in March 2017 when I applied, because I was worried I would never work again. But then I got the Northbrook job. And then another job, and another.

When it came to do my taxes for 2017, I made a horrible discovery. There is a limit on how much you can earn if you take early retirement. If you earn more than I think about $12,000 for the year, they will reduce your benefit by

$1 for every $1 over. That meant I was now *in debt to Social Security*. I not only needed to immediately stop receiving benefits, I had to pay some back!

2019

February 1, 2019

Scan day! Sadly, this turned into an almost identical repeat of what happened over a year ago (January 15, 2018). The lab was scheduled at 7 am, and the MRI, which was downstairs from the lab, was at 7:30. I did not schedule it that way, Emory did. But my doctor's appointment was not until 1:30. So, Holly and I were planning on what we could do for the estimated three to four hours between appointments. Shopping was the top of her list.

Again, I was there before the lab opened downtown. This time, they had my records. But for whatever reason, they were running really slow. I wasn't called back for the lab until almost 7:30. Fearing the worst, I sent Holly down to the MRI to explain the situation and why I was running late. It didn't help.

When I finally got down there at 7:45, they had given my slot away. While upsetting, I had plenty of time to get it done before my doctor's appointment. They said they would try to work me in.

Two hours later, they finally get me back for the CT Scan, which only takes five minutes. When it was done, I was supposed to go in for the MRI. But they were having equipment problems. I was placed back in the patient waiting room. Holly, though, was in the main waiting room and since they took my phone, I couldn't tell her what was going on. I should not have worried, though, Holly was fast asleep.

An hour later, I am ushered back to the MRI. No problem. It's 10:30. I still have three hours before my Doctor's appointment. So, Holly doesn't get to shop as much. Saves money . . .

But that's not the end of the story. The MRI continued to have problems. It would run about five minutes of scans, then overheat. The total time for the scans is normally about forty-five minutes, which is a long time to spend in a cocoon, especially when you're claustrophobic. But my discomfort was only going to grow. It turns out there was a problem with the cooling system. The technician tried to make a go of it. We would do about five minutes of scans, then five minutes of cooling, then repeat. But after about an hour and a half, she finally gave up. She then said they would try to work me in downstairs. I was ushered back to the patient waiting room.

Fortunately, they were able to work me – about thirty minutes later. I grabbed my clothes out of the locker and we collected Holly from the main waiting room, then headed downstairs to the main floor and the in-patient MRI. I got to enjoy showing off my elegant dress to all we passed in the halls and elevator.

The good news was they were able to use the partial scan that I had already done, so we did not have to start over from scratch. The rest went smoothly.

When it was all over, it was time to head over to the main campus. I looked at my watch. It was now almost 1:30. Not only did we not get our shopping trip in, but my dreams of a Romeo's lunch had evaporated as we were now *late* for my doctor's appointment. And when we were done with the doctor's visit (after a 45-minute wait), I had to wait another hour and half to get into infusion. By the time we were done, it was after six. At least we got to eat at Romeo's for dinner!

Fortunately, it was all just a humorous (although not at the time) annoyance. The scans again showed no growth. And while we did not see Dr. Bilen during the office visit (Greta was a capable replacement), I did run into him in the infusion lab. But only because I had gone back to the lab after reaching the car, because I forgot the parking validation ticket. But I was so glad I did as Dr. Bilen indicated that perhaps after two more treatments, we would finally stop.

February 10, 2019
Just one more quick update before I put this baby to bed. I got a call from Howard. Apparently, he is having to take Paul to court as he did not fulfill his obligations, plus he billed him an unexpected extra $600,000, plus he put a lien on the property. The course, by the way, finally opened to rave reviews in September, about a year later than Paul had originally promised. But the project was not complete. The driving range, which I had planned to open first, was not finished – still. Maybe there is such a thing as poetic justice.

March 15, 2019 – Ring Da Bell
My six-week visit to Dr. Bilen today was eventful. It is his opinion that it is time to conclude the treatments. That is to say, he feels I am cancer free! The spots on the MRIs are unchanged and are consistent with being scar tissue rather than active tumors. The only way to tell for sure is to do a biopsy, but he feels that is not needed, especially since we will be repeating the scans every three months for the foreseeable future.

Holly came with me today, in anticipation of receiving this news and celebrating! And while Dr. Bilen cancelled today's treatment, it did not stop us from visiting the infusion center. This is because I really, really wanted to ring that bell! The bell, which is probably in every infusion center in the country, is rung when a patient has finished their last treatment because they have beaten cancer. It not only commemorates the occasion for the patient and his family, but also gives hope to those being treated at that time.

April 2019
This will be my last entry in the Epilogue. With Holly's blessing, I have made the decision to transition to a full-time career as a writer. In addition to this book, I have resurrected two other works that I am now feverishly editing: *From Dusty Plains to Wartime Planes* – which is my dad's memoir about growing up impoverished in western Kansas during the dust bowl, then going on to a fascinating career as a pilot during World War II; and *Prime Directive: Earth*, a young adult science fiction that asks, 'What if the Prime Directive was reversed, where Earth is in trouble and aliens are being prevented from helping.'

The fact the golf consulting opportunities have virtually disappeared, has nothing to do with my decision . . . well, maybe a little. I take it as a sign. Wish me luck!

May 2019
Okay, I know I promised April would be the last. But I had to share this story. If you remember, my previous scan in February took nearly three hours to complete – a nightmare for someone with claustrophobia. Well, it happened again this time.

As was the case in February, I had a three-hour window between when the 45-minute MRI was scheduled and my doctor's appointment. This time, though, instead of having the MRI done on the eighth floor of the downtown Emory hospital, they scheduled me for the main center on the first floor.

I had my labs done first, then the CT. Everything was fine. Then I was put in the MRI.

I must have a negative vibe that triggers an adverse reaction with the equipment. Well whatever the reason, the machine broke again while I was in it. Once again, a 45-minute exam took over three hours to complete. Only this time, most of it was spent *in* the machine. Not fun.

We at least stopped to get fast food on the way to Dr. Bilen's, knowing they would need time to get the results anyway. And again, the news was good. Just another story to tell.

Postscript

What can I conclude from all that I have gone through? Besides God having a nasty sense of humor? I wish I knew. I do know my faith has become even stronger. And I am *extremely* grateful for my extended life, which I view as being miraculous, given the circumstances.

I owe my life now to a lot of people. Certainly, my brother-in-law, Michael, who referred me to Emory comes to mind. Dr. Bilen tops the list, along with the wonderful staff at Emory. My family and friends, and especially Holly have contributed immensely, both with their love and by strengthening my will to live.

I know my faith and strong will to live are among the reasons I am here now. But I also realize there have been many who have as strong a faith, as strong a will to live who failed to survive the battle. Why me?

One could say I'm just really lucky. I certainly have beaten some very long odds, winning the lottery of life. But to say it was luck is to say that there was no purpose to my survival. I like to think it was more than that.

I believe faith alone is not enough. You can't expect God to do all the work for you. You must contribute *your* effort as well. Do everything you can, then give Him a reason to help.

Believe me, I am extremely thankful for having cheated death. I'm just not certain why I am still here.

Having stage IV cancer had a profound effect on my life. Beating it has had another. I deal with survivor's guilt and I struggle to justify my continued existence. I have taken it as an opportunity to work on improving myself. That is the least I can do to pay back the tremendous favor I have received. And I believe I am making progress, although I know I have a long way to go.

One of the ways I have tried to do this is by attempting to take the "sole out of soul." By that I mean, thinking less about what is best for myself and more about what is best for others. I know I have been selfish in my life and I want to change that. It's not easy.

But is there more? Is there another purpose that I'm missing?

Perhaps that purpose was to write this book, and by so doing, help a lot of people. But then if that's case, now that the book is completed, does that mean that I am now literally writing my death sentence? I certainly hope not.

Other titles by BLKDOG Publishing that you may enjoy:

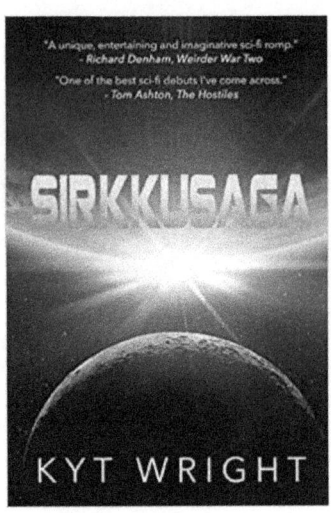

Sirkkusaga
By Kyt Wright

A saga – a long story of heroic achievement, especially a medieval prose narrative in Old Norse or a long, involved story, account, or series of incidents often named for the principal character.

Several hundred years after an world-shattering war, two of the surviving nations, the Reignweald and the Dominion have fought themselves to a standstill, both remaining determined to control of what's left of it.

Sirki Vigsdottir, a songstress who performs under the name Freya in folk-rock group *The Harvest* is beautiful, self-centered woman who is fond of drink and a recovering addict to boot, not the sort of girl a boy brings home to mother.

Following an attack from an unexpected quarter, abilities awaken within Sirki, who begins a journey of self-discovery. These new found skills attract the attention of both the Psi, a mysterious group of telepaths headed by the fearsome Mina and an equally sinister government department; the ACG.

Sirki, learning the real truth of her origin, is dragged into plotting between the queen and the Government, finding herself in constant danger as Bren, fighting for the nation, becomes an important part of her life. As it becomes clear that her life of self-indulgence is over, Sirki wonders if her newfound powers are a blessing or a curse.

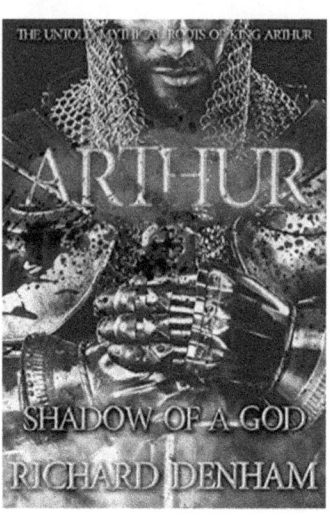

Arthur: Shadow of a God
By Richard Denham

King Arthur has fascinated the Western world for over a thousand years and yet we still know nothing more about him now than we did then. Layer upon layer of heroics and exploits has been piled upon him to the point where history, legend and myth have become hopelessly entangled.

In recent years, there has been a sort of scholarly consensus that 'the once and future king' was clearly some sort of Romano-British warlord, heroically stemming the tide of wave after wave of Saxon invaders after the end of Roman rule. But surprisingly, and no matter how much we enjoy this narrative, there is actually next-to-nothing solid to support this theory except the wishful thinking of understandably bitter contemporaries. The sources and scholarship used to support the 'real Arthur' are as much tentative guesswork and pushing 'evidence' to the extreme to fit in with this version as anything involving magic swords, wizards and dragons. Even Archaeology remains silent. Arthur is, and always has been, the square peg that refuses to fit neatly into the historians round hole.

Arthur: Shadow of a God gives a fascinating overview of Britain's lost hero and casts a light over an often-overlooked and somewhat inconvenient truth; Arthur was almost certainly not a man at all, but a god. He is linked inextricably to the world of Celtic folklore and Druidic traditions. Whereas tyrants like Nero and Caligula were men who fancied themselves gods; is it not possible that Arthur was a god we have turned into a man? Perhaps then there is a truth here. Arthur, 'The King under the Mountain'; sleeping until his return will never return, after all, because he doesn't need to. Arthur the god never left in the first place and remains as popular today as he ever was. His legend echoes in stories, films and games that are every bit as imaginative and fanciful as that which the minds of talented bards such as Taliesin and Aneirin came up with when the mists of the 'dark ages' still swirled over Britain – and perhaps that is a good thing after all, most at home in the imaginations of children and adults alike – being the Arthur his believers want him to be.

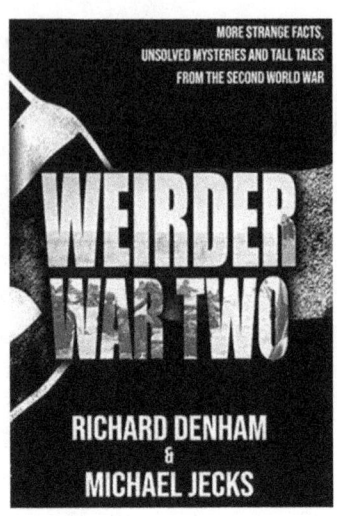

Weirder War Two
By Richard Denham & Michael Jecks

Did a Warner Bros. cartoon prophesize the use of the atom bomb? Did the Allies really plan to use stink bombs on the enemy? Why did the Nazis make their own version of Titanic and why were polar bear photographs appearing throughout Europe?

The Second World War was the bloodiest of all wars. Mass armies of men trudged, flew or rode from battlefields as far away as North Africa to central Europe, from India to Burma, from the Philippines to the borders of Japan. It saw the first aircraft carrier sea battle, and the indiscriminate use of terror against civilian populations in ways not seen since the Thirty Years War. Nuclear and incendiary bombs erased entire cities. V weapons brought new horror from the skies: the V1 with their hideous grumbling engines, the V2 with sudden, unexpected death. People were systematically starved: in Britain food had to be rationed because of the stranglehold of U-Boats, while in Holland the German blockage of food and fuel saw 30,000 die of starvation in the winter of 1944/5. It was a catastrophe for millions.

At a time of such enormous crisis, scientists sought ever more inventive weapons, or devices to help halt the war. Civilians were involved as never before, with women taking up new trades, proving themselves as capable as their male predecessors whether in the factories or the fields.

The stories in this book are of courage, of ingenuity, of hilarity in some cases, or of great sadness, but they are all thought-provoking - and rather weird. So whether you are interested in the last Polish cavalry charge, the Blackout Ripper, Dada, or Ghandi's attempt to stop the bloodshed, welcome to the Weirder War Two!

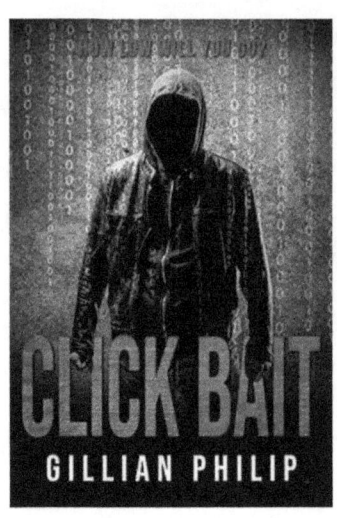

**Click Bait
By Gillian Philip**

A funny joke's a funny joke. Eddie Doolan doesn't think twice about adapting it to fit a tragic local news story and posting it on social media.

It's less of a joke when his drunken post goes viral. It stops being funny altogether when Eddie ends up jobless, friendless and ostracized by the whole town of Langburn. This isn't how he wanted to achieve fame.

Under siege from the press and facing charges not just for the joke but for a history of abusive behavior on the internet, Eddie grows increasingly paranoid and desperate. The only people still speaking to him are Crow, a neglected kid who relies on Eddie for food and company, and Sid, the local gamekeeper's granddaughter. It's Sid who offers Eddie a refuge and an understanding ear.

But she also offers him an illegal shotgun…

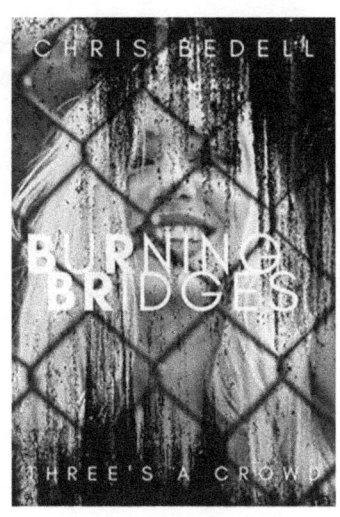

**Burning Bridges
By Chris Bedell**

They've always said that three's a crowd...

24-year-old Sasha didn't anticipate her identical twin Riley killing herself upon their reconciliation after years of estrangement. But Sasha senses an opportunity and assumes Riley's identity so she can escape her old life.

Playing Riley isn't without complications, though. Riley's had a strained relationship with her wife and stepson so Sasha must do whatever she can to make her newfound family love and accept her. If Sasha's arrangement ends, then she'll have nothing protecting her from her past. However, when one of Sasha's former clients tracks her down, Sasha must choose between her new life and the only person who cared about her.

But things are about to become even more complicated, as a third sister, Katrina, enters the scene...

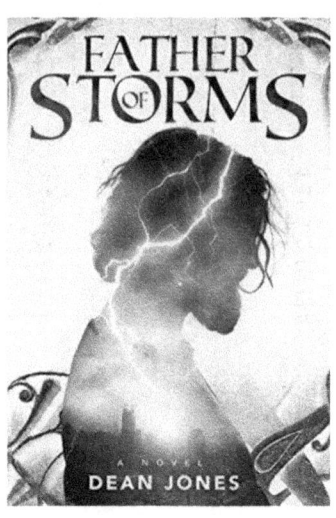

Father of Storms
By Dean Jones

Imagine losing everything you loved as well as the future you'd wished for so long to come true.

Seth was born with the gift to manipulate energy, unfortunately his skills mark him as a target for one who wishes to control everything. So began a life running from those who would seek to command him, a life that spans over a thousand years waiting for the day when all will be once again as it was.

Captured in modern day London, Seth needs the help of his companions, the Mara, to show him who he is through dreams of his past, so he can save the family he has waited so long to have. A warrior bred for battle must fight once more but this time the battlefield is his mind. Can Seth win, or will he finally lose who he is and become the weapon of the man who started his nightmare all those years ago? *Father of Storms* is a story told through time, a tale of love and hope where there seems to be none and above all it is a reminder that if you believe, truly believe then even from the darkest places, good things come to those who wait.

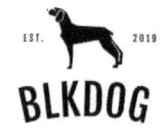

www.blkdogpublishing.com

www.ingramcontent.com/pod-product-compliance
Lightning Source LLC
Chambersburg PA
CBHW020741100426
42735CB00037B/158